Drug Charts
In Basic Pharmacology

Second Edition

Drug Charts In Basic Pharmacology

Second Edition

ISBN 0-942447-26-3

Printed in the United States of America

Printing: 1 2 3 4 5 6

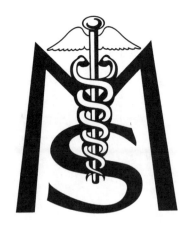

Drug Charts
In Basic Pharmacology

Second Edition

Jonathan D. Baum, M.D., M.M.B.[a]
Resident in Obstetrics and Gynecology

Andrew P. Ferko, Ph.D.[b]
Associate Professor of Pharmacology

G. John DiGregorio, M.D., Ph.D.[b]
Professor of Pharmacology and Medicine

Edward J. Barbieri, Ph.D.[b]
Associate Professor of Pharmacology

Joseph R. DiPalma, M.D., D.Sc. (Hon.)[b]
Professor Emeritus of Pharmacology and Medicine

[a] Department of Obstetrics and Gynecology
New York University Downtown Hospital
New York, New York

[b] Department of Pharmacology
Division of Toxicology
Allegheny University of the Health Sciences
Center City Campus
Philadelphia, Pennsylvania

Medical Surveillance Inc.
West Chester
1998

PREFACE

The **Second Edition of Drug Charts in Basic Pharmacology** is designed as a concise source of basic pharmacology and drug information. The chart format is useful in organizing the vast number of pharmacologic agents used in medicine. The First Edition of Drug Charts in Basic Pharmacology was a popular quick reference for busy students and medical personnel. The Second Edition provides a much expanded index including both generic and common trade names (in CAPS) for each agent. Two chapters have been added to the Drug Information section: Food and Drug Administration's Pregnancy Categories and Known or Suspected Teratogens. The alphabetical listing of commonly prescribed drugs has also been updated for quick classification of agents. The Brief Drug Description section provides an alphabetical listing of a few key facts describing an agent or class of agents.

Drug Charts in Basic Pharmacology should be used with the **Handbook of Commonly Prescribed Drugs, 12th Edition** by DiGregorio and Barbieri. Each topic is placed in a chart format for quick reference. The charts are concise, detailed and user friendly. It should not be considered as an official therapeutic document. If there is a discrepancy in the therapeutic category, preparation or indication, the reader is advised to obtain official and more complete information from the pharmaceutical manufacturer.

We hope you find **Drug Charts in Basic Pharmacology** as useful as we and our students have in the past.

The Authors

TABLE OF CONTENTS

PAGE

ix

DRUG INFORMATION

AGENTS AND THERAPEUTIC CATEGORIES

ACEBUTOLOL (anti-anginal, antiarrhythmic, antihypertensive agent)

ACETAMINOPHEN (non-opioid analgesic, antipyretic)

ACETAZOLAMIDE (diuretic, antiglaucoma)

ACETOHEXAMIDE (hypoglycemic)

ACETYLCHOLINE (cholinomimetic)

ACETYLCYSTEINE (mucolytic)

ACTH (corticosteroid)

ACYCLOVIR (antiviral)

ADENOSINE (IV antiarrhythmic)

ALBUTEROL (bronchodilator)

ALCLOMETASONE (corticosteroid)

ALDESLEUKIN (immunosuppressant)

ALFENTANIL (opioid analgesic)

ALLOPURINOL (antigout agent)

ALPRAZOLAM (antianxiety)

ALTEPLASE, RECOMBINANT (thrombolytic)

ALTRETAMINE (antineoplastic)

ALUMINUM HYDROXIDE (antacid)

AMANTADINE (antiviral, antiparkinsonian)

AMBENONIUM (cholinomimetic)

AMCINONIDE (corticosteroid)

AMIKACIN (systemic antibacterial)

AMILORIDE (diuretic)

AMINOCAPROIC ACID (coagulant)

AMINOPHYLLINE (bronchodilator)

AMIODARONE (antiarrhythmic)

AMITRIPTYLINE (tricyclic antidepressant)

AMLODIPINE (antihypertensive, antianginal)

AMOBARBITAL (sedative-hypnotic)

AMODIAQUINE (antimalarial)

AMOXAPINE (antidepressant)

AMOXICILLIN (systemic antibacterial)

AMPHETAMINES (mixed acting adrenergic agonist)

AMPHOTERICIN B (antifungal)

AMPICILLIN (systemic antibacterial)

AMRINONE (inotropic agent)

AMYL NITRATE (antianginal)

ANISTREPLASE (thrombolytic)

ANTHRALIN (antipsoriasis agent)

ARSENIC (heavy metal)

ASPARAGINASE (antineoplastic)

ASPIRIN (non-opioid analgesic, antipyretic)

ASTEMIZOLE (antihistamine)

ATENOLOL (beta adrenergic blocker)

ATORVASTATIN (hypolipidemic)

ATOVAQUONE (antiprotozoal)

ATRACURIUM (skeletal muscle relaxant)

ATROPINE (anticholinergic)

ATTAPULGITE (antidiarrheal)

AURANOFIN (immunosuppressant)

AUROTHIOGLUCOSE (immunosuppressant)

AZATADINE (antihistamine)

AZATHIOPRINE (immunosuppressant)

AZITHROMYCIN (systemic antibacterial)

AZTREONAM (monobactam)

BACAMPICILLIN (systemic antibacterial)

BACITRACIN (antibacterial, topical)

BACLOFEN (skeletal muscle relaxant)

BACTRIM (systemic antibacterial)

BECLOMETHASONE (corticosteroid)

BENAZEPRIL (antihypertensive)

BENDROFLUMETHIAZIDE (diuretic, antihypertensive)

BENZATHINE PENICILLIN (antibacterial)

BENZOCAINE (local anesthetic)

BENZOYL PEROXIDE (antiacne agent)

BENZPHETAMINE (anorexiant)

BENZQUINAMIDE (antiemetic)

BENZTHIAZIDE (diuretic, antihypertensive)

BENZTROPINE (anticholinergic)

BEPRIDIL (antianginal)

BETAMETHASONE (corticosteroid)

BETAXOLOL (antihypertensive, antiglaucoma agent)

BETHANECHOL (cholinomimetic)

BIPERIDEN (antiparkinsonian)

BISACODYL (irritant laxative)

BISMUTH SUBSALICYLATE (antidiarrheal)

BISOPROLOL (antihypertensive)

BITOLTEROL MESYLATE (bronchodilator)

BLEOMYCIN (antineoplastic)

BRETYLIUM (antiarrhythmic)

BROMOCRIPTINE (antiparkinsonian)

BROMPHENIRAMINE (antihistamine)

BUMETANIDE (diuretic)

BUPRENORPHINE (opioid analgesic)

BUPROPION (antidepressant)

BUSPIRONE (antianxiety)

BUSULFAN (antineoplastic)

BUTABARBITAL (sedative hypnotic)

BUTAMBEN (local anesthetic)

BUTOCONAZOLE (topical antifungal)

BUTORPHANOL (opioid analgesic)

CADMIUM (heavy metal)

CAFFEINE (CNS stimulant)

CALCIFEDIOL (hypercalcemic agent)

CALCITONIN (hypocalcemic agent)

CALCITRIOL (hypercalcemic agent)

CALCIUM CARBONATE (antacid)

CALCIUM SALTS (calcium supplement)

CAPSAICIN (analgesic, topical)

1

AGENTS AND THERAPEUTIC CATEGORIES

CAPTOPRIL (antihypertensive, post-MI drug,
    congestive heart failure agent))
CARBACHOL (cholinomimetic)
CARBAMAZEPINE (antiepileptic)
CARBENICILLIN (antibacterial)
CARBOPLATIN (antineoplastic)
CARISOPRODOL (skeletal m. relaxant)
CARMUSTINE (antineoplastic)
CARTEOLOL (antihypertensive)
CARVEDILOL (antihypertensive)
CASTOR OIL (irritant laxative)
CEFACLOR (antibacterial)
CEFADROXIL (systemic antibacterial)
CEFAMANDOLE (systemic antibacterial)
CEFAZOLIN (systemic antibacterial)
CEFIXIME (systemic antibacterial)
CEFMETAZOLE (systemic antibacterial)
CEFONICID (systemic antibacterial)
CEFOPERAZONE (systemic antibacterial)
CEFOTAXIME (systemic antibacterial)
CEFOTETAN (systemic antibacterial)
CEFOXITIN (systemic antibacterial)
CEFPODOXIME (systemic antibacterial)
CEFPROZIL (systemic antibacterial)
CEFTAZIDIME (systemic antibacterial)
CEFTRIAXONE (systemic antibacterial)
CEFUROXIME (systemic antibacterial)
CEPHALEXIN (systemic antibacterial)
CEPHALOTHIN (systemic antibacterial)
CEPHAPIRIN (systemic antibacterial)
CEPHRADINE (systemic antibacterial)
CHLORAL HYDRATE (sedative-hypnotic)
CHLORAMBUCIL (antineoplastic)
CHLORAMPHENICOL (antibacterial)
CHLORDIAZEPOXIDE (antianxiety)
CHLORMEZANONE (antianxiety)
CHLOROGUANIDE (antimalarial)
CHLOROQUINE (antimalarial)
CHLOROTHIAZIDE (diuretic, antihypertensive)
CHLOROTRIANISENE (estrogen, antineoplastic)
CHLORPHENESIN (skeletal m. relaxant)
CHLORPHENIRAMINE (antihistamine)
CHLORPROMAZINE (antipsychotic)
CHLORPROPAMIDE (hypoglycemic)
CHLORPROTHIXENE (antipsychotic)
CHLORTHALIDONE (diuretic, antihypertensive)
CHLORZOXAZONE (skeletal m. relaxant)
CHOLESTYRAMINE (hypolipidemic)
CICLOPIROX (antifungal)
CILASTATIN (penicillin adjunct agent)
CIMETIDINE (histamine H2 blocker)
CINOXACIN (urinary anti-infective)
CIPROFLOXACIN (antibacterial)

CISAPRIDE (GI stimulant)
CISPLATIN (antineoplastic)
CLARITHROMYCIN
  (systemic antibacterial)
CLAVULANATE (penicillin adjunct agent)
CLEMASTINE (systemic antihistamine)
CLIDINIUM (anticholinergic)
CLINDAMYCIN (systemic antibacterial)
CLIOQUINOL (antifungal, antibacterial)
CLOBETASOL (topical corticosteroid)
CLOCORTOLONE (topical corticosteroid)
CLOFIBRATE (hypolipidemic)
CLOMIPHENE (ovulation stimulant)
CLOMIPRAMINE (antidepressant)
CLONAZEPAM (antiepileptic)
CLONIDINE (antihypertensive)
CLORAZEPATE (antianxiety)
CLOTRIMAZOLE (antifungal, topical)
CLOXACILLIN (systemic antibacterial)
CLOZAPINE (antipsychotic)
COCAINE (psychotomimetic drug)
COCAINE HCL (local anesthetic)
CODEINE (opioid analgesic)
COLCHICINE (anti-gout)
COLESTIPOL (hypolipidemic)
COLISTIMETHATE (systemic antibacterial)
COLISTIN (systemic antibacterial)
CROMOLYN (antiallergic, antiasthmatic)
CROTAMITON (scabicide)
CYCLIZINE (antihistamine, antiemetic)
CYCLOBENZAPRINE (skeletal m. relaxant)
CYCLOPHOSPHAMIDE (antineoplastic)
CYCLOSPORINE (immunosuppressant)
CYPROHEPTADINE
  (antihistamine, antipruritic)
CYTARABINE (antineoplastic)
DACARBAZINE (antineoplastic)
DACTINOMYCIN (antineoplastic)
DANAZOL (androgen)
DANTROLENE (skeletal m. relaxant)
DAPSONE (leprostatic)
DAUNORUBICIN (antineoplastic)
DECAMETHONIUM (anti-glaucoma)
DEFEROXAMINE (iron chelating agent)
DEMECLOCYCLINE (systemic antibacterial)
DESIPRAMINE (antidepressant)
DESMOPRESSIN
  (posterior pituitary hormone)
DESONIDE (topical corticosteroid)
DESOXIMETASONE (topical corticosteroid)
DEXAMETHASONE (corticosteroid)
DEXCHLORPHENIRAMINE
  (systemic antihistamine)

2

DEXTROMETHORPHAN (antitussive)
DEZOCINE (opioid analgesic)
DIAZEPAM (antianxiety)
DIAZOXIDE (IV antihypertensive)
DIBUCAINE (local anesthetic)
DICLOFENAC (systemic antiinflammatory)
DICLOXACILLIN (systemic antibacterial)
DICUMAROL (oral anticoagulant)
DICYCLOMINE (anticholinergic)
DIDANOSINE (ddI, antiviral)
DIENESTROL (non-steroidal estrogen)
DIETHYLPROPION (anorexiant)
DIETHYLSTILBESTROL (estrogen)
DIFLORASONE (topical corticosteroid)
DIFLUNISAL
   (non-opioid analgesic, antiinflammatory)
DIGITALIS (inotropic agent for congestive
    heart failure)
DIGITOXIN (see Digitalis)
DIGOXIN (see Digitalis)
DIHYDROTACHYSTEROL (hypercalcemic)
DILTIAZEM (antihypertensive, antianginal,
   antiarrhythmic agent)
DIMENHYDRINATE (antivertigo, antiemetic)
DIMERCAPROL (chelating agent)
DINOPROSTONE (cervical ripening agent)
DIPHENHYDRAMINE (antihistamine)
DIPHENOXYLATE (antidiarrheal)
DIPYRIDAMOLE
   (platelet aggregation inhibitor)
DISOPYRAMIDE (antiarrhythmic)
DISULFIRAM (antialcoholic)
DIVALPROEX (antiepileptic, antimaniacal,
   antimigraine)
DOBUTAMINE (adrenergic agonist)
DOCUSATE SODIUM (laxative, emollient)
DONEPEZIL (anti-Alzheimer's dementia)
DOPAMINE (adrenergic agonist)
DOXACURIUM (neuromuscular blocker)
DOXAZOSIN (α adrenergic blocker)
DOXEPIN (antidepressant)
DOXORUBICIN (antineoplastic)
DOXYCYCLINE (antibacterial, antimalarial)
DOXYLAMINE (sedative)
DRONABINOL
   (antiemetic, appetite stimulant)
DROPERIDOL (antianxiety)
DYPHYLLINE (bronchodilator)
ECONAZOLE (antifungal)
ECHOTHIOPHATE (antiglaucoma)
EDETATE CALCIUM DISODIUM (chelator)
EDROPHONIUM (cholinomimetic)
EFLORNITHINE (antiprotozoal)

EMETINE (amebicide)
ENALAPRIL (antihypertensive, heart failure drug)
ENALAPRILAT (antihypertensive)
ENFLURANE (general anesthetic)
ENOXACIN (systemic antibacterial)
ENOXAPARIN (anticoagulant)
EPHEDRINE (mixed adrenergic agonist)
EPINEPHRINE (direct adrenergic agonist)
ERGOCALCIFEROL (hypercalcemic)
ERGONOVINE (alpha adrenergic blocker)
ERGOTAMINE (antimigraine)
ERYTHROMYCIN (antibacterial)
ESMOLOL (antiarrhythmic)
ESTAZOLAM (hypnotic)
ESTRADIOL, ESTRONE (estrogen)
ESTRAMUSTINE (antineoplastic)
ESTROGENS, CONJUGATED (estrogen)
ESTROPIPATE (estrogen, antiosteoporotic)
ETHACRYNIC ACID (diuretic)
ETHAMBUTOL (tuberculostatic)
ETHANOL (alcohol)
ETHCHLORVYNOL (sedative-hypnotic)
ETHINYL ESTRADIOL (estrogen)
ETHIONAMIDE (tuberculostatic)
ETHOTOIN (antiepileptic)
ETHOSUXIMIDE (antiepileptic)
ETHYLENE GLYCOL (alcohol)
ETIDOCAINE (analgesic, local)
ETIDRONATE (bone stabilizer)
ETODOLAC
   (antiinflammatory, non-opioid analgesic)
ETOPOSIDE (antineoplastic)
ETRETINATE (antpsoriasis agent)
FAMOTIDINE (histamine H2 blocker)
FANSIDAR (antimalarial)
FELODIPINE (antihypertensive)
FENFLURAMINE (anorexiant)
FENOPROFEN
   (antiinflammatory, non-opioid analgesic)
FENTANYL (opioid analgesic, IV anesthetic)
FERROUS SULFATE (hematinic)
FINASTERIDE (androgen hormone inhibitor)
FLECAINIDE (antiarrhythmic)
FLOXURIDINE (antineoplastic)
FLUCONAZOLE (antifungal)
FLUCYTOSINE (antifungal)
FLUDROCORTISONE
   (systemic corticosteroid)
FLUMAZENIL (benzodiazepine antagonist)
FLUNISOLIDE (corticosteroid)
FLUOCINOLONE (topical corticosteroid)
FLUOCINONIDE (topical corticosteroid)

3

AGENTS AND THERAPEUTIC CATEGORIES

FLUOROMETHOLONE
  (topical corticosteroid)
FLUOROURACIL (antineoplastic)
FLUOXETINE (antidepressant)
FLUOXYMESTERONE (androgen)
FLUPHENAZINE (antipsychotic)
FLURANDRENOLIDE
  (topical corticosteroid)
FLURAZEPAM (hypnotic)
FLURBIPROFEN (antiinflammatory)
FLUTAMIDE (androgen hormone inhibitor)
FLUTICASONE (topical corticosteroid)
FLUVASTATIN (hypolipidemic)
FOLIC ACID (anti-anemic)
FOSFOMYCIN (urinary anti-infective)
FOSINOPRIL (antihypertensive)
FURAZOLIDONE (systemic antibacterial)
FUROSEMIDE (diuretic, antihypertensive agent)
GALLAMINE (skeletal m. relaxant)
GEMFIBROZIL (hypolipidemic)
GENTAMICIN (systemic antibacterial)
GLIMEPIRIDE (hypoglycemic)
GLIPIZIDE (hypoglycemic)
GLYBURIDE (hypoglycemic)
GLYCERIN (laxative)
GOLD (heavy metal)
GOLD SODIUM THIOMALATE
  (antirheumatic)
GRISEOFULVIN (antifungal)
GUAIFENESIN (expectorant)
GUANABENZ (antihypertensive)
GUANADREL (antihypertensive)
GUANETHIDINE (antihypertensive)
GUANFACINE (antihypertensive)
HALAZEPAM (antianxiety)
HALCINONIDE (topical corticosteroid)
HALOBETASOL (topical corticosteroid)
HALOPERIDOL (antipsychotic)
HALOPROGIN (antifungal)
HALOTHANE (general anesthetic)
HEPARIN (anticoagulant)
HEROIN (abuse, drug of)
HOMATROPINE (anticholinergic)
HYDRALAZINE (antihypertensive)
HYDROCHLOROTHIAZIDE (diuretic,
  antihypertensive agent)
HYDROCORTISONE (corticosteroid)
HYDROFLUMETHIAZIDE
  (diuretic, antihypertensive)
HYDROMORPHONE (opioid analgesic)
HYDROXYCHLOROQUINE (antimalarial)
HYDROXYUREA (antineoplastic)

HYDROXYZINE (antianxiety, sedative, anti-
  pruritic agent)
HYOSCYAMINE
  (anticholinergic, antispasmodic)
IBUPROFEN (non-opioid analgesic)
IDARUBICIN (antineoplastic)
IDOXURIDINE (antiviral)
IMIPENEM (carbapenam, antibacterial)
IMIPRAMINE (antidepressant)
INDAPAMIDE (diuretic, antihypertensive)
INDOMETHACIN (antiinflammatory)
INSULIN (hypoglycemic)
INTERFERON ALFA-2a,b (antineoplastics)
INTERFERON BETA (immunosuppressant)
INTERFERON GAMMA
  (immunosuppressant)
IODOQUINOL (amebicide)
IPRATROPIUM (anticholinergic)
IRON (heavy metal)
IRON DEXTRAN (hematinic)
ISOCARBOXAZID (antidepressant)
ISOETHARINE (bronchodilator)
ISOFLURANE (general anesthetic)
ISONIAZID (tuberculostatic)
ISOPROTERENOL (adrenergic agonist, ß)
ISOSORBIDE (antianginal)
ISOTRETINOIN (antiacne agent)
ISRADIPINE (antihypertensive)
ITRACONAZOLE (antifungal, systemic)
KANAMYCIN (systemic antibacterial)
KETAMINE (general anesthetic)
KETOCONAZOLE (antifungal, topical)
KETOPROFEN
  (antiinflammatory, non-opioid analgesic)
KETOROLAC (non-opioid analgesic)
LABETALOL (antihypertensive)
LACTULOSE (laxative)
LEAD (heavy metal)
LEUCOVORIN (anti-anemic)
LEVOBUNOLOL (antiglaucoma agent)
LEVOCABASTINE (antiallergic)
LEVODOPA (antiparkinsonian)
LEVODOPA-CARBIDOPA (antiparkinsonian)
LEVONORGESTREL (implant contraceptive)
LEVORPHANOL (opioid analgesic)
LEVOTHYROXINE (thyroid hormone)
LIDOCAINE
  (local anesthetic, antiarrhythmic)
LINCOMYCIN (systemic antibacterial)
LINDANE (antiparasitic, scabicide)
LIOTHYRONINE (thyroid hormone)
LIOTRIX (thyroid hormone)

4

AGENTS AND THERAPEUTIC CATEGORIES

LISINOPRIL (antihypertensive, heart failure,
  post-MI agent)
LITHIUM (antimaniacal)
LOBELINE (smoking deterrent)
LODOXAMIDE (antiallergic)
LOMEFLOXACIN (antibacterial)
LOMUSTINE (antineoplastic)
LOPERAMIDE (antidiarrheal)
LORACARBEF (systemic antibacterial)
LORATADINE (antihistamine)
LORAZEPAM (antianxiety)
LOSARTAN (antihypertensive)
LOVASTATIN (hypolipidemic)
LOXAPINE (antipsychotic)
LSD (psychotomimetic drug)
LYPRESSIN (posterior pituitary hormone)
MAGALDRATE (antacid)
MAGNESIUM CITRATE (laxative, osmotic)
MAGNESIUM HYDROXIDE (antacid)
MALATHION (insecticide)
MALT SOUP EXTRACT (bulk laxative)
MANNITOL (diuretic)
MAPROTILINE (antidepressant)
MARIJUANA (psychotomimetic drug)
MAZINDOL (anorexiant)
MEBENDAZOLE (anthelmintic)
MECAMYLAMINE (antihypertensive agent)
MECHLORETHAMINE (antineoplastic)
MECLIZINE (antihistamine)
MECLOCYCLINE (antiacne agent)
MECLOFENAMATE (antiinflammatory)
MEDROXYPROGESTERONE (progestin)
MEDRYSONE (topical corticosteroid)
MEFENAMIC ACID (non-opioid analgesic)
MEFLOQUINE (antimalarial)
MEGESTROL (antineoplastic, appetite stimulant)
MELPHALAN (antineoplastic)
MEPERIDINE (opioid analgesic)
MEPHENYTOIN (antiepileptic)
MEPHOBARBITAL (antiepileptic, sedative)
MEPIVACAINE (local anesthetic)
MEPROBAMATE (antianxiety)
MERCAPTOPURINE (antineoplastic)
MERCURY (heavy metal)
MESALAMINE (bowel antiinflammatory)
MESORIDAZINE (antipsychotic)
MESTRANOL (estrogen)
METAPROTERENOL (bronchodilator)
METHACHOLINE (cholinomimetic)
METHADONE (opioid analgesic)
METHAMPHETAMINE (anorexiant)
METHANOL (alcohol)
METHDILAZINE (systemic antihistamine)

METHENAMINE (urinary anti-infective)
METHICILLIN (antibacterial)
METHIMAZOLE (antithyroid)
METHOCARBAMOL (skeletal m. relaxant)
METHOTREXATE (antimetabolite)
METHSCOPOLAMINE (anticholinergic)
METHSUXIMIDE (antiepileptic)
METHYCLOTHIAZIDE
  (diuretic, antihypertensive)
METHYLDOPA (antihypertensive)
METHYLDOPATE (antihypertensive)
METHYLERGONOVINE (oxytocic)
METHYLPHENIDATE (CNS stimulant)
METHYLPREDNISOLONE (corticosteroid)
METHYLTESTOSTERONE (androgen)
METHYSERGIDE (antimigraine agent)
METIPRANOLOL (antiglaucoma agent)
METOCLOPRAMIDE
  (GI stimulant, antiemetic)
METOCURINE (neuromuscular blocker)
METOLAZONE (antihypertensive, diuretic)
METOPROLOL (antihypertensive, antianginal,
  post-MI drug)
METRIFONATE (anthelminthic)
METRONIDAZOLE (amebicide, antibacterial,
  antitrichomonal agent)
METYRAPONE (corticosteroid)
METYROSINE (antihypertensive)
MEXILETINE (antiarrhythmic)
MEZLOCILLIN (antibacterial)
MICONAZOLE (antifungal)
MIDAZOLAM (sedative-hypnotic)
MILRINONE (inotropic agent)
MINERAL OIL (laxative, lubricant)
MINOCYCLINE (systemic antibacterial)
MINOXIDIL (hair growth stimulator,
  antihypertensive agent)
MISOPROSTOL (antiulcer)
MOLINDONE (antipsychotic)
MOMETASONE (topical corticosteroid)
MORICIZINE (antiarrhythmic)
MORPHINE (opioid analgesic)
MUPIROCIN (antibacterial, topical)
MUROMONAB-CD3 (immunosuppressant)
MUSCARINE (cholinomimetic)
NABUMETONE (antiinflammatory)
NADOLOL (antihypertensive, anti-anginal)
NAFCILLIN (antibacterial)
NAFTIFINE (antifungal)
NALBUPHINE (opioid analgesic)
NALIDIXIC ACID (urinary anti-infective)
NALOXONE (opioid antagonist)

5

AGENTS AND THERAPEUTIC CATEGORIES

NALTREXONE (opioid antagonist)
NANDROLONE (anabolic steroid)
NAPHAZOLINE (nasal decongestant)
NAPROXEN (non-opioid analgesic)
NATAMYCIN (antifungal, topical)
NEDOCROMIL (antiasthmatic)
NEOMYCIN (antibacterial, topical)
NEOSTIGMINE (cholinomimetic)
NETILMICIN (systemic antibacterial)
NICARDIPINE (antihypertensive, anti-anginal)
NICLOSAMIDE (anthelminthic)
NICOTINE (smoking deterrent)
NICOTINE POLACRILEX
   (smoking deterrent)
NICOTINIC ACID (hypolipidemic)
NIFEDIPINE (antihypertensive, antianginal)
NITROFURANTOIN (urinary anti-infective)
NITROGLYCERIN (antianginal)
NITROPRUSSIDE (antihypertensive)
NITROUS OXIDE (general anesthetic)
NIZATIDINE (histamine H2 blocker)
NOREPINEPHRINE (vasoconstrictor)
NORETHINDRONE (progestin)
NORFLOXACIN (antibacterial, topical)
NORGESTREL (oral contraceptive)
NORTRIPTYLINE (antidepressant)
NYSTATIN (antifungal)
OFLOXACIN (systemic antibacterial)
OLSALAZINE (bowel antiinflammatory)
OMEPRAZOLE (gastric acid pump inhibitor)
ONDANSETRON (antiemetic)
ORPHENADRINE (skeletal m. relaxant)
OXACILLIN (systemic antibacterial)
OXAMNIQUINE (anthelminthic)
OXANDROLONE (anabolic steroid)
OXAPROZIN (antiinflammatory)
OXAZEPAM (antianxiety)
OXICONAZOLE (antifungal, topical)
OXIDIZED CELLULOSE (coagulant)
OXTRIPHYLLINE (bronchodilator)
OXYBUTYNIN (urinary antispasmodic)
OXYCODONE (opioid analgesic)
OXYMETAZOLINE
   (ocular and nasal decongestant)
OXYMORPHONE (opioid analgesic)
OXYTETRACYCLINE
   (systemic antibacterial)
OXYTOCIN (posterior pituitary hormone)
PAMIDRONATE (bone stabilizer)
PANCURONIUM (skeletal m. relaxant)
PAPAVERINE (vasodilator)
PARAMETHADIONE (antiepileptic)
PARALDEHYDE (sedative-hypnotic)

PARATHION (cholinomimetic)
PAROMOMYCIN (amebicide)
PAROXETINE (antidepressant)
PEMOLINE (CNS stimulant)
PENBUTOLOL (antihypertensive)
PENCICLOVIR (antiviral)
PENICILLAMINE (chelating agent)
PENICILLIN G (systemic antibacterial)
PENICILLIN V (systemic antibacterial)
PENTAERYTHRITOL TETRANITRATE
   (antianginal)
PENTAMIDINE (antiprotozoal)
PENTAZOCINE (opioid analgesic)
PENTOBARBITAL (sedative-hypnotic)
PENTOXIFYLLINE (hemorheologic agent)
PERGOLIDE (antiparkinsonian)
PERMETHRIN (scabicide)
PERPHENAZINE (antipsychotic, antiemetic)
PHENACEMIDE (antiepileptic)
PHENAZOPYRIDINE (urinary analgesic)
PHENCYCLIDINE (psychotomimetic drug)
PHENDIMETRAZINE (anorexiant)
PHENELZINE (antidepressant)
PHENINDAMINE (systemic antihistamine)
PHENINDIONE (anticoagulant)
PHENOBARBITAL (sedative-hypnotic)
PHENOL (local anesthetic)
PHENOLPHTHALEIN (contact laxative)
PHENOXYBENZAMINE (antihypertensive)
PHENTERMINE (anorexiant)
PHENTOLAMINE (adrenergic blocker, α)
PHENYLEPHRINE (adrenergic agonist, α)
PHENYTOIN (antiepileptic)
PHOSPHATE SALT (hypocalcemic)
PHYSOSTIGMINE (cholinomimetic)
PHYTONADIONE (vitamin K_1)
PILOCARPINE (cholinomimetic)
PIMOZIDE (antipsychotic)
PINDOLOL (adrenergic blocker, ß)
PIPERCURONIUM (neuromuscular blocker)
PIPERACILLIN (beta-lactam, penicillin)
PIRBUTEROL (bronchodilator)
PIROXICAM (antiinflammatory)
PLICAMYCIN (hypocalcemic)
POLYMYXIN B (systemic antibacterial)
POLYTHIAZIDE (diuretic, antihypertensive)
POTASSIUM CHLORIDE (expectorant)
PRAMOXINE
   (local anesthetic, antihemorrhoidal)
PRAVASTATIN (hypolipidemic)
PRAZIQUANTEL (anthelminthic)
PRAZOSIN (selective $\alpha 1$ blocker)
PREDNICARBATE (topical corticosteroid)

6

PREDNISOLONE (corticosteroid)
PREDNISONE (corticosteroid)
PRIMAQUINE (antimalarial)
PRIMIDONE (antiepileptic)
PROBENECID (antigout agent)
PROCAINAMIDE (antiarrhythmic)
PROCARBAZINE (antineoplastic)
PROCAINE (analgesic, local)
PROCAINE PENICILLIN (penicillin, depot)
PROCHLORPERAZINE (antiemetic)
PROCYCLIDINE (antiparkinsonian)
PROGESTERONE (progestin)
PROMAZINE (antipsychotic)
PROMETHAZINE (antihistamine)
PROPAFENONE (antiarrhythmic)
PROPANTHELINE (anticholinergic)
PROPOXYPHENE (opioid analgesic)
PROPRANOLOL (adrenergic blocker, ß)
PROPYLTHIOURACIL (antithyroid)
PROTAMINE SULFATE (heparin antagonist)
PROTRIPTYLINE (antidepressant)
PSEUDOEPHEDRINE (adrenergic agonist)
PSYLLIUM (laxative, bulk)
PTH (hypocalcemic agent)
PYRANTEL PAMOATE (anthelminthic)
PYRAZINAMIDE (tuberculostatic)
PYRIDOSTIGMINE (cholinomimetic)
PYRILAMINE (antihistamine)
PYRIMETHAMINE (antimalarial)
QUAZEPAM (sedative-hypnotic)
QUINAPRIL (antihypertensive)
QUINESTROL (estrogen)
QUINIDINE (antiarrhythmic)
QUININE (antimalarial)
RADIOACTIVE IODINE (antithyroid)
RAMIPRIL (antihypertensive)
RANITIDINE (histamine H2 blocker)
RESERPINE (antihypertensive)
RIBAVIRIN (antiviral)
RIFABUTIN (tuberculostatic)
RIFAMPIN (tuberculostatic)
RIMANTADINE (antiviral)
RITODRINE (adrenergic agonist, ß)
SALSALATE (antiinflammatory)
SCOPOLAMINE (anticholinergic)
SECOBARBITAL (sedative-hypnotic)
SELEGILINE (antiparkinsonian)
SELENIUM SULFIDE
  (antiseborrheic, antifungal)
SENNA CONCENTRATE (irritant laxative)
SERTRALINE (antidepressant)
SILVER SULFADIAZINE
  (antibacterial, topical)

SIMETHICONE (antiflatulent)
SIMVASTATIN (hypolipidemic)
SODIUM BICARBONATE (antacid)
SODIUM NITROPRUSSIDE (antihypertensive)
SODIUM POLYSTYRENE SULFONATE
  (potassium binding resin)
SOMAN (cholinomimetic)
SOTALOL (antiarrhythmic)
SPECTINOMYCIN (systemic antibacterial)
SPIRONOLACTONE (diuretic)
STANOZOLOL (anabolic steroid)
STIBOGLUCANATE (antiprotozoal)
STREPTOKINASE (thrombolytic)
STREPTOMYCIN (tuberculostatic)
STREPTOZOCIN (antineoplastic)
SUCCINYLCHOLINE (skeletal m. relaxant)
SUCRALFATE (antiulcer)
SUFENTANIL (opioid analgesic)
SULBACTAM (penicillin, adjunct agent)
SULCONAZOLE (antifungal, topical)
SULFACETAMIDE (antibacterial, topical)
SULFADIAZINE (systemic antibacterial)
SULFAMETHIZOLE (systemic antibacterial)
SULFAMETHOXAZOLE
  (systemic antibacterial)
SULFANILAMIDE (antifungal)
SULFASALAZINE (bowel antiinflammatory)
SULFINPYRAZONE (antigout agent)
SULFISOXAZOLE (antibacterial, topical)
SULINDAC (antiinflammatory)
SUMATRIPTAN (antimigraine agent)
TAMOXIFEN (antineoplastic)
TEMAZEPAM (sedative-hypnotic)
TERAZOSIN (adrenergic blocker, α)
TERBINAFINE (antifungal, topical)
TERBUTALINE (adrenergic agonist, ß)
TERCONAZOLE (antifungal, topical)
TERFENADINE (systemic antihistamine)
TESTOLACTONE (androgen)
TESTOSTERONE CYPIONATE (androgen)
TESTOSTERONE PROPIONATE (androgen)
TETRACAINE (analgesic, local)
TETRACYCLINE (antibacterial)
TETRAHYDROZOLINE (decongestant)
THEOPHYLLINE (bronchodilator)
THIABENDAZOLE (anthelmintic)
THIETHYLPERAZINE (antiemetic)
THIOGUANINE (antineoplastic)
THIOPENTAL (general anesthetic)
THIORIDAZINE (antipsychotic)
THIOTHIXENE (antipsychotic)
THYROID DESICCATED (thyroid hormone)
TICARCILLIN (antibacterial, penicillin)

7

AGENTS AND THERAPEUTIC CATEGORIES

TICLOPIDINE (platelet aggregation inhibitor)
TIMOLOL (adrenergic blocker, ß)
TIOCONAZOLE (topical antifungal)
TOBRAMYCIN (systemic antibacterial)
TOCAINIDE (antiarrhythmic)
TOLAZAMIDE (hypoglycemic)
TOLBUTAMIDE (hypoglycemic)
TOLMETIN (systemic antiinflammatory)
TOLNAFTATE (antifungal, topical)
TRANYLCYPROMINE (antidepressant)
TRAZODONE (antidepressant)
TRETINOIN (antiacne agent)
TRIAMCINOLONE (corticosteroid)
TRIAMTERENE (diuretic)
TRIAZOLAM (sedative-hypnotic)
TRICHLORMETHIAZIDE
  (diuretic, antihypertensive)
TRIFLUOPERAZINE (antipsychotic)
TRIFLURIDINE (antiviral)
TRIHEXYPHENIDYL (antiparkinsonian)
TRIMEPRAZINE (antihistamine, antipruritic)
TRIMETHADIONE (antiepileptic)
TRIMETHOBENZAMIDE (antiemetic)
TRIMETHOPRIM (systemic antibacterial)
TRIMIPRAMINE (antidepressant)
TRIPELENNAMINE (antihistamine)
TROGLITAZONE (hypoglycemic)
TROLEANDOMYCIN
  (systemic antibacterial)
TROPICAMIDE (anticholinergic)
TUBOCURARINE (skeletal m. relaxant)
UROKINASE (thrombolytic)
VALPROIC ACID (antiepileptic)
VALSARTAN (antihypertensive)
VANCOMYCIN (systemic antibacterial)
VASOPRESSIN
  (posterior pituitary hormone)
VECURONIUM (skeletal m. relaxant)
VERAPAMIL (antihypertensive)
VIDARABINE (antiviral)
VINBLASTINE (antineoplastic)
VINCRISTINE (antineoplastic)
VITAMIN B12 (anti-anemia)
WARFARIN SODIUM (anticoagulant)
XYLOMETAZOLINE (nasal decongestant)
YOHIMBINE (adrenergic blocker, α2)
ZAFIRLUKAST (antiasthmatic)
ZIDOVUDINE (AZT, antiviral)
ZINC OXIDE (skin protectant)
ZOLPIDEM (hypnotic)

THERAPEUTIC CATEGORIES

ABUSE, DRUGS OF

barbiturates
benzodiazepines
heroin
cocaine
solvents

ADRENERGIC AGONISTS, DIRECT ACTING

albuterol (ß2)
clonidine (α2 > α1)
dobutamine (ß1 > ß2)
epinephrine (α,ß)
isoetharine (ß2 > ß1)
isoproterenol (ß)
metaproterenol (ß2 > ß1)
norepinephrine (α)
oxymetazoline
phenylephrine (α1 > α2)
ritodrine (ß2)
terbutaline (ß2 > ß1)
tetrahydrozoline

ADRENERGIC AGONISTS, MIXED ACTING

amphetamines
dopamine (D1, D2 > ß1 > α)
ephedrine (α, ß)
pseudoephedrine (α, ß)

ADRENERGIC BLOCKERS, ALPHA

doxazosin (α1)
phenoxybenzamine (α)
phentolamine (α) (M, H2)
prazosin (α1)
terazosin (α1)
yohimbine (α2)

ADRENERGIC BLOCKERS, BETA

acebutolol (ß1 > ß2)
atenolol (ß1 > ß2)
betaxolol
bisoprolol
carteolol
esmolol (ß1 > ß2)
labetalol (α and ß blocker)
metoprolol (ß1 > ß2)
nadolol
penbutolol

pindolol
propranolol
sotalol
timolol

ADRENERGIC NEURONAL BLOCKERS

guanethidine
guanadrel
metyrosine
reserpine

ALCOHOLS, THE

ethanol
ethylene glycol
isopropyl alcohol
methanol

AMEBICIDES

emetine
iodoquinol
metronidazole
paromomycin

AMINOGLYCOSIDES, ANTIBACTERIAL

amikacin
gentamicin
neomycin
netilmicin
streptomycin
tobramycin

ANABOLIC STEROIDS

nandrolone decanoate
nandrolone phenpropionate
oxandrolone
oxymetholone
stanozolol

ANALGESICS, NON-OPIOID

acetaminophen
aspirin
diflunisal
etodolac
fenoprofen calcium
ibuprofen
ketoprofen
ketorolac tromethamine

THERAPEUTIC CATEGORIES

meclofenamate sodium
mefenamic acid
naproxen

ANALGESICS, OPIOID

alfentanil
buprenorphine
butorphanol
codeine
dezocine
fentanyl
hydromorphone
levorphanol
meperidine
methadone
morphine
nalbuphine
oxycodone
oxymorphone
pentazocine
propoxyphene

ANALGESICS, TOPICAL

capsaicin

ANDROGEN HORMONE INHIBITORS

cyproterone
flutamide
finasteride

ANDROGENS

danazol
methyl testosterone
oxymetholone
testosterone
testosterone cypionate
testosterone propionate
testolactone

ANESTHETICS, GENERAL

diethylether
enflurane
fentanyl
halothane
isoflurane
ketamine
meperidine

nitrous oxide
thiopental

ANESTHETICS, LOCAL

benzocaine
cocaine
cyclomethycaine
dibucaine
etidocaine
lidocaine
mepivacaine
procaine
tetracaine

ANOREXIANTS

amphetamine sulfate
benzphetamine
diethylpropion
fenfluramine
mazindol
methamphetamine
phendimetrazine tartrate
phentermine
phentermine resin

ANTACIDS

aluminum hydroxide
calcium carbonate
magnesium hydroxide
sodium bicarbonate

ANTHELMINTICS

mebendazole
niclosamide
oxamniquine
praziquantel
pyrantel pamoate
thiabendazole

ANTIACNE AGENTS

benzoyl peroxide
clindamycin phosphate
erythromycin
isotretinoin
meclocycline sulfosalicylate
tretinoin

THERAPEUTIC CATEGORIES

ANTIALCHOLIC

disulfiram

ANTIALLERGICS

cromolyn sodium
levocabastine
lodoxamide tromethamine

ANTIANGINALS

atenolol
diltiazem
erythrityl tetranitrate
isosorbide nitrate
metoprolol
nifedipine
nitroglycerin
pentaerythritol tetranitrate
propranolol
timolol
verapamil

ANTIANXIETY AGENTS

alprazolam
buspirone
chlordiazepoxide
clorazepate
diazepam
hydroxyzine
lorazepam
meprobamate
oxazepam
prazepam

ANTIARRHYTHMICS

amiodarone (III)
bretylium (III)
esmolol (III)
lidocaine (Ib)
mexiletine (Ib)
procainamide (Ia)
propranolol (II)
quinidine (Ia)
tocainide (Ib)
verapamil (IV)

ANTIARTHRITIC

aurothioglucose

ANTIASTHMATICS

cromolyn sodium
nedocromil sodium
theophylline
zafirlukast

ANTIBACTERIALS, SYSTEMIC

amikacin
amoxicillin
ampicillin
azithromycin
aztreonam
bacampicillin
carbenicillin
cefaclor
cefadroxil
cefamandole
cefazolin
cefixime
cefmetazole
cefonicid
cefoperazone
cefotaxime
cefotetan
cefoxitin
cefpodoxime
cefprozil
ceftazidime
ceftizoxime
ceftriaxone
cefuroxime
cephalexin
cephalothin
cephaprin
cephradine
chloramphenicol
ciprofloxacin
clarithromycin
clindamycin
cloxacillin
colistimethate
colistin
demeclocycline
dicloxacillin
doxycycline
enoxacin
erythromycin

11

THERAPEUTIC CATEGORIES

furazolidone
gentamicin
kanamycin
lincomycin
lomefloxacin
loracarbef
methicillin
metronidazole
mezlocillin
minocycline
nafcillin
netilmicin
nitrofurantoin
ofloxacin
oxacillin
oxytetracycline
penicillin G benzathine
penicillin G procaine
penicillin V
piperacillin
polymyxin
spectinomycin
sulfamethizole
sulfamethoxazole
sulfisoxazole
tetracycline
ticarcillin
tobramycin
trimethoprim
troleandomycin
vancomycin

ANTIBACTERIALS, TOPICAL

acetic acid
bacitracin
chloramphenicol
chlortetracycline
ciprofloxacin
clindamycin phosphate
clioquinol
erythromycin
gentamicin sulfate
metronidazole
mupirocin
neomycin sulfate
norfloxacin
ofloxacin
silver sulfadiazine
sulfacetamide sodium
sulfisoxazole diolamine
tetracycline
tobramycin

ANTICHOLINERGICS

atropine
benztropine
botulinus toxin
dicyclomine
hemicholinium
homatropine
ipratropium
methscopolamine
propantheline
scopolamine
tropicamide

ANTICOAGULANTS

dicumarol
enoxaparin
heparin
warfarin sodium

ANTIDEPRESSANTS

amitriptyline
amoxapine
desipramine
doxepin
fluoxetine
imipramine
isocarboxazid
maprotiline
nortriptyline
phenelzine
protriptyline
sertraline
tranylcypromine
trazodone
trimipramine

ANTIDIARRHEALS

attapulgite
bismuth subsalicylate
diphenoxylate
loperamide

ANTIEMETICS

benzquinamide
buclizine
chlorpromazine
cyclizine
dimenhydrinate

THERAPEUTIC CATEGORIES

diphenhydramine
dronabinol
hydroxyzine
metoclopramide
ondansetron
perphenazine
prochlorperazine
prochlorperazine edisylate
promethazine
scopolamine
thiethylperazine maleate
trimethobenzamide

ANTIENURETIC AGENT

desmopressin acetate

ANTIEPILEPTICS and ANTICONVULSANTS

acetazolamide
carbamazepine
clonazepam
clorazepate
diazepam
divalproex
ethotoin
felbamate
mephenytoin
mephobarbital
methsuximide
paramethadione
phenacemide
phenobarbital
phenytoin
primidone
trimethadione
valproic acid

ANTIFLATULENTS

simethicone

ANTIFUNGALS, SYSTEMIC

amphotericin B
fluconazole
flucytosine
griseofulvin
itraconazole
ketoconazole
miconazole

ANTIFUNGALS, TOPICAL

acetic acid
amphotericin B
butoconazole nitrate
ciclopirox olamine
clioquinol
clotrimazole
econazole nitrate
haloprogin
ketoconazole
miconazole nitrate
naftifine
natamycin
nystatin
oxiconazole nitrate
selenium sulfide
sulconazole nitrate
sulfanilamide
terbinafine
terconazole
tioconazole
tolnaftate

ANTIGLAUCOMA AGENTS

acetazolamide
betaxolol
carteolol
epinephrine
isoflurophate
levobunolol
metipranolol
pilocarpine
timolol

ANTIGOUT AGENTS

allopurinol
colchicine
probenecid
sulfinpyrazone
NSAIDs

ANTIHEMORRHOIDALS

dibucaine

ANTIHISTAMINES, SYSTEMIC

astemizole
chlorpheniramine
cyclizine

13

THERAPEUTIC CATEGORIES

dimenhydrinate
diphenhydramine
loratadine
meclizine
promethazine
terfenadine

ANTIHISTAMINES, TOPICAL

diphenhydramine

ANTIHYPERTENSIVES

acebutolol
amlodipine
atenolol
benazepril
bendroflumethiazide
benzthiazide
betaxolol
bisoprolol
captopril
carteolol
chlorothiazide
chlorthalidone
clonidine
diazoxide
diltiazem
doxazosin
enalapril
enalaprilat
felodipine
fosinopril
furosemide
guanabenz
guanadrel
guanethidine
guanfacine
hydralazine
hydrochlorothiazide
hydroflumethiazide
indapamide
isradipine
labetalol
lisinopril
losartan
methyclothiazide
methyldopa
methyldopate
metolazone
metoprolol
minoxidil
nadolol

nicardipine
nifedipine
penbutolol
phenoxybenzamine
phentolamine
pindolol
polythiazide
prazosin
propranolol
quinapril
ramipril
reserpine
sodium nitroprusside
spironolactone
terazosin
timolol
torsemide
trichlormethiazide
trimethaphan
valsartan
verapamil

ANTIINFLAMMATORY AGENTS, BOWEL

mesalamine
olsalazine sodium
sulfasalazine

ANTIINFLAMMATORY AGENTS, SYSTEMIC

aspirin
diclofenac sodium
diflunisal
etodolac
fenoprofen calcium
flurbiprofen
ibuprofen
indomethacin
ketoprofen
meclofenamate sodium
nabumetone
naproxen
oxaprozin
phenylbutazone
piroxicam
salsalate
sulindac
tolmetin sodium

ANTIINFLAMMATORY AGENTS, TOPICAL

diclofenac sodium
flurbiprofen sodium

14

THERAPEUTIC CATEGORIES

ketorolac tromethamine

ANTIMALARIALS

amodiaquine
chloroguanide
chloroquine
fansidar
hydroxychloroquine
mefloquine
primaquine
pyrimethamine
quinine
sulfonamide
sulfone
tetracycline
trimethoprim

ANTIMANIACALS

lithium carbonate
lithium citrate

ANTIMIGRAINE AGENTS

ergotamine tartrate
methysergide maleate
propranolol
sumatriptan succinate
timolol

ANTINEOPLASTICS

altretamine
asparaginase
bleomycin
busulfan
carboplatin
carmustine
chlorambucil
chlorotrianisene
cisplatin
cyclophosphamide
cytarabine
dacarbazine
dactinomycin
diethylstilbestrol
doxorubicin
estradiol
estramustine
etoposide
floxuridine
fluorouracil

flutamide
hydroxyurea
idarubicin
interferon alfa-2a
interferon alfa-2b
interferon alfa-n3
lomustine
mechlorethamine
medroxyprogesterone
megestrol
melphalan
mercaptopurine
methyltestosterone
pegaspargase
plicamycin
procarbazine
streptozocin
tamoxifen
testolactone
testosterone
thioguanine
vinblastine
vincristine

ANTIOSTEOPOROTICS

calcitonin-salmon
estropipate

ANTIPARASITICS

lindane
malathion

ANTIPARKINSONIANS

amantadine
benztropine
biperiden
bromocriptine
diphenhydramine
levodopa
levodopa-carbidopa
pergolide
procyclidine
selegiline
trihexyphenidyl

ANTIPROTOZOALS

atovaquone
eflornithine
pentamidine isethionate

15

THERAPEUTIC CATEGORIES

ANTIPRURITICS

cyproheptadine
hydroxyzine
hydroxyzine pamoate
trimeprazine tartrate

ANTIPSORIASIS AGENTS

anthralin
etretinate

ANTIPSYCHOTICS

chlorpromazine
chlorprothixene
clozapine
fluphenazine
haloperidol
loxapine
mesoridazine
molindone
perphenazine
pimozide
prochlorperazine
promazine
promethazine
risperidone
thioridazine
trifluoperazine

ANTIPYRETICS

acetaminophen
aspirin
ibuprofen

ANTIRHEUMATICS

auranofin
gold sodium thiomalate

ANTISEBORRHEICS

selenium sulfide

ANTISPASMODICS

hyoscyamine sulfate

ANTITHYROID DRUGS

methimazole

propylthiouracil
radioactive iodine

ANTITRICHOMONALS

metronidazole

ANTITUSSIVES

codeine sulfate
dextromethorphan
diphenhydramine

ANTIULCER AGENTS

cimetidine
famotidine
misoprostol
nizatidine
ranitidine
sucralfate

ANTIVERTIGO AGENTS

buclizine
dimenhydrinate
meclizine

ANTIVIRALS, SYSTEMIC

acyclovir
amantadine
didanosine
penciclovir
rimantadine
ribavirin
valacyclovir
vidarabine
zidovudine

ANTIVIRALS, TOPICAL

acyclovir
idoxuridine
trifluridine
vidarabine monohydrate

APPETITE STIMULANTS

dronabinol

THERAPEUTIC CATEGORIES

BENZODIAZEPINE ANTAGONIST

flumazenil

BETA-LACTAMS, CEPHALOSPORIN

cefaclor
cefadroxil
cefamandole
cefazolin
cefixime
cefmetazole
cefonicid
cefoperazone
cefotaxime
cefotetan
cefoxitin
cefpodoxime
cefprozil
ceftazidime
ceftizoxime
ceftriaxone
cefuroxime
cephalexin
cephalothin
cephapirin
cephradine

BETA-LACTAMS, PENICILLIN

amoxicillin
amoxicillin/clavulanate
ampicillin
ampicillin/sulbactam
cloxacillin
dicloxacillin
methicillin
mezlocillin
nafcillin
oxacillin
penicillin G
penicillin V
piperacillin/tazobactam
piperacillin
ticarcillin
ticarcillin/clavulanate

BONE STABILIZERS

etidronate disodium
pamidronate disodium

BRONCHODILATORS

albuterol
aminophylline
dyphylline
epinephrine
ipratropium
isoetharine
isoproterenol
metaproterenol
terbutaline
theophylline

CALCIUM CHANNEL BLOCKERS

amlodipine
bepridil
diltiazem
felodipine
isradipine
nicardipine
nifedipine
nimodipine
verapamil

CALCIUM SUPPLEMENTS

calcium carbonate
calcium glubionate
calcium gluconate

CARBAPENAM, ANTIBACTERIAL

imipenem

CARDIAC GLYCOSIDES

digitoxin
digoxin

CERVICAL RIPENING AGENT

dinoprostone

CHELATING AGENTS

edetate calcium disodium
deferoxamine
dimercaprol
penicillamine

17

THERAPEUTIC CATEGORIES

CHOLINOMIMETICS

acetylcholine
ambenonium
bethanechol
carbachol
echothiophate
edrophonium
isoflurophate
malathion
methacholine
muscarine
neostigmine
parathion
physostigmine
pilocarpine
pyridostigmine
soman

CNS STIMULANTS

amphetamine sulfate
caffeine
dextroamphetamine sulfate
methylphenidate
pemoline

COAGULANTS

aminocarpoic acid
oxidized cellulose

CONTRACEPTIVES, IMPLANT

levonorgestrel

CONTRACEPTIVES, INJECTABLE

medroxyprogesterone acetate

CONTRACEPTIVES, INTRAUTERINE

progesterone

CONTRACEPTIVES, ORAL

diethylstilbestrol
ethinyl estradiol
levonorgestrel
medroxyprogesterone (depot)
mestranol
mifepristone (RU 486)
norethindrone

norethindrone acetate
norgestrel

CORTICOSTEROIDS, SYSTEMIC

ACTH
dexamethasone
fludrocortisone
hydrocortisone
prednisolone
prednisone
methylprednisolone
triamcinolone

CORTICOSTEROIDS, TOPICAL

alclometasone
amcinonide
beclomethasone
betamethasone benzoate
betamethasone valerate
clobetasol propionate
clocortolone
desonide
desoximetasone
dexamethasone sodium phosphate
diflorasone
flunisolide
fluocinolone
fluocinonide
fluorometholone
flurandrenolide
fluticasone propionate
halcinonide
halobetasol propionate
hydrocortisone
hydrocortisone acetate
hydrocortisone valerate
medrysone
mometasone
prednicarbate
prednisolone acetate
prednisolone sodium phosphate
triamcinolone

DECONGESTANTS, NASAL

ephedrine sulfate
naphazoline
oxymetazoline
phenylephrine
tetrahydrozoline
xylometazoline

18

THERAPEUTIC CATEGORIES

DECONGESTANTS, OCULAR

oxymetazoline
tetrahydrozoline

DECONGESTANTS, SYSTEMIC

phenergan
pseudoephedrine

DIURETICS

acetazolamide
amiloride
bumetanide
chlorothiazide
chlorthalidone
ethacrynic acid
furosemide
hydrochlorothiazide
indapamide
mannitol
metolazone
spironolactone
triamterene

ESTROGENS

chlorotrianisene
conjugated estrogen
dienestrol
diethylstilbestrol
estradiol
ethinyl estradiol
mestranol
quinestrol

EXPECTORANTS

ammonium chloride
guaifenesin
potassium iodide

FLUOROQUINOLONES, ANTIBACTERIAL

ciprofloxacin
lomefloxacin
norfloxacin
ofloxacin
pefloxacin
rufloxacin

GASTRIC ACID PUMP INHIBITOR

omeprazole

GI STIMULANTS

cisapride
metoclopramide

GONADOTROPIN INHIBITOR

danazol

GRAM NEGATIVE, ANTIBACTERIAL

amikacin
ciprofloxacin
gentamicin
lomefloxacin
neomycin
netilmicin
norfloxacin
ofloxacin
spectinomycin
streptomycin
tobramycin

HAIR GROWTH STIMULATOR

minoxidil

HEAVY METALS, THE

arsenic
cadmium
gold
iron
lead
mercury

HEMATINICS

ferrous sulfate
iron dextran injection

HEMORHEOLOGIC AGENT

pentoxifylline

HEPARIN ANTAGONIST

protamine sulfate

THERAPEUTIC CATEGORIES

HISTAMINE H2-BLOCKERS

cimetidine
famotidine
nizatidine
ranitidine

HYPERGLYCEMIC AGENT

diazoxide

HYPOCALCEMIC AGENTS

calcitonin
etidronate
glucocorticoid
inorganic phosphates (KPO4)
loop diuretics
plicamycin

HYPOGLYCEMIC AGENTS

acetohexamide
chlorpropamide
glimepiride
glipizide
glyburide
tolazamide
tolbutamide
troglitazone

HYPOLIPIDEMICS

atorvastatin
cholestyramine
clofibrate
colestipol
lovastatin
nicotinic acid
pravastatin
simvastatin
gemfibrozil
probucol
vitamin C, E

IMMUNOSUPPRESSANTS

aldesleukin (IL-2)
azathioprine
cyclophosphamide
cyclosporine
interferon alfa
interferon beta

interferon gamma
lymphocyte immune globulin
muromonab-CD3

IMMUNOSUPPRESSANTS, RHEUMATOID ARTHRITIS

auranofin
aurothioglucose
gold sodium thiomalate
hydroxychloroquine

INOTROPIC AGENTS

amrinone lactate
digitoxin
digoxin
milrinone

INSULINS, THE

insulin injection
isophane insulin
lente
protamine zinc insulin
semilente
ultralente

LAXATIVES

glycerin
lactulose
mineral oil (lubricant)

LAXATIVES, BULK

psyllium

LAXATIVES, EMOLLIENT

docusate sodium

LAXATIVES, IRRITANT (CONTACT)

castor oil
phenolphthalein

LAXATIVES, SALINE

magnesium citrate
magnesium hydroxide

THERAPEUTIC CATEGORIES

LEPROSTATICS

clofazimine
dapsone

MINERALOCORTICOIDS

fludrocortisone acetate

MONOBACTAM ANTIBACTERIAL

aztreonam

MUCOLYTIC

acetylcysteine sodium

MYDRIATIC-CYCLOPLEGICS

atropine sulfate
scopolamine

NEUROMUSCULAR BLOCKERS

atracurium besylate
doxacurium chloride
metrocurine iodide
pancuronium bromide
pipercuronium bromide
succinylcholine chloride
tubocurarine chloride
vecuronium bromide

NICOTINIC RECEPTOR AGONISTS

hexamethonium
mecamylamine
nicotine
nicotine polacrilex

NSAIDs

aspirin
piroxicam
naproxen
ibuprofen
indomethacin
ketoprofen
ketorolac
non-acetylated salicylates

OPIOID AGONIST-ANTAGONIST, MIXED ACTING

buprenorphine
butorphanol
nalbuphine
pentazocine

OPIOID ANTAGONISTS

naloxone
naltrexone

OVULATION STIMULANTS

clomiphene citrate

OXYTOCIC AGENTS

ergonovine maleate
methylergonovine

PENICILLIN, ADJUNCT AGENTS

cilastatin (dipeptidase inhibitor)
clavulanic acid (ß-lactamase inhibitors)
probenecid (↓ penicillin excretion)
sulbactam (ß-lactamase inhibitors)

PLATELET AGGREGATION INHIBITORS

dipyridamole
ticlopidine

POST-MYOCARDIAL INFARCTION DRUGS

atenolol
metoprolol
propranolol
timolol

POSTERIOR PITUITARY HORMONES

desmopressin
lypressin
oxytocin
vasopressin

POTASSIUM SUPPLEMENTS

potassium chloride
potassium gluconate

THERAPEUTIC CATEGORIES

POTASSIUM REMOVING RESINS

sodium polystyrene sulfonate

PROGESTINS

medroxyprogesterone acetate
norethindrone
norethindrone acetate

PSYCHOTOMIMETIC DRUGS

lysergic acid diethylamide (LSD)
marijuana (Δ^9-tetrahydrocannabinol)
phencyclidine (PCP)

SCABICIDES

crotamiton
lindane
permethrin

SEDATIVES and HYPNOTICS

butabarbital
chloral hydrate
doxylamine
estazolam
ethchlorvynol
flurazepam
hydroxyzine
hydroxyzine pamoate
mephobarbital
midazolam
pentobarbital
phenobarbital
promethazine
quazepam
secobarbital
temazepam
triazolam
zolpidem

SKELETAL MUSCLE RELAXANTS

atracurium
baclofen
cyclobenzaprine
dantrolene
diazepam
gallamine
pancuronium
succinylcholine

tubocurarine
vecuronium

SKIN PROTECTANT

zinc oxide

SMOKING DETERRENTS

lobeline sulfate
nicotine
nicotine polacrilex

STOOL SOFTENERS

docusate calcium
docusate sodium

SULFONAMIDES, ANTIBACTERIAL

sulfacetamide
sulfadiazine
sulfamethizole
sulfamethoxazole
sulfasalazine
sulfisoxazole

SYMPATHOMIMETICS

dobutamine
dopamine
epinephrine
phenylephrine

THROMBOLYTICS

alteplase, recombinant
anistreplase

streptokinase
urokinase

THYROID HORMONES

levothyroxine (L-T4)
liothyronine (L-T3)
liotrix
thyroid

TUBERCULOSTATICS

capreomycin
cyclosporine

ethambutol (1st line)
ethionamide
isoniazid (1st line)
kanamycin
para-aminosalicylic acid
pyrazinamide (1st line)
rifampin (1st line)
streptomycin (1st line)

URINARY ANALGESICS

phenazopyridine

URINARY ANTI-INFECTIVES

cinoxacin
ciprofloxacin
fosfomycin
methenamine
nalidixic acid
nitrofurantoin
norfloxacin
ofloxacin

URINARY ANTISPASMODICS

oxybutynin chloride

VASODILATORS

isoxsuprine
papaverine

VITAMINS & VITAMIN SUPPLEMENTS

calcifediol
calcitriol
dihydrotachysterol
phytonadione

BRIEF DRUG DESCRIPTIONS

ACARBOSE: hypoglycemic agent

ACEBUTOLOL: $\beta1 > \beta2$ blocker; antihypertensive, antiarrhythmic

ACETAMINOPHEN: non-opioid analgesic, antipyretic, NOT antiinflammatory

ACETAZOLAMIDE: diuretic, antiepileptic, anti-glaucoma drug, inhibits carbonic anhydrase

ACETOHEXAMIDE: 1st generation oral hypoglycemic; used in NIDDM; ↑ Ca influx, insulin efflux

ACETYLCHOLINE: miotic (direct acting cholinomimetic)

ACETYLCYSTEINE: mucolytic; acetaminophen overdose antidote

ACTH: diagnosis of adrenocortical insufficiency (corticotropin)

ACYCLOVIR: antiviral; topical, po, IV; acyclo-GTP blocks viral DNA polymerase; **prodrug**

ADENOSINE: IV antiarrhythmic; depresses sinus node automaticity and ↓ AV nodal conduction

ALBUTEROL: selective ß2 adrenergic agonist; bronchodilator

ALCLOMETASONE: mild (class IV) topical corticosteroid

ALDESLEUKIN: IL-2; used to treat metastatic renal cell carcinoma; very toxic

ALENDRONATE: bone stabilizer

ALFENTANIL: opioid analgesic; 100x's the potency of morphine

ALLOPURINOL: antigout agent; xanthine oxidase inhibitor that decreases uric acid; used to treat hyperuricemia or gout

ALPRAZOLAM: benzodiazepine anxiety agent; short acting

ALTEPLASE, RECOMBINANT: thrombolytic

ALTRETAMINE: antineoplastic used in ovarian, small cell lung, cervical and breast carcinomas

ALUMINUM HYDROXIDE: antacid; constipating

AMANTADINE: antiparkinsonian (increases DA release, blocks re-uptake of DA); antiviral (inhibits influenza A virus)

AMBENONIUM: cholinomimetic used in myasthenia gravis

AMCINONIDE: potent (class II) topical corticosteroid

AMIKACIN: systemic aminoglycoside antibacterial; binds 30s and 50s; blocks initiation, causes misreads

AMILORIDE: K^+ sparing diuretic

24

BRIEF DRUG DESCRIPTIONS

AMINOCAPROIC ACID: hemostatic; inhibits dissolution of clots

AMINOPHYLLINE: oral or IM bronchodilator; adenosine receptor antagonist

AMIODARONE: antiarrhythmic; prolongs repolarization

AMITRIPTYLINE: tricyclic antidepressant

AMLODIPINE: antihypertensive; antianginal (calcium channel blocker)

AMOBARBITAL: sedative hypnotic (nonspecific effect on membranes; GABA-like effect on neurons)

AMODIAQUINE: antimalarial effective against rbc stage (4-aminoquinoline)

AMOXAPINE: 2nd generation antidepressant

AMOXICILLIN: aminopenicillin systemic antibacterial; spectrum covers gram negatives

AMPHETAMINES: mixed acting adrenergic drug; used for attention deficit disorder, narcolepsy, and obesity

AMPHOTERICIN B: antifungal; po, topical, IV, intrathecal; binds ergosterol, will NOT cross blood brain barrier (BBB)

AMPICILLIN: aminopenicillin systemic antibacterial; spectrum covers gram negatives; undergoes *enterohepatic circulation*

AMRINONE: inotropic agent; phosphodiesterase inhibitor, increases cAMP

AMYL NITRATE: antianginal available as inhalant capsule

ANASTROZOLE: antineoplastic

ANISTREPLASE: thrombolytic (anisoylated plasminogen streptokinase anistreplase, APSAC)

ANTHRALIN: antipsoriasis agent; reduces epidermal cell DNA synthesis and mitotic activity of hyperplastic epidermis

APROTININ: systemic hemostatic agent

ARSENIC: pentavalent heavy metal form uncouples oxidative phosphorylation, trivalent form ties up sulfhydryl groups

ASPARAGINASE: antineoplastic; decreased asparagine in neoplastic cells

ASPIRIN: non-opioid analgesic; antiinflammatory; antipyretic (acetyl salicylic acid, ASA)

ASTEMIZOLE: non-sedative antihistamine

ATENOLOL: ß1 > ß2 blocker; antihypertensive, antianginal, and post-MI drug

ATORVASTATIN: hypolipidemic; HMG-CoA Reductase inhibitor

BRIEF DRUG DESCRIPTIONS

ATOVAQUONE: antiprotozoal

ATRACURIUM: nondepolarizing curariform; used for laryngoscopy and bronchoscopy

ATROPINE: antimuscarinic; used in organophosphate poisoning, and to induce cycloplegia

ATTAPULGITE: antidiarrheal

AURANOFIN: disease modifying agent used in rheumatoid arthritis

AUROTHIOGLUCOSE: disease modifying agent used in rheumatoid arthritis

AZATADINE: antihistamine

AZATHIOPRINE: immunosuppressant; prodrug metabolized to 6-MP; affects B cells > T cells; prevents graft reject

AZELAIC ACID: anti-acne agent

AZITHROMYCIN: macrolide systemic antibacterial; po for *Streptococci*, community acquired pneumonia, Lyme disease

AZTREONAM: monobactam systemic antibacterial; covers *B. fragilis*, *Pseudomonas*; IM, IV

BACAMPICILLIN: systemic antibacterial

BACITRACIN: topical antibacterial; used in triple ointment with neomycin and polymyxin B

BACLOFEN: spasmolytic; central acting skeletal m. relaxant at spinal cord; GABA derivative

BACTRIM: sulfamethoxazole-trimethoprim; systemic antibacterial

BECLOMETHASONE: inhalant corticosteroid

BENAZEPRIL: antihypertensive; ACE inhibitor

BENDROFLUMETHIAZIDE: diuretic; antihypertensive

BENZATHINE PENICILLIN: penicillin antibacterial depot form; used in treatment of syphilis

BENZOCAINE: topical local anesthetic (sodium influx inhibitor)

BENZOYL PEROXIDE: topical antiacne agent; bacteriostatic against *Propionibacterium acnes*

BENZPHETAMINE: anorexiant; secondary agent for use in obesity

BENZQUINAMIDE: antiemetic; used in postoperative nausea and vomiting

BENZTHIAZIDE: diuretic; antihypertensive

BENZTROPINE: antiparkinsonian; antimuscarinic

BEPRIDIL: antianginal; calcium channel blocker

BRIEF DRUG DESCRIPTIONS

BETAMETHASONE: systemic and topical corticosteroid

BETAXOLOL: β adrenergic blocker; antihypertensive, antiglaucoma agent

BETHANECHOL: direct acting cholinomimetic; used for post operative urinary retention

BICALUTAMIDE: antineoplastic agent

BIPERIDEN: antiparkinsonian; centrally active anticholinergic agent

BISACODYL: irritant laxative

BISMUTH SUBSALICYLATE: antidiarrheal

BISOPROLOL: antihypertensive

BITOLTEROL MESYLATE: ß2 adrenergic agonist; bronchodilator (more potent than albuterol)

BLEOMYCIN: antibiotic antineoplastic agent; bleomycin lung (serious side effect)

BRETYLIUM: class III antiarrhythmic; last resort, prolongs repolarization

BRIMONIDINE: anti-glaucoma agent

BROMOCRIPTINE: antiparkinsonian (direct DA agonist)

BROMPHENIRAMINE: antihistamine

BUDESONIDE: inhalational corticosteroid

BUMETANIDE: loop diuretic

BUPRENORPHINE: potent opioid analgesic (mixed opioid agonist-antagonist; agonist at μ)

BUPROPION: antidepressant; stimulant rather than sedative activity

BUSPIRONE: antianxiety; LSD overdose (↓ 5-HT activity at 5-HT$_{1A}$ receptors)

BUSULFAN: alkylating antineoplastic agent; used in CML, polycythemia vera, BM transplant

BUTABARBITAL: sedative-hypnotic

BUTAMBEN: local anesthetic; used on skin to relieve pruritus and burning; water insoluble

BUTENAFINE: topical antifungal

BUTOCONAZOLE: topical antifungal; used for local treatment of vulvovaginal Candidiasis

BUTORPHANOL: potent opioid analgesic (mixed opioid agonist-antagonist)

CADMIUM: binds tissues avidly, kidney and lung toxicity; resistant to chelator therapy

CAFFEINE: CNS stimulant

BRIEF DRUG DESCRIPTIONS

CALCIFEDIOL: hypocalcemic agent; used for osteomalacia; ↑ serum calcium; ↓ PTH

CALCITONIN-SALMON: hypocalcemic agent; used for Paget's disease, bone mineral loss; increases   bone resorption

CALCITRIOL: hypercalcemic agent; increases serum calcium; decreases PTH

CALCIUM CARBONATE: good antacid, but causes acid rebound at high dose

CALCIUM SALTS: ↑ serum calcium (calcium carbonate, citrate, gluconate; hypercalcemic agents)

CAPSAICIN: topical analgesic; used in post-herpetic neuralgia and diabetic neuropathy (interferes with substance P)

CAPTOPRIL: ACE inhibitor; antihypertensive, post-MI drug, drug for heart failure

CARBACHOL: direct acting cholinomimetic; produces prolonged miosis

CARBAMAZEPINE: antiepileptic; used in tonic-clonic, cortical focal, and psychomotor epilepsy (blocks sodium channels)

CARBENICILLIN: beta-lactam antibacterial; covers gram negatives; *Pseudomonas, Proteus, Enterobacter* species

CARBIDOPA: antiparkinsonian (inhibits peripheral DOPA decarboxylase)

CARBOPLATIN: alkylating antineoplastic; testicular carcinoma, ovarian carcinoma; less nephrotoxic than cisplatin

CARISOPRODOL: skeletal m. relaxant

CARMUSTINE: antineoplastic; alkylates and crosslinks DNA; cell cycle nonspecific

CARTEOLOL: β-adrenergic blocker; antihypertensive

CARVEDIOLOL: β- and α-adrenergic blocker; antihypertensive and drug for heart failure

CASTOR OIL: irritant (contact) laxative; ricinoleic acid is active agent component

CEFACLOR: 2nd generation po cephalosporin antibacterial; covers *H. flu*

CEFADROXIL: 1st generation po cephalosporin antibacterial; covers gram positives

CEFAMANDOLE: 2nd generation cephalosporin antibacterial; covers *H. flu*

CEFAZOLIN: 1st generation cephalosporin antibacterial; covers gram positives

CEFEPIME: antibacterial

CEFIXIME: 3rd generation po cephalosporin antibacterial; covers gram negatives

CEFMETAZOLE: 2nd generation cephalosporin antibacterial; covers *B. fragilis, H. flu*

BRIEF DRUG DESCRIPTIONS

CEFONICID: 2nd generation cephalosporin antibacterial; covers *H. flu*

CEFOPERAZONE: 3rd generation cephalosporin antibacterial; covers gram negatives

CEFOTAXIME: 3rd generation cephalosporin antibacterial; covers gram negatives

CEFOTETAN: 2nd generation cephalosporin antibacterial; covers *H. flu*

CEFOXITIN: 2nd generation cephalosporin antibacterial; covers *B. fragilis, H. flu*

CEFPODOXIME: 3rd generation po cephalosporin antibacterial; covers gram negatives

CEFPROZIL: 2nd generation po cephalosporin antibacterial; covers *B. fragilis, H. flu*

CEFTAZIDIME: 3rd generation cephalosporin; covers *Serratia, Proteus, Pseudomonas, B. burgdorferi, N. gonorrhea*

CEFTIBUTEN: antibacterial; cephalosporin

CEFTIZOXIME: 3rd generation cephalosporin antibacterial; covers gram negatives

CEFTRIAXONE: 3rd generation cephalosporin, same as ceftazidime; undergoes *enterohepatic circulation*

CEFUROXIME: 2nd generation cephalosporin antibacterial; covers *B. fragilis, H. flu*

CEPHALEXIN: 1st generation po cephalosporin antibacterial; covers gram positives

CEPHALOTHIN: 1st generation IM cephalosporin antibacterial; covers gram positives

CEPHAPIRIN: 1st generation IM cephalosporin antibacterial; covers gram positives

CEPHRADINE: 1st generation cephalosporin antibacterial; covers gram positives

CETIRIZINE: anthistamine; low sedative activity

CHLORAL HYDRATE: non-barbiturate sedative hypnotic; "Mickey Finn" in combination with ethanol

CHLORAMBUCIL: nitrogen mustard antineoplastic; drug of choice in palliative treatment of chronic lymphocytic leukemia

CHLORAMPHENICOL: antibacterial; binds 50S (*Salmonella, H. flu, S. typhi*, anaerobic, and Rickettsial infections)

CHLORDIAZEPOXIDE: benzodiazepine antianxiety drug (long acting)

CHLORMEZANONE: antianxiety

CHLOROGUANIDE: antifolate antimalarial

CHLOROQUINE: antimalarial effective against rbc stage (4-aminoquinoline)

29

BRIEF DRUG DESCRIPTIONS

CHLOROTHIAZIDE: thiazide diuretic with action on the early segment of renal distal tubules; antihypertensive

CHLOROTRIANISENE: nonsteroidal estrogen; used in prostatic carcinoma

CHLORPHENESIN: skeletal m. relaxant; used to treat the pain of local muscle spasm

CHLORPHENIRAMINE: antihistamine

CHLORPROMAZINE: antipsychotic (HIGH sedation; HIGH α blocking)

CHLORPROPAMIDE: 1st generation oral hypoglycemic used in NIDDM; ↑ Ca influx and insulin efflux

CHLORPROTHIXENE: antipsychotic (thioxanthene)

CHLORTHALIDONE: thiazide-like diuretic that acts on the early segment of renal distal tubules; antihypertensive

CHLORZOXAZONE: skeletal m. relaxant; used to treat local muscle spasms

CHOLESTYRAMINE: hypolipidemic agent; cholesterol binding resin

CICLOPIROX: antifungal; as effective as clotrimazole

CIDOFOVIR: systemic antiviral

CILASTATIN: antibacterial adjunct for imipenem (dipeptidase inhibitor)

CIMETIDINE: histamine H2 blocker

CINOXACIN: urinary anti-infective

CIPROFLOXACIN: fluoroquinolone systemic and topical antibacterial; inhibits DNA gyrase; used for uncomplicated gonorrhea, UTI

CISAPRIDE: GI stimulant

CISPLATIN: alkylating antineoplastic; testicular carcinoma, ovarian carcinoma; 2nd line for all carcinoma

CLARITHROMYCIN: macrolide systemic antibacterial; po

CLAVULANIC ACID: used with ampicillin, IV, IM; with amoxicillin, po (ß-lactamase inhibitor)

CLEMASTINE: systemic antihistamine

CLIDINIUM: anticholinergic antispasmodic; irritable bowel syndrome

CLINDAMYCIN: antibacterial; binds to 50S subunit; blocks translocation; associated with pseudomembraneous colitis (PMC); covers most gram positives and anaerobic gram negatives

CLIOQUINOL: antifungal; antibacterial

BRIEF DRUG DESCRIPTIONS

CLOBETASOL: super-potent (class I) topical corticosteroid

CLOCORTOLONE: mid-strength (class IV) topical corticosteroid

CLOFAZIMINE: leprostatic; used in combination with other antimycobacterial drugs to treat *Mycobacterium avium* in AIDS

CLOFIBRATE: hypolipidemic agent; fibric acid derivative, ↓ LDL synthesis by liver, ↓ TGs

CLOMIPHENE: antiestrogen used in infertility; competes with endogenous estrogen; ↑ FSH & LH

CLOMIPRAMINE: antidepressant; more potent 5-HT uptake blocking property than imipramine

CLONAZEPAM: antiepileptic benzodiazepine; absence seizures

CLONIDINE: antihypertensive (central acting sympatholytic, selective α2 agonist)

CLORAZEPATE: antianxiety; long acting; **prodrug** converted by stomach

CLOTRIMAZOLE: topical antifungal; dermatophytic and mucocutaneous infections

CLOXACILLIN: penicillinase-resistant beta-lactam antibacterial; po

CLOZAPINE: antipsychotic; low-potency neuroleptic; extrapyramidal side effects are minimal

COCAINE: local anesthetic (Na influx inhibitor; intrinsic vasoconstrictor; blocks NE reuptake)

CODEINE: opioid analgesic; antitussive

COLCHICINE: acute gouty arthritis, gout prophylaxis (hyperuricemia or gout)

COLESTIPOL: hypolipidemic agent; cholesterol binding resin

COLISTIMETHATE: systemic antibacterial; relative of polymyxin antibacterials

COLISTIN: systemic antibacterial; relative of polymyxin antibacterials

CONJUGATED ESTROGEN: replacement therapy in hypogonadism; atrophic vaginitis

CROMOLYN: antiallergic, antiasthmatic; mast cell stabilizer; blocks calcium ion influx into mast cell

CROTAMITON: topical scabicide

CYCLIZINE: antiemetic, antihistamine

CYCLOBENZAPRINE: skeletal m. relaxant (central acting at CNS)

CYCLOPHOSPHAMIDE: alkylating antineoplastic; Hodgkin's and Burkitt's lymphomas, multiple myeloma, BM transplant prep agent

CYCLOSPORINE: immunosuppressant; used to prevent organ rejection in kidney, liver, and heart allogeneic transplants

BRIEF DRUG DESCRIPTIONS

CYPROHEPTADINE: antihistamine; antipruritic

CYTARABINE: antimetabolite antineoplastic used in leukemia; prodrug

DACARBAZINE: alkylating antineoplastic used in metastatic melanoma; causes severe nausea, vomiting

DACTINOMYCIN: antibiotic antineoplastic used in Wilms tumor

DALTEPARIN: anticoagulant (low molecular weight heparin)

DANAZOL: used in endometriosis; ↓ FSH, LH surge from pituitary (antiestrogen, androgen)

DANTROLENE: direct acting skeletal m. relaxant; spasmolytic; used to treat malignant hyperthermia

DAPSONE: leprostatic, *Mycobacterium leprae*; type IV hypersensitivity (DTH) and hemolysis are adverse reactions

DAUNORUBICIN: antibiotic antineoplastic used in acute myelogenous leukemia; inhibits topoisomerase

DECAMETHONIUM: nicotinic (N-II) blocker

DEFEROXAMINE: chelating agent used in iron and aluminum toxicity

DEMECLOCYCLINE: systemic antibacterial; spectrum, use and adverse effects similar to tetracycline

DESIPRAMINE: TCA (blocks 5-HT reuptake, $\alpha2$ antagonist, ↓ sensitivity of post-synaptic 5-HT and NE receptors)

DESMOPRESSIN: posterior pituitary hormone; anti-enuretic agent

DESONIDE: mild (class VI) topical corticosteroid

DESOXIMETASONE: potent (class II) topical corticosteroid

DEXAMETHASONE: long acting antiinflammatory; topical and systemic corticosteroid

DEXCHLORPHENIRAMINE: antihistamine

DEXFENFLURAMINE: anorexiant

DEXTROMETHORPHAN: antitussive (weak opioid agonist)

DEZOCINE: opioid analgesic; IM, IV

DIAZEPAM: long acting, > 20 hour duration, benzodiazepine; central acting skeletal m. relaxant; antianxiety

DIAZOXIDE: IV: antihypertensive (direct acting arterial vasodilator); po: hyperglycemic agent

BRIEF DRUG DESCRIPTIONS

DIBUCAINE:　　　　　　　　spinal anesthetic and topical anesthetic (sodium influx inhibitor)

DICHLORPHENAMIDE:　anti-glaucoma agent

DICLOFENAC:　　　　　　　systemic antiinflammatory; NSAID; for rheumatoid arthritis, osteoarthritis and ankylosing spondylitis

DICLOXACILLIN:　　　　　penicillinase-resistant systemic antibacterial

DICUMAROL:　　　　　　　oral anticoagulant; inhibits clotting factors II, VII, IX, and X [vitamin K dependent]

DICYCLOMINE:　　　　　　anticholinergic antispasmodic; used in irritable bowel syndrome

DIDANOSINE:　　　　　　　formerly called dideoxyinosine (ddI); 2nd choice if AZT cannot be tolerated (antiviral)

DIENESTROL:　　　　　　　nonsteroidal estrogen; used to treat hypoestrogenic vaginal atrophy

DIETHYLPROPION:　　　　anorexiant

DIETHYLSTILBESTROL:　　nonsteroidal estrogen; postcoital contraceptive; used in treatment of prostatic carcinoma

DIFLORASONE:　　　　　　potent (class II) to super-potent (class I) topical corticosteroid

DIFLUNISAL:　　　　　　　non-opioid analgesic; antiinflammatory; antipyretic; long duration of action

DIGITALIS:　　　　　　　　cardiac glycoside; positive inotropic agent, Na-K ATPase inhibitor, decreases heart rate at SAN, increases refractory period at AVN

DIGOXIN:　　　　　　　　　same as digitalis

DIHYDROTACHYSTEROL:　hypercalcemic agent; used for hypoparathyroidism

DILTIAZEM:　　　　　　　　antihypertensive, antianginal, antiarrhythmic (IV only); calcium channel blocker

DIMENHYDRINATE:　　　　antiemetic, antivertigo, used to prevent motion sickness (antihistamine)

DIMERCAPROL:　　　　　　chelating agent used for lead, high level mercury, arsenic and gold toxicities

DINOPROSTONE:　　　　　prostaglandin E_2, used to ripen cervix for labor inductions

DIPHENHYDRAMINE:　　　antiemetic; antivertigo; antitussive; sedating antihistamine

DIPHENOXYLATE:　　　　　antidiarrheal (opioid agonist, preparation includes atropine)

DIPYRIDAMOLE:　　　　　　antiplatelet agent; used as warfarin adjunct and for secondary prevention of MI

DIRITHROMYCIN:　　　　　antibacterial

DISOPYRAMIDE:　　　　　　class Ia antiarrhythmic; prolongs refractoriness and slows conduction

DISULFIRAM:　　　　　　　antialcoholic; aldehyde dehydrogenase inhibitor

33

BRIEF DRUG DESCRIPTIONS

DIVALPROEX: antiepileptic, antimaniacal, antimigraine drug (similar to valproic acid)

DOBUTAMINE: sympathomimetic pressor agent (direct acting ß1 > ß2 adrenergic agonist)

DOCUSATE SODIUM: emollient laxative

DONEPEZIL: cholinesterase inhibitor (used in dementia of Alzheimer's type)

DOPAMINE: mixed acting adrenergic agonist; pressor agent used to increase renal perfusion and in the treatment of shock (affinity: D > ß1 > α)

DORZOLAMIDE: anti-glaucoma agent

DOXACURIUM: neuromuscular blocker; adjunct to anesthesia

DOXAZOSIN: selective α1 adrenergic blocker; used for benign prostatic hypertrophy (BPH)

DOXEPIN: tricyclic antidepressant (TCA)

DOXORUBICIN: antibiotic antineoplastic; inhibits topisomerase

DOXYCYCLINE: antibacterial; antimalarial; NOT used in pregnancy, nursing women or children

DOXYLAMINE: antihistamine; used as a sedative

DROPERIDOL: antianxiety agent; preoperative medication; adjunct to general anesthesia

DYPHYLLINE: oral and IM bronchodilator; adenosine receptor antagonist

ECHOTHIOPHATE: irreversible cholinesterase inhibitor (indirect-acting cholinomimetic); anti-glaucoma agent

ECONAZOLE: topical antifungal used for dermatophytic skin infections

EDETATE CALCIUM DISODIUM: chelating agent used in lead and cadmium toxicity

EDROPHONIUM: reversible indirect acting cholinomimetic used in the diagnosis of myasthenia gravis; anticurare

EFLORNITHINE: antiprotozoal

EMETINE: amebicide, *Entamoeba histolytica*

ENALAPRIL: antihypertensive, heart failure drug; ACE inhibitor; prodrug

ENALAPRILAT: antihypertensive; ACE inhibitor

ENFLURANE: stage 3 complete inhalant general anesthetic

ENOXACIN: fluoroquinolone systemic antibacterial

ENOXAPARIN: anticoagulant

BRIEF DRUG DESCRIPTIONS

EPHEDRINE: nasal and ocular decongestant (mixed acting α,ß adrenergic agonist)

EPINEPHRINE: direct acting adrenergic α, ß agonist; systemic allergy; asthma; ER cardiac stimulant; local anesthetic adjunct

ERGOCALCIFEROL: hypercalcemic agent; increases serum calcium; increases serum phosphate

ERGONOVINE: 5-HT agonist with α adrenergic blocker activity; used in post-partum bleeding (intrinsic vasoconstrictor)

ERGOTAMINE: 5-HT agonist with α adrenergic blocker activity; used in migraines; stabilizes vasospasm by vasoconstriction

ERYTHROMYCIN: antibacterial; covers *Mycoplasma, Legionella, Chlamydia*; antiacne; binds 50S blocks translocation

ESMOLOL: class II antiarrhythmic

ESTAZOLAM: hypnotic

ESTRADIOL: estrogen antineoplastic; alters tumor growth environment

ESTRAMUSTINE: nitrogen mustard antineoplastic; promotes microtubule disassembly; anti-gonadotropin effects

ESTROPIPATE: antiosteoporotic estrogen

ETHACRYNIC ACID: loop diuretic; teratogenic

ETHAMBUTOL: tuberculostatic; decreases renal excretion of uric acid; decreases red-green acuity

ETHANOL: non-specific CNS depressant; causes euphoria, disinhibitory effects

ETHCHLORVYNOL: non-barbiturate sedative-hypnotic

ETHINYL ESTRADIOL: synthetic estrogen; used as componenet of oral contraceptives

ETHIONAMIDE: tuberculostatic; about one-tenth as active as isoniazid

ETHOSUXIMIDE: antiepileptic used in absence seizures; may block T-type calcium channels

ETHOTOIN: antiepileptic

ETHYLENE GLYCOL: alcohol component of antifreeze; nephrotoxic

ETIDOCAINE: infiltration or field block anesthetic; sodium influx inhibitor

ETIDRONATE: used in Paget's disease of bone; slows osteoclast activity

ETODOLAC: non-opioid analgesic; antiinflammatory

ETOPOSIDE: plant alkaloid antineoplastic used in testicular cancer, small cell lung carcinoma

BRIEF DRUG DESCRIPTIONS

ETRETINATE: antipsoriasis agent; inhibits keratinization, proliferation and differentiation of epithelial tissues

FAMCICLOVIR: antiviral

FAMOTIDINE: histamine H2 blocker; antiulcer agent

FANSIDAR: antimalarial; combination of sulfadoxine-pyrimethamine; Stevens Johnson syndrome is serious side effect

FELBAMATE: antiepileptic

FELODIPINE: antihypertensive; calcium channel blocker; vasodilator

FENFLURAMINE: anorexiant; primary action is to promote satiety rather than inhibit food-seeking behavior

FENOPROFEN: non-opioid analgesic; antiinflammatory

FENTANYL: opioid analgesic; IV anesthetic

FERROUS SULFATE: anti-anemic agent; used to treat microcytic anemia, restores iron storage, may take 3-6 months to resolve anemia)

FEXOFENADINE: antihistamine; low sedative activity

FINASTERIDE: androgen hormone inhibitor used in prostate CA; blocks negative feedback of testosterone on pituitary

FLECAINIDE: class Ic antiarrhythmic

FLOXURIDINE: antineoplastic

FLUCONAZOLE: antifungal

FLUCYTOSINE: antifungal; thymidylate synthetase inhibitor; amphotericin B synergist; **prodrug**

FLUDROCORTISONE: systemic corticosteroid; high mineralocorticoid activity

FLUMAZENIL: benzodiazepine antagonist; acts on alpha subunit of $GABA_A$/benzodiazepine receptor chloride channel

FLUNISOLIDE: inhalant corticosteroid; antimediator

FLUOCINONIDE: potent (class II) topical corticosteroid

FLUOROMETHOLONE: topical ophthalmic corticosteroid

FLUOROURACIL: antimetabolite antineoplastic used in breast cancer, basal cell carcinoma and topically for keratosis

FLUOXETINE: 2nd generation antidepressant; selective 5-HT blocker

BRIEF DRUG DESCRIPTIONS

FLUOXYMESTERONE: androgen; used for anabolic therapy

FLUPHENAZINE: antipsychotic, depot (piperazine phenothiazine; high EPR and potency)

FLURANDRENOLIDE: mid-strength (class IV) topical corticosteroid

FLURAZEPAM: sedative hypnotic; long acting benzodiazepine; prodrug

FLURBIPROFEN: antiinflammatory; available po and as ophthalmic solution

FLUTAMIDE: androgen hormone inhibitor used in prostate CA; blocks negative feedback of testosterone on pituitary

FLUTICASONE: topical corticosteroid; used as an antiinflammatory drug (skin) and for COPD (by aerosol)

FLUVASTATIN: hypolipidemic; HMG CoA Reductase inhibitor

FLUVOXAMINE: antidepressant

FOLIC ACID: anti-anemic used for macrocytic anemia

FOSCARNET: systemic antiviral for CMV retinitis and Herpes simplex infections

FOSFOMYCIN: single dose urinary anti-infective agent

FOSPHENYTOIN: antiepileptic; prodrug to phenytoin

FOSINOPRIL: antihypertensive; ACE inhibitor; prodrug

FURAZOLIDONE: antigiardial antibacterial

FUROSEMIDE: loop diuretic; antihypertensive; agent used in acute pulmonary edema

GABAPENTIN: antiepileptic

GALLAMINE: skeletal m. relaxant (non-depolarizing curariform; muscarinic blocker)

GANCICLOVIR: systemic antiviral for CMV infections

GEMFIBROZIL: hypolipidemic; fibric acid derivative, ↓ LDL synthesis by liver, ↓ TGs

GENTAMICIN: aminoglycoside antibacterial; binds 30s and 50s; blocks initiation, causes misreadings in the genetic code

GLIMEPIRIDE: 2nd generation oral hypoglycemic; used in NIDDM; increases calcium influx and insulin efflux

GLIPIZIDE: 2nd generation oral hypoglycemic; used in NIDDM; increases calcium influx and insulin efflux

GLYBURIDE: 2nd generation oral hypoglycemic; used in NIDDM; increases calcium influx and insulin efflux

BRIEF DRUG DESCRIPTIONS

GLYCERIN: laxative

GOLD SODIUM THIOMALATE: disease modifying agent used in rheumatoid arthritis; immunosuppressant

GOLD: used in rheumatoid arthritis, treatment for toxicity: dimercaprol, penicillamine

GRANISETRON: antiemetic

GRISEOFULVIN: systemic antifungal; dermatophytic infections ONLY; deposited in skin, hair, nails; blocks fungal mitosis

GUAIFENESIN: expectorant

GUANABENZ: antihypertensive (central acting sympatholytic, selective $\alpha2$ agonist)

GUANADREL: antihypertensive (adrenergic neuronal blocker)

GUANETHIDINE: antihypertensive (adrenergic neuronal blocker)

GUANFACINE: antihypertensive (central acting sympatholytic, selective $\alpha2$ agonist)

HALAZEPAM: benzodiazepine used for generalized anxiety disorder

HALCINONIDE: potent (class II) topical corticosteroid

HALOBETASOL: topical corticosteroid

HALOPERIDOL: antipsychotic (low sedation, slow extrapyramidal reaction (EPR) onset)

HALOPROGIN: synthetic topical antifungal used for superficial dermatophytic (tinea) infections

HALOTHANE: stage 3 complete general anesthetic

HEPARIN: in vivo and in vitro anticoagulant, accelerates antithrombin III binding to Xa & IIa

HEROIN: drug of abuse (diacetylmorphine, opioid agonist)

HOMATROPINE: anticholingeric agent used to induce mydriasis

HYDRALAZINE: antihypertensive (direct acting arterial vasodilator)

HYDROCHLOROTHIAZIDE: thiazide diuretic; acts on the early segment of renal distal tubules; antihypertensive

HYDROCORTISONE: systemic corticosteroid used in adrenocortical insufficiency; mid-strength (class IV, V) topical corticosteroid

HYDROFLUMETHIAZIDE: antihypertensive, diuretic

HYDROMORPHONE: opioid analgesic, 8x's potency of morphine (opioid agonist)

HYDROXYCHLOROQUINE: antimalarial; works on the rbc stage; 4-aminoquinoline; disease modifying agent used in rheumatoid arthritis

38

BRIEF DRUG DESCRIPTIONS

HYDROXYUREA:	antineoplastic; inhibits ribonucleoside diphosphate reductase; S phase specific
HYDROXYZINE:	antianxiety agent, antihistamine (for sedation and pruritis)
HYOSCYAMINE:	anticholinergic antispasmodic; used in irritable bowel syndrome
IBUPROFEN:	non-opioid analgesic; antiinflammatory; antipyretic (NSAID)
IBUTILIDE:	antiarrhythmic
IDARUBICIN:	antineoplastic used in acute myelogenous leukemia
IDOXURIDINE:	herpes simplex keratitis; ophthalmic antiviral
IMIPENEM:	carbapenam systemic antibacterial with broad spectrum; IM, IV; used with cilastatin used as adjunct
IMIPRAMINE:	tricyclic antidepressant (TCA)
INDAPAMIDE:	thiazide-like diuretic that acts on the early segment of renal distal tubules; antihypertensive
INDOMETHACIN:	nonsteroidal antiinflammatory drug
INSULIN:	hypoglycemic; replacement therapy in IDDM and insulin requiring type II diabetics
INSULIN LISPRO:	hypoglycemic agent; short-acting insulin derivative
INTERFERON ALFA-2A:	antineoplastic
INTERFERON ALFA-2B:	antineoplastic
INTERFERON ALFA-N3:	antineoplastic
INTERFERON BETA-1A:	used to treat mutiple sclerosis
INTERFERON BETA-1B:	used to treat mutiple sclerosis
INTERFERON GAMMA:	antiviral; antineoplastic
IODOQUINOL:	amebicide; *Entamoeba histolytica*
IPRATROPIUM:	inhaled bronchodilator (anticholinergic, does not block mucociliary escalator)
IRON DEXTRAN:	anti-anemic; used for microcytic anemia, restores iron storage, takes 3-6 months
IRON:	free form VERY toxic, causes cardiovascular collapse; chelate with deferoxamine
ISOCARBOXAZID:	MAOI antidepressant (down regulates post-synaptic ß2)
ISOETHARINE:	inhaled bronchodilator (direct ß2 > ß1 adrenergic agonist)
ISOFLURANE:	inhalation general anesthetic

39

BRIEF DRUG DESCRIPTIONS

ISONIAZID: 1st line tuberculostatic; used in prophylaxis and treatment

ISOPROTERENOL: bronchodilator; cardiac stimulant, ↑ SP, ↓ DP, ↑ PP (direct ß adrenergic agonist)

ISOSORBIDE: antianginal (organic nitrate)

ISOTRETINOIN: antiacne agent; reduces sebaceous gland cell size, decreases sebum production

ISRADIPINE: antihypertensive; calcium channel blocker; vasodilator

ITRACONAZOLE: systemic antifungal; interferes with ergosterol synthesis

KANAMYCIN: systemic antibacterial; used to treat susceptible aerobic gram-negative bacilli, primarily Enterobacteriaceae

KETAMINE: induction agent (dissociative anesthetic)

KETOCONAZOLE: 2nd line dermatophytic; use in mucocutaneous and some systemic fungi

KETOPROFEN: non-opioid analgesic; antiinflammatory; rheumatoid arthritis, ankylosing spondylitis, acute gout, osteoarthritis

KETOROLAC: non-opioid analgesic (injectable and oral NSAID)

LABETALOL: antihypertensive (α1 blocker, non-selective ß blocker)

LACTULOSE: laxative

LAMIVUDINE: antiviral

LAMOTRIGINE: antiepileptic

LANSOPRAZOLE: anti-ulcer agent; gastric acid pump inhibitor

LATANOPROST: fluoroquinolone antibacterial

LEAD: may cause lead colic, treatment is chelation with edetate calcium disodium, dimercaprol, and penicillamine

LEUCOVORIN: macrocytic anemia, active form of folic acid (anti-anemic)

LEVOBUNOLOL: antiglaucoma agent; long acting nonselective ß adrenergic blocker

LEVOCABASTINE: antiallergic

LEVODOPA: antiparkinsonian (replaces diminished DA)

LEVONORGESTREL: implant contraceptive

LEVORPHANOL: synthetic opioid analgesic, 4-8x's more potent than morphine after IM injection

LEVOTHYROXINE: thyroid hormone; L-T4; used to treat hypothyroidism

BRIEF DRUG DESCRIPTIONS

LIDOCAINE: local anesthetic, class lb antiarrhythmic; decreases depolarization, shortens repolarization, slows conduction

LINCOMYCIN: systemic antibacterial, similar to clindamycin; binds 50S, blocks translocation

LINDANE: antiparasitic, scabicide; shampoo very effective killing adult head and pubic lice

LIOTHYRONINE: thyroid hormone; L-T3; used to treat hypothyroidism

LIOTRIX: L-T3 and L-T4; long term thyroid replacement in hypothyroidism

LISINOPRIL: antihypertensive, drug for heart failure, post-MI drug; ACE inhibitor

LITHIUM CARBONATE: antimaniacal; used to treat manic phase of bipolar disease

LODOXAMIDE: ophthalmic antiallergic

LOMEFLOXACIN: urinary tract infections; fluoroquinolone antibacterial

LOMUSTINE: alkylating antineoplastic; meningeal leukemia, brain, GI, small cell lung carcinoma; HIGH lipid solubility

LOPERAMIDE: antidiarrheal (opioid agonist)

LORACARBEF: 2nd generation po cephalosporin antibacterial; covers gram positives

LORATADINE: antihistamine; low sedative activity

LORAZEPAM: antianxiety (short acting benzodiazepine, duration 3-20 hours)

LOSARTAN: angiotensin II receptor (type AT_1) inhibitor (antihypertensive)

LOVASTATIN: hypolipidemic; HMG CoA Reductase inhibitor, prodrug, ↓ LDL, ↑ HDL, ↓ TGs

LOXAPINE: antipsychotic (dibenzoxazepine)

LSD: lysergic acid diethylamide (psychotomimetic, hallucinogen)

LYPRESSIN: posterior pituitary hormone

MAFENIDE: sulfonamide antibacterial; used topically to treat infections due to burns

MAGALDRATE: antacid

MAGNESIUM CITRATE: osmotic laxative

MAGNESIUM HYDROXIDE: laxative; antacid

MAGNESIUM SULFATE: anticonvulsant (injectable)

MALATHION: insecticide; irreversible cholinesterase inhibitor (indirect acting cholinomimetic)

MALT SOUP EXTRACT: bulk laxative

BRIEF DRUG DESCRIPTIONS

MANNITOL: osmotic diuretic

MAPROTILINE: 2nd generation antidepressant

MARIJUANA: antiemetic; psychotomimetic drug of abuse (Δ^9-tetrahydrocannabinol)

MAZINDOL: anorexiant; blocks neuronal uptake of norepinephrine and synaptically released dopamine

MEBENDAZOLE: *Enterobius vermicularis, Ascaris lumbricoides, Trichuris trichuria, Necator species* (roundworms);

MECAMYLAMINE: antihypertensive (anti-depolarizing ganglionic blocker)

MECHLORETHAMINE: alkylating antineoplastic; Hodgkin's lymphoma; vesicant on skin; VERY toxic

MECLIZINE: antihistamine, antivertigo agent; used for motion sickness

MECLOCYCLINE: topical antibacterial used as antiacne agent

MECLOFENAMATE: non-opioid analgesic; antiinflammatory

MEDROXYPROGESTERONE: synthetic progestin; replacement therapy; dosed with estrogen replacement regimen; endometriosis

MEDRYSONE: ophthalmic corticosteroid

MEFENAMIC ACID: non-opioid analgesic

MEFLOQUINE: antimalarial that acts on the rbc stage; quinoline methanol

MEGESTROL: synthetic progestin; used as an antineoplastic agent in the palliative treatment of advanced carcinoma of breast or endometrium, and as an appetite stimulant in patients with AIDS

MELPHALAN: nitrogen mustard antineoplastic, cell cycle nonspecific; used in palliative treatment of multiple myeloma

MEPERIDINE: opioid analgesic; high antimuscarinic properties

MEPHENYTOIN: antiepileptic; effective in partial (focal) seizures but may be bone marrow toxic

MEPHOBARBITAL: sedative, antiepilecptic; enhances GABA, decreases glutamic acid

MEPIVACAINE: local anesthetic used in peripheral nerve blocks (sodium influx inhibitor)

MEPROBAMATE: antianxiety agent

MERCAPTOPURINE: antimetabolite antineoplastic; use in acute and chronic leukemia; use with allopurinol

MERCURY: toxicity: cardiovascular collapse and organic psychosis, treat with dimercaprol (high), penicillamine (low)

BRIEF DRUG DESCRIPTIONS

MESALAMINE: bowel antiinflammatory; enema form use for ulcerative colitis limited to left colon

MESORIDAZINE: effective, low potency antipsychotic

MESTRANOL: prodrug; estrogen replacement (synthetic estrogen)

METAPROTERENOL: bronchodilator (direct acting ß2 > ß1 adrenergic agonist)

METAXOLONE: centrally-acting skeletal m. relaxant

METFORMIN: hypoglycemic agent

METHACHOLINE: used in diagnosis of bronchial hyperactivity (direct acting cholinomimetic)

METHADONE: long acting opioid agonist; used in morphine addiction maintenance therapy

METHAMPHETAMINE: anorexiant

METHANOL: an alcohol that is metabolized to formic acid which is toxic, causing blindness

METHDILAZINE: systemic antihistamine

METHENAMINE: urinary anti-infective; in acid is hydrolyzed to ammonia and formaldehyde which kills bacteria and fungi

METHICILLIN: penicillinase-resistent beta-lactam antibacterial

METHIMAZOLE: antithyroid drug; inhibits thyroid peroxidase, blocks iodide ⁻ OI⁻ and coupling reaction

METHOCARBAMOL: skeletal m. relaxant; adjunct to rest and physical therapy to alleviate the pain of local muscle spasm

METHOTREXATE: antimetabolite antineoplastic agent for choriocarcinoma, NHL, head, neck, breast, lung carcinomas

METHSCOPOLAMINE: antimuscarinic agent; used to reduce hypermotility of the bowel

METHSUXIMIDE: antiepileptic

METHYCLOTHIAZIDE: antihypertensive, diuretic

METHYL TESTOSTERONE: androgen with duration 8-12 hours

METHYLCELLULOSE: bulk laxative

METHYLDOPA: antihypertensive; prodrug; central acting, selective α2 agonist

METHYLDOPATE: IV antihypertensive; ethyl ester derivative of methyldopa

METHYLERGONOVINE: oxytocic

METHYLPHENIDATE: CNS stimulant

43

BRIEF DRUG DESCRIPTIONS

METHYLPREDNISOLONE: short acting systemic corticosteroid, used as antiinflammatory

METHYLTESTOSTERONE: androgen

METHYSERGIDE: ergot alkaloid with 5-HT antagonist activity; used in migraine prophylaxis

METIPRANOLOL: antiglaucoma agent, beta adrenergic blocker

METOCLOPRAMIDE: GI stimulant; antiemetic

METOCURINE: neuromuscular blocker

METOLAZONE: thiazide-like diuretic that acts on early segment of renal distal tubules; antihypertensive

METOPROLOL: ß1 > ß2 blocker; antihypertensive, antianginal, and post-MI drug

METRIFONATE: *Schistosoma haematobium and S. mansoni* (blood flukes) not responding to praziquantel (anthelminthic)

METRONIDAZOLE: antibacterial, amebicide, antitrichomonal drug (systemic use); antiacne agent (topical use)

METYRAPONE: blocks cortisol production; diagnosis of HT-pituitary dysfunction (corticosteroid)

METYROSINE: inoperable pheochromocytoma (tyrosine hydroxylase inhibitor, adrenergic neuronal blocker)

MEXILETINE: class Ib antiarrhythmic; slightly depresses depolarization, shortens repolarization, slows conduction

MEZLOCILLIN: gram negative antibacterial: *Pseudomonas, Proteus, Enterobacter*; undergoes *enterohepatic circulation*

MICONAZOLE: dermatophytic antifungal; used to treat mucocutaneous and some systemic fungi

MIDAZOLAM: sedative-hypnotic

MIDODRINE: α-adrenergic agonist; used to treat orthostatic hypotension

MIFEPRISTONE (RU 486): abortifacient agent, used in Europe, controversial in United States

MILRINONE: inotropic agent; phosphodiesterase inhibitor, increases cAMP

MINERAL OIL: lubricant laxative

MINOCYCLINE: systemic antibacterial; tetracycline analog; use limited by vestibular toxicity

MINOXIDIL: antihypertensive: direct acting arterial vasodilator, prodrug; hair growth stimulator (topical use)

MIRTAZAPINE: antidepressant

BRIEF DRUG DESCRIPTIONS

MISOPROSTOL: antiulcer; PG derivative; decreases gastric acid; aborticant

MIVACURIUM: neuromuscular blocker

MOEXIPRIL: antihypertensive; ACE inhibitor

MOLINDONE: antipsychotic, high extrapyramidal reaction (EPR) with quick onset

MOMETASONE: potent (class III) topical corticosteroid

MORICIZINE: class Ib antiarrhythmic; shortens refractory period, with little effect on conduction in normal tissue

MORPHINE: opioid analgesic, used for post-operative pain control

MUPIROCIN: topical antibacterial; used in impetigo due to *Staphylococci aureus* and *Streptococcus pyogenes*

MUROMONAB-CD3:   immunosuppressant used in renal graft rejection; blocks all T cell function (OKT3)

MUSCARINE: direct acting cholinomimetic

MYCOPHENOLATE: immunosuppressant

NABUMETONE: antiinflammatory

NADOLOL: β-blocker; antihypertensive; antianginal; long acting drug

NAFCILLIN: antibacterial; used to treat methicillin sensitive *Staphylococci aureus* (MSSA); undergoes *enterohepatic circulation*; available IM, IV, po

NAFTIFINE: topical antifungal; squalene epoxidase inhibitor

NALBUPHINE: opioid analgesic (mixed opioid agonist-antagonist)

NALIDIXIC ACID: urinary anti-infective; inhibits the A subunit of bacterial DNA gyrase

NALMEFENE: opioid antagonist; used in opioid-induced respiratory depression and known or suspected opioid overdosage

NALOXONE: opioid antagonist; use in opioid-induced respiratory depression

NALTREXONE: opioid antagonist; use in post opioid-withdrawal prophylaxis

NANDROLONE: anabolic steroid; adverse effects: cholestatic hepatitis, hepatocellular carcinoma; increases LDL, decreases HDL

NAPHAZOLINE: nasal decongestant, ocular decongestant; α-adrenergic agonist

NAPROXEN: non-opioid analgesic, antiinflammatory (longer acting NSAID)

NATAMYCIN: topical (ophthalmic) antifungal

BRIEF DRUG DESCRIPTIONS

NEDOCROMIL: antiasthmatic

NEFAZODONE: antidepressant

NEOMYCIN: aminoglycoside antibacterial (topical only); binds 30s and 50s subunits; blocks initiation, causing misreads in the genetic code

NEOSTIGMINE: reversible cholinesterase inhibitor (indirect-acting cholinomimetic); used to treat Myasthenia gravis and to reverse curariform-induced neuromuscular blockade

NETILMICIN: aminoglycoside systemic antibacterial; binds 30s and 50s subunits; blocks initiation, causing misreads in the genetic code

NEVIRAPINE: antiviral

NICARDIPINE: antihypertensive, anti-anginal; calcium channel blocker; vasodilator

NICLOSAMIDE: anthelmintic; used to treat cestode (tapeworm) infestation

NICOTINE POLACRILEX: used as smoking deterrent (depolarizing ganglionic stimulant; chemoreceptor trigger zone, CTZ)

NICOTINE: used as smoking deterrent (depolarizing ganglionic stimulant; chemoreceptor trigger zone, CTZ)

NICOTINIC ACID: niacin; hypolipidemic; decreases TGs, slight decreases LDL

NIFEDIPINE: antihypertensive; antianginal; calcium channel blocker vasodilator

NISOLDIPINE: antihypertensive; calcium channel blocker

NITROFURANTOIN: urinary anti-infective; mechanism of action is unclear

NITROGLYCERIN: antianginal, vasodilator, common side effect is headache (emergency cardiac agent)

NITROPRUSSIDE: antihypertensive (direct acting arterial and venous vasodilator)

NITROUS OXIDE: inhalation general anesthetic; incomplete anesthetic

NIZATIDINE: anti-ulcer agent; histamine H2-receptor antagonist

NOREPINEPHRINE: α-adrenergic receptor agonist; used in acute hypotension; shock; ↑ systolic and diastolic blood pressures

NORETHINDRONE: progestin; oral contraceptive component; C19 nortestosterone

NORFLOXACIN: fluoroquinolone antibacterial (systemic and ophthalmic); inhibits DNA gyrase; used to treat urinary tract infection

NORGESTREL: oral contraceptive

NORTRIPTYLINE: tricyclic antidepressant (TCA)

BRIEF DRUG DESCRIPTIONS

NSAIDs   non-steroidal antiinflammatory drugs

NYSTATIN: oral or topical antifungal, NOT used IV; dermatophytic, mucocutaneous infections

OFLOXACIN: fluoroquinolone antibacterial (systemic and ophthalmic); uncomplicated *Neisseria gonorrhea* and *Chlamydia trachomatis*

OLSALAZINE: bowel antiinflammatory

OMEPRAZOLE: gastric acid pump inhibitor; used as an anti-ulcer agent; blocks H-K ATPase which provides total block of gastric acid secretion

ONDANSETRON: antiemetic

ORPHENADRINE: skeletal m. relaxant

OXACILLIN: penicillinase-resistent beta-lactam systemic antibacterial

OXAMNIQUINE: anthelmintic; alternative agent for *Schistosoma mansoni*; alkylates worm DNA

OXANDROLONE: anabolic steroid with adverse effects: cholestatic hepatitis, hepatocellular carcinoma; increases LDL, decreases HDL

OXAPROZIN: antiinflammatory

OXAZEPAM: benzodiazepine antianxiety drug, short acting

OXICONAZOLE: topical antifungal

OXIDIZED CELLULOSE: hemostatic agent

OXTRIPHYLLINE: bronchodilator

OXYBUTYNIN: urinary antispasmodic

OXYCODONE: opioid analgesic (opioid agonist)

OXYMETAZOLINE: nasal and ocular decongestant; direct acting adrenergic agonist

OXYMORPHONE: opioid analgesic (opioid agonist)

OXYTETRACYCLINE: systemic antibacterial; effective against gram positive, gram negative, aerobic and anaerobic organisms

OXYTOCIN: posterior pituitary hormone; used for induction of labor or stimulation of labor in uterine dysfunction

PAMIDRONATE: bone stabilizer

PANCURONIUM: skeletal m. relaxant (non-depolarizing curariform; muscarinic blocker)

PAPAVERINE: vasodilator

BRIEF DRUG DESCRIPTIONS

PARALDEHYDE: used in alcohol withdrawal (non-barbiturate sedative hypnotic)

PARAMETHADIONE: antiepileptic

PARATHION: irreversible cholinesterase inhibitor (indirect acting cholinomimetic); used as an insecticide

PAROMOMYCIN: amebicide; an aminoglycoside antibacterial effective against *Entamoeba histolytica*

PAROXETINE: antidepressant; selective serotonin (5-HT) reuptake blocker

PEGASPARGASE: antineoplastic

PEMOLINE: CNS stimulant

PENBUTOLOL: β-adrenergic receptor blocker; antihypertensive

PENICILLAMINE: chelating agent used in lead, low level mercury, arsenic and gold toxicity

PENICILLIN G: injectable systemic antibacterial

PENICILLIN V: po systemic antibacterial used for Streptococcal, Pneumococcal, Neisserial, Treponemal, *E. coli* infection

PENCICLOVIR: antiviral (used in recurrent herpes labialis a.k.a. cold sores)

PENTAERYTHRITOL TETRANITRATE: antianginal (organic nitrate)

PENTAMIDINE: antiprotozoal effective against *Pneumocystis carinii* pneumonia

PENTAZOCINE: opioid analgesic (mixed opioid agonist-antagonist)

PENTOBARBITAL: sedative hypnotic (non-specific effect on membrane; GABA-like effect on neurons)

PENTOSAN POLYSULFATE: urinary analgesic

PENTOXIFYLLINE: hemorheologic agent; used in intermittent claudication

PERGOLIDE: antiparkinsonian; a synthetic ergoline with direct dopaminergic activity; has both D1 and D2 receptor activity

PERMETHRIN: scabicide; high ovicidal activity; single application effective against head lice infestation

PERPHENAZINE: antipsychotic; antiemetic

PHENACEMIDE: last resort antiepileptic; high toxicity

PHENAZOPYRIDINE: urinary analgesic

PHENCYCLIDINE (PCP):   psychotomimetic drug of abuse; hallucinogen

BRIEF DRUG DESCRIPTIONS

PHENDIMETRAZINE: anorexiant; suppresses the appetite and stimulates the CNS; causes euphoria, potential for abuse

PHENELZINE: MAOI, antidepressant (down regulates post-synaptic ß2)

PHENINDAMINE: systemic antihistamine

PHENINDIONE: oral anticoagulant; inhibits clotting factors II, VII, IX, and X (vitamin K dependent)

PHENOBARBITAL: sedative-hypnotic; antiepileptic (GABA-like effect on neurons; enhances GABA, ↓ glutamic acid)

PHENOL: local anesthetic

PHENOLPHTHALEIN: contact laxative

PHENOXYBENZAMINE: antihypertensive; used in pheochromocytoma (non-selective non-equilibrium α adrenergic blocker)

PHENTERMINE: anorexiant

PHENTOLAMINE: antihypertensive; used in pheochromocytoma (non-selective α adrenergic blocker)

PHENYLEPHRINE: direct acting adrenergic agonist ($\alpha 1 > \alpha 2$); used as a decongestant and vasoconstrictor

PHENYTOIN: antiepileptic used in tonic-clonic, cortical focal, psychomotor seizures (↓ PTP, sodium channel blocker)

PHOSPHATE SALTS: inorganic hypocalcemic; used to treat hypophosphatemic rickets and osteomalacia

PHYSOSTIGMINE: reversible cholinesterase inhibitor (indirect acting cholinomimetic); antiglaucoma agent and antidote in overdose of antimuscarinic agents

PHYTONADIONE: vitamin K_1

PILOCARPINE: direct acting cholinomimetic; used as miotic and antiglaucoma agent

PIMOZIDE: antipsychotic; used in Tourette's disorder

PINDOLOL: non-selective ß-adrenergic blocker; antihypertensive, antianginal, antiarrhythmic, antiglaucoma, and antimigraine agent with intrinsic sympathomimetic activity

PIPERACILLIN: gram negative antibacterial; *Pseudomonas, Proteus, and Enterobacter* species

PIPECURONIUM: neuromuscular blocker; adjunct to anesthesia

PIRBUTEROL: selective ß2 agonist; used as a bronchodilator

PIROXICAM: non-opioid analgesic, antiinflammatory (long acting NSAID)

PLICAMYCIN: antineoplastic; hypocalcemia agent used in severe hypercalcemia associated with carcinoma; kills osteoclasts

POLYMYXIN B: antibacterial; effective against many aerobic gram negative bacilli, excellent for *Pseudomonas aeruginosa*

POLYTHIAZIDE: antihypertensive, diuretic

POTASSIUM CHLORIDE: potassium supplement

POTASSIUM GLUCONATE: potassium supplement

PRALIDOXIME: antidote for irreversible cholinesterase inhibitors

PRAMOXINE: local anesthetic; antihemorrhoidal

PRAVASTATIN: hypolipidemic; HMG CoA reductase inhibitor, decreases LDL, increases HDL, and decreases TGs

PRAZIQUANTEL: anthelmintic; effective agent against blood flukes: *Schistosoma haematobium, mansoni, japonicum*

PRAZOSIN: selective α1-adrenergic blocker; used for the treatment of hypertension and for benign prostatic hypertrophy

PREDNICARBATE: topical corticosteroid

PREDNISOLONE: systemic corticosteroid; also has ophthalmic applications

PREDNISONE: systemic corticosteroid; inhibits leukocyte migration; short acting antiinflammatory

PRIMAQUINE: antimalarial effective against tissue stage (8-aminoquinoline)

PRIMIDONE: antiepileptic used in tonic-clonic, cortical focal, and psychomotor epilepsy (blocks sodium channels)

PROBENECID: antigout agent; uricosuric, blocks uric acid reabsorption, decreases penicillin excretion; NOT antiinflammatory

PROCAINAMIDE: class la antiarrhythmic that depresses depolarization, prolongs repolarization, and slows conduction

PROCAINE PENICILLIN: depot form penicillin; used in gonorrhea

PROCAINE: infiltration local anesthetic; an ester; short acting, sodium influx inhibitor

PROCARBAZINE: antineoplastic; use in Hodgkin's disease with mechlorethamine, vincristine and prednisone (MOPP regimen)

PROCHLORPERAZINE: antiemetic; piperazine phenothiazine with low extrapyramidal reaction (EPR) at antiemetic dose

50

BRIEF DRUG DESCRIPTIONS

PROCYCLIDINE: antiparkinsonian; centrally acting anticholinergic agent

PROGESTERONE: natural progestin that increases vascularization, glands, and glycogen of uterus, and decreases uterine contraction; used as an intrauterine contraceptive

PROMAZINE: antipsychotic; aliphatic phenothiazine with low extrapyramidal reaction

PROMETHAZINE: phenothiazine antihistamine; sedative; antiemetic

PROPAFENONE: class Ic antiarrhythmic; slows conduction, little effect on refractory period

PROPANTHELINE: antimuscarinic; used to treat GI hypermotility

PROPOXYPHENE: opioid analgesic (weak opioid agonist)

PROPRANOLOL: β-adrenergic blocker; antihypertensive; antianginal; antiarrhythmic, antimigraine drug with membrane stabilizing activity and highest lipid solubility

PROPYLTHIOURACIL: antithyroid drug; thyroid peroxidase inhibitor; blocks T4 → T3 outside thyroid

PROTAMINE SULFATE: heparin antagonist; very positively charged molecule

PROTRIPTYLINE: tricyclic antidepressant (TCA)

PSEUDOEPHEDRINE: mixed acting adrenergic agonist; used as a decongestant

PSYLLIUM HYDROPHILIC
    MUCILLOID: bulk laxative

PARATHYROID HORMONE: hypercalcemic agent; stimulates osteoclast and increases serum calcium

PYRANTEL PAMOATE: anthelmintic; *Enterobius vermicularis*; depolarizing neuromuscular blocker

PYRAZINAMIDE: 1st line tuberculostatic; unknown mechanism; hepatotoxic, causes hyperuricemia

PYRIDOSTIGMINE: reversible cholinesterase inhibitor (indirect acting cholinomimetic); used to treat Myasthenia gravis

PYRILAMINE: antihistamine

PYRIMETHAMINE: antimalarial; inhibits DHF reductase; pyrimethamine + sulfadoxine = Fansidar

QUAZEPAM: benzodiazepine sedative

QUINAPRIL: antihypertensive agent; ACE inhibitor

QUINESTROL: synthetic estrogen used in replacement therapy; prodrug

QUINIDINE: class Ia antiarrhythmic; depresses depolarization, prolongs repolarization, slows conduction

QUININE: antimalarial effective against rbc stage (quinoline methanol)

BRIEF DRUG DESCRIPTIONS

RADIOACTIVE IODINE: I^{131} ß particles (electrons) cause thyroid ablation; gamma rays for monitoring

RAMIPRIL: antihypertensive agent, heart failure drug; ACE inhibitor

RANITIDINE: anti-ulcer agent; histamine H2-receptor antagonist

RESERPINE: antihypertensive (adrenergic neuronal blocker)

RETEPLASE, RECOMBINANT: thrombolytic

RIBAVIRIN: antiviral; used in respiratory syncytial virus in infants and children

RIFABUTIN: tuberculostatic; reverse transcriptase inhibitor

RIFAMPIN: 1st line tuberculostatic; DNA-dependent RNA polymerase inhibitor; causes orange secretions

RIMANTADINE: antiviral; similar to amantadine, inhibits growth of influenza A

RIMEXOLONE: corticosteroid for ophthalmic use

RISPERIDONE: antipsychotic

RITODRINE: selective ß2-adrenergic agonist; used to treat premature labor (tocolytic agent)

RITONAVIR: antiviral

SALMETEROL: bronchodilator; long-acting selective β2-adrenergic agonist

SALSALATE: antiinflammatory (salicylsalicylic acid)

SAQUINAVIR: antiviral

SCOPOLAMINE: antimuscarinic; used for motion sickness, as an adjunct to general anesthesia, and as a mydriatic-cycloplegic in ophthalmology

SECOBARBITAL: sedative hypnotic (non-specific effect membranes; enhances GABA)

SELEGILINE: antiparkinsonian, protective against MPTP (inhibits MAO-B in CNS)

SELENIUM SULFIDE: antiseborrheic; antifungal

SENNA CONCENTRATE: irritant laxative

SERTRALINE: antidepressant; selective serotonin (5-HT) reuptake blocker

SILVER SULFADIAZINE: topical sulfonamide antibacterial; of choice for infected burns and grafts

SIMETHICONE: antiflatulent

SIMVASTATIN: hypolipidemic; HMG CoA reductase inhibitor that is a prodrug that decreases LDL, increases HDL, and decreases triglycerides

BRIEF DRUG DESCRIPTIONS

SODIUM BICARBONATE: antacid

SODIUM NITROPRUSSIDE: IV antihypertensive, drug for heart failure

SODIUM POLYSTYRENE SULFONATE: potassium removing resin

SOMAN: aging war gas (irreversible indirect acting cholinomimetic)

SOTALOL: class III antiarrhythmic (ß-adrenergic blocker)

SPECTINOMYCIN: aminoglycoside systemic antibacterial; binds 30s ONLY, blocks initiation, and causes misreads

SPIRONOLACTONE: K^+ sparing diuretic; antihypertensive also used in hirsutism, hyperaldosteronism, and precocious puberty

STANOZOLOL: anabolic steroid

STAVUDINE: antiviral

STIBOGLUCANATE: antiflagellate; used in Leishmaniasis infection

STREPTOKINASE: thrombolytic; activates plasminogen; allergic reaction is adverse effect

STREPTOMYCIN: 1st line tuberculostatic used IM, IV (aminoglycoside systemic antibacterial)

STREPTOZOCIN: antineoplastic; a nitrosurea; cell cycle phase non-specific

SUCCINYLCHOLINE: non-depolarizing curariform skeletal m. relaxant used in laryngoscopy, orthopedics, and electroshock therapy

SUCRALFATE: antiulcer agent that binds to active ulcer site; blocks penetration of acid

SUFENTANIL: opioid analgesic, MOST potent opioid (625 times more potent than morphine)

SULBACTAM: used with ampicillin, IV (ß-lactamase inhibitor)

SULCONAZOLE: topical antifungal

SULFACETAMIDE: dihydropteroate synthetase inhibitor; ophthalmologic solution (sulfonamide antibacterial)

SULFADIAZINE: dihydropteroate synthetase inhibitor; topical for burns (sulfonamide antibacterial)

SULFAMETHIZOLE: systemic sulfonamide antibacterial; used to treat acute, uncomplicated UTI

SULFAMETHOXAZOLE: systemic sulfonamide antibacterial; used in urinary tract infection

SULFANILAMIDE: sulfonamide antibacterial; antifungal; used in vaginal cream or suppository

SULFASALAZINE: dihydropteroate synthetase inhibitor; used in inflammatory bowel disease (sulfonamide)

53

BRIEF DRUG DESCRIPTIONS

SULFINPYRAZONE: antigout agent; uricosuric used in tophaceous gout and hyperuricemia

SULFISOXAZOLE: dihydropteroate synthetase inhibitor (sulfonamide antibacterial)

SULINDAC: antiinflammatory; analog of indomethacin with similar analgesic and antipyretic activity

SUMATRIPTAN: antimigraine agent; IM and po available

SUPROFEN: ophthalmic antiinflammatory

TACRINE: drug for Alzheimer's disease; cholinesterase inhibitor

TACROLIMUS: immunosuppressant

TAMOXIFEN: antineoplastic used in breast cancer (antiestrogen)

TEMAZEPAM: benzodiazepine hypnotic; intermediate duration of effect

TERAZOSIN: selective α1-adrenergic receptor blocker; antihypertensive and used for benign prostatic hyperplasia (BPH)

TERBINAFINE: topical antifungal

TERBUTALINE: bronchodilator (direct acting ß2 > ß1 adrenergic agonist)

TERCONAZOLE: antifungal; used for vulvovaginal candidiasis

TERFENADINE: antihistamine with low sedative activity; contraindication with erythromycin and antifungals due to possiblility of serious arrhythmia

TESTOLACTONE: antineoplastic used for breast cancer (androgenic activity)

TESTOSTERONE CYPIONATE: depot form; duration 1-2 weeks (androgen)

TESTOSTERONE PROPIONATE: androgen; duration 8-10 hours

TESTOSTERONE: androgen; teratogen; contraindicated in prostate cancer

TETRACAINE: topical and spinal anesthetic (sodium influx inhibitor)

TETRACYCLINE: systemic antibacterial; binds 30S, blocks aminoacyl-tRNA access to A site; *enterohepatic circulation*

TETRAHYDROZOLINE: nasal and ocular decongestant (direct acting adrenergic agonist)

THEOPHYLLINE: oral bronchodilator; adenosine receptor antagonist

THIABENDAZOLE: anthelmintic

THIETHYLPERAZINE: antiemetic

BRIEF DRUG DESCRIPTIONS

THIOGUANINE: antineoplastic; prodrug metabolized to 6-TGRP, inhibits aminotransferase step in purine synthesis

THIOPENTAL: general anesthetic used as induction agent (IV barbiturate)

THIORIDAZINE: antipsychotic (HIGHEST anticholinergic; HIGH α blocking; LOWEST EPR)

THIOTHIXENE: antipsychotic

THYROID DESICCATED: thyroid hormone used in hypothyroid replacement therapy

TICARCILLIN: gram negative penicillin systemic antibacterial; covers *Pseudomonas, proteus, enterobacter* species

TICLOPIDINE: platelet aggregation inhibitor

TIMOLOL: non-selective β-adrenergic blocker; antihypertensive, post-MI agent; antimigraine drug, and antiglaucoma agent (topical)

TIOCONAZOLE: topical antifungal

TIZANIDINE: skeletal m. relaxant

TOBRAMYCIN: topical and systemic aminoglycoside antibacterial; binds 30s and 50s subunits, blocks initiation, and causes misreads in the genetic code

TOCAINIDE: class lb antiarrhythmic; slightly depresses depolarization, shortens repolarization, slows conduction

TOLAZAMIDE: 1st generation oral hypoglycemic; used to treat NIDDM (increases calcium ion influx and increases insulin efflux)

TOLBUTAMIDE: 1st generation oral hypoglycemic; used to treat NIDDM (increases calcium ion influx and increases insulin efflux)

TOLMETIN: systemic antiinflammatory

TOLNAFTATE: topical antifungal

TORSEMIDE: loop diuretic; antihypertensive

TRAMADOL: centrally-acting analgesic

TRANDOLAPRIL: antihypertensive; ACE inhibitor

TRANEXAMIC ACID: systemic hemostatic

TRANYLCYPROMINE: MAOI antidepressant (down regulates post-synaptic $\beta2$)

TRAZODONE: 2nd generation antidepressant

TRETINOIN: antiacne agent

BRIEF DRUG DESCRIPTIONS

TRIAMCINOLONE: systemic and topical corticosteroid; intermediate action antiinflammatory; inhalation corticosteroid

TRIAMTERENE: K^+ sparing diuretic

TRIAZOLAM: benzodiazepine hypnotic; short acting

TRICHLORMETHIAZIDE: antihypertensive, diuretic

TRIFLUOPERAZINE: antipsychotic (piperazine phenothiazine; HIGH potency and EPR)

TRIFLURIDINE: ophthalmologic antiviral of choice for herpes simplex keratitis

TRIHEXYPHENIDYL: antiparkinsonian (antimuscarinic)

TRIMEPRAZINE: antihistamine, antipruritic

TRIMETHADIONE: antiepileptic

TRIMETHOBENZAMIDE: antiemetic

TRIMETHOPRIM: antibacterial; dihydrofolate reductase inhibitor used in the prophylaxis for and treatment of *Pneumocystis carinii* and urinary tract infections

TRIMETREXATE: antiparasitic; must be administered with concurrent leucovorin

TRIMIPRAMINE: tricyclic antidepressant (TCA)

TRIPELENNAMINE: antihistamine

TROGLITAZONE: oral antihyperglycemic agent that decreases insulin resistence

TROLEANDOMYCIN: systemic macrolide antibacterial; relative of erythromycin, offers no advantage over erythromycin

TROPICAMIDE: anticholinergic; used to induce mydriasis, cycloplegia

TUBOCURARINE: skeletal m. relaxant; exists in NH_4+ form, non-depolarizing curariform

UREA: osmotic diurectic

UROKINASE: thrombolytic; non-antigenic, and does not induce allergic reactions associated with streptokinase

VALACYCLOVIR: antiviral; used for Herpes infections

VALPROIC ACID: antiepileptic used in absence seizures; inhibits GABA transaminase and succinic semialdehyde DH

VALSARTAN: antihypertensive; angiotensin II receptor (type AT_1) inhibitor

VANCOMYCIN: systemic antibacterial effective against methicillin resistant *Staphylococci aureus* (MRSA)

56

BRIEF DRUG DESCRIPTIONS

VASOPRESSIN: posterior pituitary hormone used in central diabetes insipidus; acts on V1 and V2 receptors

VECURONIUM: skeletal m. relaxant; used during intubation (non-depolarizing curariform)

VENLAFAXINE: antidepressant

VERAPAMIL: antianginal; antihypertensive; class IV antiarrhythmic (calcium channel blocker, vasodilator)

VIDARABINE: topical antiviral; used for herpes simplex keratitis

VINBLASTINE: plant alkaloid antineoplastic used in testicular cancer and lymphoma

VINCRISTINE: plant alkaloid antineoplastic used in acute lymphocytic leukemia (ALL)

VITAMIN B12:   macrocytic anemia (anti-anemia)

WARFARIN SODIUM: oral anticoagulant; inhibit clotting factors II, VII, IX, and X (all vitamin K dependent)

XYLOMETAZOLINE: nasal decongestant

YOHIMBINE: selective α2-adrenergic blocker

ZAFIRLUKAST: anti-asthmatic agent; cysteinyl leukotriene inhibitor

ZALCITABINE: antiviral

ZIDOVUDINE (AZT):   antiviral; used in HIV infection; prodrug metabolized to tri-PO4-AZT; inhibits RNA dependant DNA polymerase

ZINC OXIDE: skin protectant

ZOLPIDEM: hypnotic

DRUGS WITH UNUSUAL PROPERTIES OR EFFECTS

AGENT	THERAPEUTIC CATEGORY	PROPERTY/SIDE EFFECT
CEFAMANDOLE CEFOTETAN	Beta-lactam cephalosporins, 2nd generation	Disulfiram reaction
CIMETIDINE	Histamine H2 blocker	Gynecomastia
CYCLOSPORINE	Immunosuppressant	Hirsutism Gingival Hyperplasia
CHLORAMPHENICOL	Antibacterial, systemic	Grey baby syndrome
DACARBAZINE	Antineoplastic	Flu-like syndrome
DIAZOXIDE	Antihypertensive	Thiazide-like structure
ETHACRYNIC ACID	Diuretic (loop)	Teratogen
ETHAMBUTOL	Tuberculostatic	↓ red-green vision
FLUOROQUINOLONES	Antibacterial, systemic	Cartilage erosion and arthropathy in immature animals
KETOCONAZOLE	Antifungal	Gynecomastia
HYDRALAZINE	Antihypertensive	Lupus-like syndrome
HYDROXYCHLOROQUINE	Antimalarial; used in rheumatoid arthritis and systemic lupus erythematosus	Retinopathy; Ophthalmologic exam is indicated during long term use
LSD	Psychotomimetic	Teratogen
MEBENDAZOLE	Anthelmintic	Teratogen
MEFLOQUINE	Antimalarial	Cinchonism
METHYLDOPA	Antihypertensive	Positive Coombs test; lupus-like syndrome
MISOPROSTOL	Antiulcer	Abortifacient
MOXALACTAM	Beta-lactam cephalosporin, 3rd gen	Disulfiram reaction

DRUGS WITH UNUSUAL PROPERTIES OR EFFECTS

AGENT	THERAPEUTIC CATEGORY	PROPERTY/SIDE EFFECT
PHENYTOIN	Antiepileptic	Gingival hyperplasia
PROCAINAMIDE	Antiarrhythmic	Lupus-like syndrome
QUINIDINE	Antihypertensive	Cinchonism
QUININE	Antimalarial	Cinchonism
RIFAMPIN	Tuberculostatic	Orange secretions
SELEGILINE	Antiparkinsonian	Positive drug screen for amphetamines
TESTOSTERONE	Androgen	Teratogen
TETRACYCLINE	Antibacterial, systemic	Tooth discoloration
WARFARIN	Anticoagulant	Teratogen

Notes

MISCELLANEOUS DRUG FACTS

DRUGS AVAILABLE IN DEPOT FORM:

Benzathine penicillin (syphilis)
Fluphenazine (antipsychotic)
Leuprolide (GnRH agonist)
Medroxyprogesterone (contraceptive)
Procaine penicillin (gonorrhea)
Testosterone cypionate (androgen)

DRUGS THAT UNDERGO ENTEROHEPATIC CIRCULATION:

Ampicillin
Ceftriaxone
Glutethimide
Metolazone (diuretic)

Mezlocillin
Nafcillin
Rifampin (tuberculostatic)
Tetracycline

AGENTS THAT MUST BE CONVERTED TO ACTIVE FORM (PRODRUGS):

Acyclovir (antiviral)
Azathioprine (immunosuppressive)
Clorazepate (antianxiety)
Cytarabine (antineoplastic)
Enalapril (ACE inhibitor)
Flucytosine (antifungal)
Flurazepam (sedative-hypnotic)
Fosinopril (ACE inhibitor)
Insulin
Lovastatin (hypolipidemic)

Mestranol (synthetic estrogen)
Methyldopa (antihypertensive)
Metronidazole (amebicide)
Minoxidil (antihypertensive)
Prazepam (antianxiety)
Quinestrol (synthetic estrogen)
Δ^9 tetrahydrocannabinol (theoretical)
Simvastatin (hypolipidemic)
Zidovudine (AZT, antiviral)

DRUGS ASSOCIATED WITH STEVENS JOHNSON SYNDROME:

Fansidar
Gold
Phenytoin
Sulfonamides

61

FDA CATEGORY	INTERPRETATION OF DRUG CATEGORY
A	**Studies show no risk.** Human studies in pregnancy fail to show fetal risk. Possibility of fetal harm is remote.
B	**No evidence of risk in humans.** Animal studies show risk while human studies do not. OR No adequate human studies available and animal studies show no risk.
C	**Risk is not ruled out.** No adequate human studies, and animal studies either show risk or are not available. Benefits of use may justify potential risk to fetus.
D	**Positive evidence of risk to fetus.** Studies show risk to human fetus. Benefits of use may justify potential risk to fetus.
X	**Contraindicated in pregnancy.** Animal or human studies clearly show fetal risk that outweighs any possible benefit of use.

KNOWN OR SUSPECTED TERATOGENS

Alcohol	Lisinopril
Benazepril	Lithium
Busulfan	Mebendazole
Captopril	Methimazole
Carbamazepine	Methotrexate
Coumadin	Penicillamine
Cyclophosphamide	Phenytoin
Danazol	Quinapril
Diethylstilbestrol (DES)	Radioactive iodine
Enalapril	Ramipril
Etretinate	Testosterone
Fosinopril	Tetracycline
Isotretinoin	Valproic acid

Note: It is estimated that possibly 50% of over 1500 agents tested in animals are teratogenic. Approximately 30 agents are actually documented teratogens. (Shepard, TH: Human teratogenicity. Adv Pediatr 33:225, 1986)

63

Notes

DRUG CHARTS

ABUSE, DRUGS OF:

DRUG	CHARACTERISTICS/EFFECTS	ADVERSE REACTIONS	WITHDRAWAL/OVERDOSE THERAPY
BARBITURATES	Source is prescription; **euphoria with sedation**; greater tolerance than with BZs; metabolic tolerance; HIGH addiction liability with short acting agents such as Secobarbital (rarely see abuse of phenobarbital which is long acting)	Addiction and withdrawal HIGHEST with short acting agents; **status epilepticus**; treat with phenobarbital or other long acting barbiturate	Treat barbiturate withdrawal with phenobarbital or other long acting barbiturates
BENZODIAZEPINES	Source is prescription; causes **euphoria without sedation**; tolerance develops; addiction is HIGH with short acting agents (lorazepam, alprazolam); withdrawal hallmark is status epilepticus	Addiction and withdrawal HIGHEST with short acting agents; **status epilepticus**; CANNOT allow patient to go through withdrawal without treatment; MUST treat with phenytoin or a BZ such as diazepam or lorazepam	Treat benzodiazepine withdrawal with Phenytoin or long acting benzodiazepine such as Diazepam
ETHANOL	Acute effects: 100 mg/dL: decreased visual acuity, increased reaction time, locomotion problems; **200 mg/dL**: foolish behavior usually ensues, often leading to embarrassment the following morning (see RMG and DRS); **350 mg/dL**: respiratory and vasomotor center depression (death uncommon); **550 mg/dL**: decreased respiration, severe vasomotor center depression, increased intracranial pressure, acidosis, hypoglycemia, stupor, coma, respiratory depression and death; NO antidote, ethanol overdose therapy is supportive	Metabolic (dispositional) tolerance, increased bio-transformation, must increase dose to achieve same effects; **functional tolerance**, cellular adaptation in CNS to presence of alcohol Acute EtOH use: INHIBITS DMMS, additive effects of CNS depressants Chronic EtOH use: increased sER, increased enzymes, increased metabolism of benzodiazepines, barbiturates, and anesthesia	**Disulfiram (Antabuse)**: irreversibly inhibits aldehyde DH (binds sulfhydryl groups and zinc); treatment for alcoholism, curtails desire to drink; metabolized to diethyldithiocarbamate, an active metabolite; EtOH + disulfiram → **acetaldehyde syndrome** (sweating, nausea, vomiting, flushing, dizziness, decreased BP, increased HR, fainting) is UNpleasant, lasts 3-10 days until body de novo synthesizes aldehyde DH; CANNOT use alcohol in any form while taking disulfiram
HALLUCINOGENS LSD PCP MDMA STP	LSD is a tryptophan derivative (serotonin precursor); 4 ring structure; **directly excitatory on S2 receptors in limbic system**; blocks 5-HT reuptake; 50 μg dose achieves hallucinations; somatic, sensory, psychotic reactions PCP has shorter somatic effects than LSD; longer sensory and psychosis effects than LSD; treat overdose with anti psychotic agents MDMA (3,4-methylene-dioxymethamphetamine) is a psychoto-mimetic drug that is a hallucinogen; agents in this class appear to work on a specific serotonin receptor subtype STP or DOM (2,5-dimethoxy-4-methylamphetamine) is also a psychotomimetic drug that is a hallucinogen	LSD causes flashbacks is teratogenic; results in sympathetic overtone and tolerance and dependence PCP does not cause flashbacks and has no teratogenic effects; but has been associated with irreversible brain damage; sympathetic overtone; tolerance and dependence	LSD overdose is treated with Buspirone (antianxiety agent) PCP overdose treatment is supportive

66

ABUSE, DRUGS OF:

DRUG	CHARACTERISTICS/EFFECTS	ADVERSE REACTIONS	WITHDRAWAL/OVERDOSE THERAPY
HEROIN (semi-synthetic)	**Diacetylmorphine;** more potent than morphine (100 mg of morphine vs. 4-5 mg of heroin); POOR oral bioavailability; IV injection; t½ ≈ **20-60 min; cleared rapidly to 6-acetyl-morphine** and **morphine-6-glucuronide;** multiple daily doses, causes tracking (purple lines with scar tissue); **Methadone** is given orally and has long duration	**Track marks; acute toxicity:** causes respiratory death; non-sterile equipment infection: systemic Staphylococci, heart valvulitis and endocarditis, pulmonary abscess; chronic toxicity: addiction, chronic infection	**Put patient into acute withdrawal** and provide supportive measures, NO narcotic supplement, lasts 2-7 days, has 80-90% failure rate; **titration approach:** give methadon and bring patient off slowly; **Methadone maintenance:** give constant dose in order to substitute Methadone for heroin, low success rate
MARIJUANA (THC) *Cannabis sativa*	⌃9-tetrahydrocannabinol (prodrug) and 11-OH-⌃9-THC-COOH (metabolite) are active; mechanism NOT known; slow leeching out of adipose; mood changes; **potent cardiac stimulation; potent bronchodilation; blocks chemotactic trigger zone (CTZ); increases adrenal cortex output; decreases intraocular pressure; decreases testosterone production in males,** decreases sperm count; BP remains normal	Impairs attention and learning, anxiety, increased heart rate, **conjunctival vascular reaction** ("red eyes"), ataxia, nystagmus, fine tremor, dry mouth, paranoid reaction, decreased testosterone in males; chronic use: amotivational syndrome, tolerance and dependence	Abrupt cessation of marijuana after prolonged use has been associated with developement of some dependency. The dependency appears to be more psychological than physical and of considerably less intensity than observed with cocaine and amphetamines.
OPIOIDS Alfentanil Codeine Fentanyl Hydrocodone Hydromorphone Morphine Oxycodone Propoxyphene Sufentanil	Morphine is best example of this class of drugs; cause **sedation (к receptor),** general CNS depression; mental clouding; **euphoria** (may relate to being free of pain, may see dysphoria if no initial pain); non-pain sensations NOT affected; **decrease respiration; stimulate CTZ; orthostatic hypotension;** few cardiac effects; smooth m. contraction, biliary contraction (gall stones, exacerbates pain); GI muscle spasm, decreases peristalsis leads to **constipation;** miosis (pinpoint pupils); increase histamine (itching, allergic rxns); decrease body temperature; hyperglycemia; antitussive	Nausea, vomiting; decreases respiratory rate; orthostatic hypotension; skeletal m. rigidity at high dose constipation; increases histamine, itching; hypothermia; bradycardia at near toxic doses; respiratory arrest in overdose at medulla; abuse/dependence/withdrawal	Most cases of opioid withdrawal require little medication, and some patients can stop without assistance, however, relapse is almost universal; shorter acting opioids have a brief, severe withdrawal syndrome; **Clonidine,** an antihypertensive agent, reduces most of the symptoms of opioid withdrawal
STIMULANTS Amphetamines Methamphetamine Ephedrine	The Amphetamines are non-catecholamine agents with CNS stimulant and peripheral sympathomimetic activity; after oral administration patients feel more confident, alert, talkative, and have increased activity level; increases endurance and decreases fatigue; anorexic effect; IV dosage gives intial "rush"; produces euphoria and excitement Ephedrine is a better direct adrenergic agonist action than norepinephrine releasing drug; cardiovascular action: vasoconstrictor thus acts as nasal and ocular decongestant; causes release of norepinephrine from SNS neurons; more lipid soluble	Amphetamines have potential for tolerance, dependence and abuse; hyperthermia, profuse sweating, respiratory difficulty, tremor, cardiovascular effects including tachycardia, palpitation, arrhythmia, and hypertension; restlessness, dizziness, insomnia, dyskinesia, dysphoria, headache Ephedrine causes some CNS stimulation, anxiety, irritability, insomnia	Abrupt discontinuation of amphetamines after chronic use results in only mild physical withdrawal symptoms. Withdrawal effects appear to be psychological and include extreme fatigue, mental depression and strong desire for the drug

ABUSE, DRUGS OF:

DRUG	CHARACTERISTICS/EFFECTS	ADVERSE REACTIONS	WITHDRAWAL/OVERDOSE THERAPY
SOLVENTS	CNS depressants, example is NO2; commercial sources; organic compounds such as butane and glue, solvents such as gasoline; compounds with toluene base such as hexane, trichloroethylene and nitrous oxide; work through general anesthetic mechanism	Acute: hepatotoxic → hepatitis, elevated liver enzymes; chronic use: cerebral atrophy; do NOT see high addiction or withdrawal	Treat underlying liver disease; supportive respiration; over 1000 teenager deaths per year

ADRENERGIC AGONISTS, DIRECT ACTING:

DRUG	ORGAN SYSTEM EFFECTS	PHARMACOKINETICS	ADVERSE REACTIONS	THERAPEUTIC USE
ALBUTEROL (Ventolin)	Non-catecholamine with similar pharmacology as terbutaline; ß2 bronchodilator; selective agonist at ß2 receptors; COMT and MAO no effect	Po, inhalational, or subcutaneously; of longer duration than isoproterenol and EPI	Muscle tremor; **Pregnancy category C**	Bronchial Asthma Bronchitis COPD
BITOLTEROL (Tornalate)	Selective ß2 agonist on the respiratory tract; non-catecholamine structure; stimulates adenylyl cyclase to increase cAMP	**Prodrug** with active product, **colterol**; duration of action is 5-8 hours	Tremor, nervousness, palpitation, cough, throat irritation, possible tachycardia; **Pregnancy category C**	Bronchial Asthma Reversible Bronchospasm
CLONIDINE (Catapres)	α2 selective adrenergic agonist; α2 > α1		Dry mouth, drowsiness, dizziness, constipation **Pregnancy category C**	Chronic Hypertension
DOBUTAMINE (Dobutrex)	CLASSIC ß1 selective agonist; ↑ cardiac contractility, ↑ CO, ↑ HR; activity at ß1 > ß2 (dose related); synthetic derivative of dopamine	MUST give IV; large NH2-R group inhibits MAO inactivation	Hypertension, tachycardia, vent. arrhythmias, nausea, headache, anginal pain, palpitations	Refractory Congestive Heart Failure (improves myocardial function)
EPINEPHRINE (Adrenalin)	Agonist activity at α and β receptors; Cardiovascular: ↑ SP, ↑ MAP, ↑ PP, less effect on DP and TPR; vasoconstriction in skin, mucous membranes, kidney and splanchnic circulation, ↑ contractility, increases HR Respiratory: bronchodilation at ß2; pulmonary vasoconstriction and respiratory mucosal decongestant; (brief with rapid onset) Ocular: contraction of radial m. or iris, decreases intraocular pressure in glaucoma GI: decreases contractions through α & ß GU: bladder and uterine relaxation thru ß2, urethral sphincter contraction & ejaculation thru α Metabolic: ↑ glycogenolysis in liver and skeletal m.., increases lipolysis in adipose, hyperglycemia, hyperlactacidemia, hyperlipidemia, ↓ insulin and ↑ glucagon, transient hyperkalemia from liver then prolonged hypokalemia as K+ uptake by muscle	Must give parenteral dose; inactivation by MAO & COMT; rapid biotransformation	CNS stimulant effects, anxiety, irritability, insomnia; palpitation, mild tachycardia, HTN, tremor, excess dosage can promote convulsions, CVA, or ventricular arrhythmia	Bronchial Asthma Glaucoma Bronchodilator Allergic Reactions i.e., Anaphylaxis Nose Bleeds (topical) Cardiac Stimulant Used with Local Anesthetics

ADRENERGIC AGONISTS, DIRECT ACTING:

DRUG	ORGAN SYSTEM EFFECTS	PHARMACOKINETICS	ADVERSE REACTIONS	THERAPEUTIC USE
ISOETHARINE (Bronkosol)	Catecholamine that is LEAST selective agonist for ß2; activity at ß2 > ß1 receptors at therapeutic doses	Effective only through inhalation; not good orally	Tachycardia, palpitation, nausea, headache, anxiety, restlessness, insomnia, tremor	Bronchodilation
ISOPROTERENOL	Synthetic catecholamine with high selectivity for beta adrenergic receptors; LACKS significant alpha agonist activity; positive chornotropic and inotropic activity; decreased peripheral vascular resistance via beta-2 receptors; net cardiovascular effect is increase in cardiac output and stroke volume; does NOT elevate systemic arterial blood pressure (in contrast to EPI and NE); bronchodilation is another prominent effect	Parental dose; inactivation by MAO amd COMT; rapidly biotransformed; also given by inhalation	Hypotension, reflex tachycardia, nervousness, mild tremor, use as cardiostimulant may cause arrhythmias	Bronchial asthma Cardiostimulant (IV)
METAPROTERENOL (Alupent)	Non-catecholamine; Less selective than terbutaline and albuterol; agonist activity at ß2 > ß1	Oral (40% absorbed) or through inhalation; COMT has no effect	Similar to prototype direct beta acting adrenergic agonists	COPD
NOREPINEPHRINE (Noradrenaline)	Direct acting agonist activity at α and some ß2; Vasopressive, vasoconstriction at α, cardiostimulant at ß1, weaker than EPI at ß2 receptors, IV dose will ↑ SP, ↑ DP, ↑ TPR, and ↑ MAP with little change in PP, reflex bradycardia; NE has little or no stimulatory effect on CHO and lipid metabolism, in contrast to EPI	Parental dose; inactivation by MAO and COMT; rapidly biotransformed	Can cause tissue necrosis at IV infusion site; so not used as local vasoconstrictor	Hypotension Shock
OXYMETAZOLINE (Afrin)	Imidazoline derivative that relieves nasal congestion associated with rhinitis	Administered as nasal spray or intraocular	Rebound congestion; nervousness	Nasal and Ocular Decongestant
PHENYLEPHRINE (Neo-synephrine)	Synthetic non-catecholamine with dose related agonist activity at α1 > α2; Vasoconstriction, little cardiostimulation, parental dose ↑ MAP with reflex bradycardia; constricts blood vessels in mucous membranes; topical application to nasal mucosa promotes local decongestion for infectious or allergic rhinitis	Administered po, topically and by injection	Nervousness, insomnia, headache, urinary retention in patients with prostatic hypertrophy	Nasal Decongestant Pressor Amine (used in hypotension Also in Cough Preparations

70

ADRENERGIC AGONISTS, DIRECT ACTING:

DRUG	ORGAN SYSTEM EFFECTS	PHARMACOKINETICS	ADVERSE REACTIONS	THERAPEUTIC USE
PIRBUTEROL (Maxair)	Bronchodilator, related to albuterol; selective β2 stimulant	Aerosol	Tachycardia, tremor, palpitation	Bronchospasms Asthma
RITODRINE (Yutopar)	Selective ß2 agonist approved for both IV and oral administration as a uterine relaxant for treatment of premature labor	Oral and IV dosage	Pulmonary edema; hypokalemia and diabetogenic effects in mother and fetus	Premature Labor
SALMETEROL (Servent)	Selective β2 adrenergic agonist which relaxes bronchial smooth muscle	Administered by aerosol; duration of action at least 12 hours; excreted in feces	Tachycardia, tremor, palpitations, parodoxical bronchospasm; **Pregnancy category C**	Asthma Bronchospasm (NOT for acute attacks)
TERBUTALINE (Brethine) synthetic	MOST selective ß2 adrenergic agonist for bronchial smooth muscle with little activity on cardiac ß1 adrenergic receptors	Po, inhalation, or subQ; COMT and MAO no effect	Tachycardia, tremor, palpitation, nervousness	Bronchiolar spasm in COPD Bronchodilator for Asthma
TETRAHYDROZOLINE (Visine)	Imidazoline derivative applied topically; constricts dilated conjunctival vessels and whitens the eyes	Nasal and ocular preparations	Local irritation	Nasal and Ocular Decongestant

71

ADRENERGIC AGONISTS, MIXED ACTING:

DRUG	AGONIST ACTION	ORGAN SYSTEM EFFECTS	PHARMACOKINETICS	ADVERSE REACTIONS	THERAPEUTIC USE
AMPHETAMINES Dextroamphetamine Methamphetamine	α, ß	Weak direct acting adrenergic agonist, in contrast to ephedrine; **CNS stimulant;** anorexiant (appetite suppressant) in exogenous obesity (not recommended)	Tolerance develops quickly; lipid soluble	CNS effects; banned in some states and Canada as anorexiant	Narcolepsy; attention deficit disorder (ADD); exogenous obesity (not recommended)
DOPAMINE (Dopastat, Intropin)	D1 > ß1 > α	Selective D1 agonist at low dose; vasodilation through D1 receptors in kidney vasculature; ß1 adrenergic agonist at higher dose; NO ß2 adrenergic activity	Short acting; IV dose; rapid onset	Nausea/ vomiting CNS disturbances	Low IV dose vasodilates kidney in poor renal perfusion states such as shock; increased dose is cardiostimulant; higher doses produce α adrenergic agonist effect; increases BP thru vasoconstriction
EPHEDRINE	α, ß	Better direct adrenergic agonist action than NE releasing drug; cardiovascular action: vasoconstrictor thus acts as nasal and ocular decongestant; causes release of NE from SNS neurons; more lipid soluble	Oral effectiveness, substituted alpha carbon blocks MAO, COMT no effect on non-catechol ring; good bioavailability; biotransformation by DMMS through oxidative deamination	Some CNS stimulation, may see anxiety or irritability, and insomnia	Nasal and ocular decongestant; present in many cough syrups; found in many non-FDA approved athletic supplement foods; also abused for CNS effects
PSEUDOEPHEDRINE (Sudafed)	α, ß	Same properties and action as Ephedrine	Same as Ephedrine	Same as Ephedrine	Nasal decongestant

72

ADRENERGIC BLOCKERS, ALPHA:

DRUG	CLASSIFICATION and MECHANISM OF ACTION/EFFECTS	ADVERSE REACTIONS	THERAPEUTIC USE
DOXAZOSIN (Cardura)	Selective α1 blocker; acts post-synaptically; orthostatic hypotension with minimal tachycardia; acts on α1, NE still released with feedback at α2; liver metabolized	**Orthostatic hypotension** on first dose (*first dose effect*); **Pregnancy category C**	Hypertension Benign Prostatic Hypertrophy (BPH)
PHENOXYBENZAMINE	**Non-selective α adrenergic blocker**; non-equilibrium α blockade; cyclizes to ethylenimonium ion, then forms carbonium ion, this covalently bonds with α receptors; **EPI vasomotor reversal**	Postural hypotension, tachycardia, inhibition of ejaculation; **Pregnancy category C**	**Pheochromocytoma:** pre-op or for inoperable tumor, chronic treatment; will decrease vasoconstriction in peripheral vascular disease (Raynaud's disease is example); for severe HTN and tachycardia; sedative effects on CNS
PHENTOLAMINE	**Non-selective α adrenergic blocker;** competitive antagonist action at α2 blocks feedback inhibition of NE release; increases NE release on ß1 R causing tachycardia; antagonist at α1 causes vasodilation and decreases BP; **musculotropic spasmolytic** (not through α R); **sympathomimetic amine-like effect** on heart through increases NE release on ß1 and through reflex tachycardia; increases GI motility at **muscarinic receptors** of gut; increases HCl and pepsin secretion through **H2 receptors;** decreased response/dose (tolerance) can develop	Tachycardia and arrhythmia, severe hypotension, abdominal pain, exacerbation of peptic ulcer	**Acute Hypertensive Crisis Pheochromocytoma:** pre-op to control paroxysmal large increases in BP, and during surgery to prevent large increases BP while removing tumor Used during IV administration of norepinephrine to **prevent dermal necrosis**
PRAZOSIN (Minipress)	Selective α1 adrenergic blocker; acts post-synaptically; **orthostatic decreases BP** (upon standing) with minimal tachycardia; acts on α1 receptors, NE still released with feedback at α2 receptors	Dizziness, headache, drowsiness, lack of energy, weakness, palpitations, nausea; first dose effect; **Pregnancy category C**	Hypertension
TERAZOSIN (Hytrin)	Selective α1 blocker; acts post-synaptically; **orthostatic hypotension** with minimal tachycardia; acts on α1, NE still released with feedback at α2	Asthenia, postural hypotension, dizziness, somnolence, nasal congestion/rhinits, impotence; first dose effect; **Pregnancy category C**	Symptomatic benign prostatic hypertrophy Hypertension
YOHIMBINE	Presynaptic alpha-2 adrenergic receptor blocker; may have activity as aphrodisiac; mild anti-diuretic activity; often found in non-FDA approved athletic supplement foods	**Not to be used in pregnancy**	Sympathicolytic Mydriatic Has been used to treat Impotence

73

ADRENERGIC BLOCKERS, BETA:

DRUG	ORGAN SYSTEM EFFECTS	PHARMACOKINETICS	ADVERSE REACTIONS	THERAPEUTIC USE
ACEBUTOLOL (Sectral)	**Selective ß1 > ß2 adrenergic blocker;** decreases HR, contractility and renin release; decreases lipolysis in fat cells; bronchoconstricts; decreases vasodilation, reflex vasoconstriction; decreases insulin; blocks uterine relaxation; decreases glycogenolysis in liver; decreases aqueous humor in anterior chamber of eye	**Intermediate acting agent** (7-12 hours); conjugation through acetylation; half-life is 3-7 hours	**CNS:** depression, insomnia, highest with Propranolol; **Heart:** cardiac arrest; **Lung:** bronchoconstriction, decreases pulmonary function; alters blood glucose; cold extremities	Hypertension Angina (prophylactically) Arrhythmias Hyperthyroidism
ATENOLOL (Tenormin)	Selective ß1 > ß2 adrenergic blocker	**Intermediate acting agent** (7-12 hours); Atenolol (and Nadolol) have the LOWEST lipid sol among ß blockers; **excreted unchanged;** half-life is 6-7 hours	Same as Acebutolol Atenolol (and Nadolol) have LOWEST CNS adverse effects	Angina Post MI Hypertension
BETAXOLOL (Kerlone)	Cardioselective beta-adrenergic blocker, β1 > β2; does not have significant membrane stabilizing activity and has no intrinsic sympathomimetic action; local application to the eye causes decrease in elevated and normal intraocular pressure	Onset of action is 30 minutes; 12 hour duration; half-life is 14-22 hours	Eye tearing, decreased corneal sensitivity, erythema, itching, keratitis; **Pregnancy category C**	Ocular Hypertension Chronic Open-Angle Glaucoma
BISOPROLOL (Zebeta)	Synthetic beta 1 selective adrenergic blocker; has no significant membrane stabilizing activity or intrinsic sympathomimetic activity; most prominent effect is negative chronotropic effect	Administered po; half-life is 9-12 hours; 30% protein bound	Bradycardia, diarrhea, vomiting, asthenia, fatigue; **Pregnancy category C**	Hypertension
CARTEOLOL (Cartrol)	Synthetic nonselective beta adrenergic receptor blocker; has intrinsic sympathomimetic activity	Half-life is 6 hours	Asthenia, muscle cramps; **Pregnancy category C**	Hypertension
ESMOLOL (Brevibloc)	Selective ß1 > ß2 adrenergic blocker	**Ultra short acting agent** (< 1 hour); Esmolol is given **IV ONLY**	Similar to Acebutolol	Antiarrhythmic
LABETALOL (Trandate)	**Non-selective ß blocker AND selective α blocker;** NOT vasoconstriction when used to treat HTN	**Intermediate acting** (7-8 hours)	Less adverse effect of cold extremities versus beta blockers	Hypertension
METOPROLOL (Lopressor)	Selective ß1 > ß2 blocker	**Short acting agent;** half-life is 3-4 hours	Similar to Acebutolol	Same as Acebutolol

74

ADRENERGIC BLOCKERS, BETA:

DRUG	ORGAN SYSTEM EFFECTS	PHARMACOKINETICS	ADVERSE REACTIONS	THERAPEUTIC USE
NADOLOL (Corgard)	Non-selective ß blocker	**Long acting** (≈ 24 hrs); Nadolol (and Atenolol) LOWEST lipid solubility; **excreted unchanged**	Same as Acebutolol Nadolol (and Atenolol) has LOWEST CNS adverse effects	Angina Hypertension
PENBUTOLOL (Levatol)	Synthetic beta blocker; non-selective beta 1 and beta 2 blocker	Rapid and complete po absorption; half-life is 3-4 hours	Asthenia, diarrhea, nausea, dyspepsia, dizziness, fatigue, headache, insomnia, dyspnea, excessive sweating, impotence; **Pregnancy category C**	Hypertension
PINDOLOL (Visken)	Non-selective ß blocker; allegedly has **intrinsic sympathomimetic activity (ISA)** or is able to cause NE release in the myocardium	**Short acting agent** (3-4 hours)	Bizarre or many dreams, fatigue, nervousness, insomnia, nervousness, weakness, paresthesia, dyspnea, edema, chest pain, joint pain, nausea; **Pregnancy category B**	Hypertension
PROPRANOLOL (Inderal)	Non-selective ß blocker; high **membrane stabilizing activity (MSA)** thus has use as anti-arrhythmic agent	**Short acting agent** (3-4 hours); HIGHEST lipid sol; **95% ppb**, highest drug-drug interaction	Same; Propranolol has HIGHEST CNS adverse effect	Angina Arrhythmia Hypertension Migraine Post MI Hyperaldosteronism
SOTALOL (Betapace)	Antiarrhythmic drug with Class II (beta-adrenoreceptor blocking) and Class III (cardiac action potential duration prolongation) properties	Oral bioavailability is 90-100%; peak plasma levels within 2.5-4 hours; does not bind to plasma protein	Contraindicated in asthma; fatigue, bradycardia, dyspnea, proarrhythmia, asthenia, dizziness; **Pregnancy category B**	Ventricular arrhythmias
TIMOLOL (Blocadren)	Non-selective ß blocker; NO significant intrinsic sympathomimetic, direct myocardial depressant or local anesthetic activity	**Short acting agent**; half-life is 3-4 hours; undergoes oxidation	Fatigue, chest pain, asthenia, bradycardia, nausea, dizziness, vertigo, paresthesia, decreased libido, dyspnea, bronchial spasm, tinnitus; **Pregnancy category C**	Hypertension Post MI Migraine prophylaxis Glaucoma

ADRENERGIC NEURONAL BLOCKERS:

DRUG	ORGAN SYSTEM EFFECTS	PHARMACOKINETICS	ADVERSE REACTIONS	THERAPEUTIC USE
GUANETHIDINE (Ismelin)	Adrenergic neuronal blocker; taken up by NE storage vesicle and displaces NE causes decreased sympathetic effects on vasculature upon NE vesicle release, decreases BP; (initial NE discharge as guanethidine fills NE vesicles)	Po, biotransformed to several inactive metabolites; excreted via kidneys	Bradycardia because NE is depleted and not available to mediate reflex tachycardia; edema, diarrhea	Severe Hypertension (onset of effect is delayed for 2-3 days)
GUANADREL (Hylorel)	Adrenergic neuronal blocker; taken up by NE storage vesicle and displaces NE causes decreased sympathetic effects on vasculature upon NE vesicle release, decreases BP	Po, administered bid; half-life is about 10 hours; excreted via kidneys	Bradycardia because NE is depleted and not available to mediate reflex tachycardia; less diarrhea than Guanethidine	Hypertension
METYROSINE (Demser)	Adrenergic neuronal blocker; **tyrosine hydroxylase** inhibitor; decreased NE and EPI in chronic adrenal (pheochromocytoma) tumors	Po, well absorbed; excreted in urine; half-lfe is 3.5 hours	Sedation, anxiety, depression, EPR, and diarrhea	Used preoperatively for Chronic Pheochromocytoma (Not used for essential hypertension)
RESERPINE	Adrenergic neuronal blocker; irreversibly blocks Mg2 + sensitive ATPase on NE storage vesicles, thus decreases NE available for release; antihypertensive; an alkaloid by structure	Takes days for onset of action	May cause severe adverse effects; long lasting depression; edema, bradycardia	Used in conjunction with diuretic agent to treat mild or moderate hypertension

76

ALCOHOLS, THE:

DRUG	CHARACTERISTICS/EFFECTS	BIOTRANSFORMATION	ADVERSE REACTIONS/USES
ETHANOL	Oral dose, some gastric, but MOST absorption in small intestine; rate peaks at 40% solution (80 proof) due to **gastric irritation, increases mucus production, pyloric spasms;** 100 mg/dL is DWI; **[lung] ≈ 0.05% of [blood];** urine excretion Mechanism of action: ↓ **cell membrane rigidity** (↑ fluidity), alters membrane enzymes, protein ion channels and NT release; NON-SPECIFIC agent; may enhance GABA effects on the CNS **Disinhibitory effect of ethanol:** inhibits inhibition of the RAS on CNS; **euphoria; hypothermia** (vasodilation at low dose → feel warm); ↓ **ADH** from posterior pituitary Acute effects: **100 mg/dL:** decreased visual acuity, increased reaction time, locomotion problems; **200 mg/dL:** uninhibited behavior often occurs; **350 mg/dL:** respiratory and vasomotor center depression (death uncommon); **550 mg/dL:** decreased respiration, severe vasomotor center depression, increased intracranial pressure, acidosis, hypoglycemia, stupor, coma, respiratory depression and death; NO antidote, ethanol overdose therapy is supportive	**Alcohol DH system** (NON microsomal, cytoplasmic, RDS, requires NAD+) takes ethanol → acetaldehyde; **aldehyde DH** (in mitochondria, requires NAD+) takes acetaldehyde → acetate; **Krebs cycle** takes acetate → CO2 + H2O; **microsomal ethanol oxidizing system (MEOS)** takes ethanol → acetaldehyde (requires NADPH and O2); MEOS is utilized with chronic use or toxic ethanol levels; **catalase system** (requires H2O2, limited function) takes ethanol → acetaldehyde	**Metabolic (dispositional) tolerance,** must ↑ dose to achieve same effects; **functional tolerance,** cellular adaptation in CNS to presence of alcohol; acute EtOH use: INHIBITS DMMS, additive effects of CNS depressants; chronic EtOH use: ↑ sER, ↑ enzymes, ↑ metabolism of BZs, barbiturates, and anesthesia; **Disulfiram (Antabuse):** irreversibly inhibits aldehyde DH (binds sulfhydryl groups and zinc); treatment for alcoholism; curtails desire to drink; metabolized to **diethyldithiocarbamate,** an active metabolite; EtOH + disulfiram → **acetaldehyde syndrome** (sweating, nausea, vomiting, flushing, dizziness, ↓ BP, ↑ HR, fainting) is UNpleasant, lasts 3-10 days until body de novo synthesizes aldehyde DH; CANNOT use alcohol in any form while taking disulfiram Naltrexone is given orally to decrease drinking of alcohol; found to be effective in reducing amount of ethanol consumption Uses: **antibacterial (70% solution);** ↓ **fever topically;** ↑ **HDL; nighttime sedative;** antidote for **methanol and ethylene glycol** poisoning
ETHYLENE GLYCOL	Dihydroxyalcohol (antifreeze); metabolized by alcohol DH; calcium oxalate crystals are **nephrotoxic**	Ethylene glycol → oxalic acid → glycolic acid + formic acid	**Symptoms of ethylene glycol poisoning:** CNS depression, convulsions, acidosis, renal damage, and respiratory failure; Treatment: gastric lavage, airway maintenance, temperature maintenance; diuresis, **ethanol** (competitively ↓ metabolism of ethylene glycol)
ISOPROPYL ALCOHOL	Isopropanol, rubbing alcohol (70% solution); **antiseptic;** **decreases body temperature** (topically); ingested or inhaled	Isopropyl alcohol → acetone	**Toxicity of isopropyl alcohol:** nausea, vomiting, dizziness, CNS depression, coma, respiratory depression; Treatment: supportive, hemodialysis
METHANOL	Methyl alcohol, wood spirit or wood alcohol; **formic acid** metabolite causes **blindness**	methanol → formaldehyde + formic acid by **alcohol DH**	**Symptoms of methanol poisoning:** visual disturbances, partial or complete blindness, CNS depression with nausea, vomiting, slowed respiration, bradycardia, and coma; Treatment: **ethanol** (competitively ↓ methanol metabolism)

AMEBICIDES:

DRUG	ORGAN SYSTEM EFFECTS	ADVERSE EFFECTS	THERAPEUTIC USE
EMETINE	Salt of an ipecac alkaloid which is amebicidal against *Entamoeba histolytica* in tissue; not active against the amoebal cyst form; Emetine blocks protein synthesis by inhibiting polypeptide chain elongation in eukaryotic cells (blocks protein synthesis in humans and parasites but not bacteria)	Precordial pain, dyspnea, tachycardia, hypotension, gallop rhythm, cardiac dilatation, congestive failure, widening of QRS complex, prolongation of PR and QT intervals, alteration of ST segment, flattening or inversion of T waves; nausea, vomiting; headache, skeletal muscle weakness, stiffness Note: these agents may cause serious cardiac effects and patients should get daily electrocardiograms during therapy	Severe intestinal and extraintestinal amebiasis
IODOQUINOL (Yodoxin)	Amebicidal against *Entamoeba histolytica* trophozoite and cyst forms	Various skin eruptions, urticaria, pruritus, nausea, vomiting, abdominal cramps, diarrhea, pruritus ani; fever, chills, headache, vertigo, thyroid enlargement; safety in pregnancy or lactation is not established	Intestinal amebiasis
METRONIDAZOLE (Flagyl)	Synthetic amebicidal agent effective against *Entamoeba histolytica*; active against both intestinal and tissue forms; effective in giardiasis, balantidiasis, *Trichomonas vaginalis*, *Gardnerella vaginalis* and many anaerobic bacterial infections	Nausea, vomiting, diarrhea, glossitis, stomatitis, anorexia, constipation, dizziness, headache, urticaria; **Pregnancy category B**	Amebiasis (intestinal and extra-intestinal) Giardiasis Trichomonas Vaginitis Bacterial Vaginosis Anaerobic Infections including *B. fragilis* *C. difficile* infections
PAROMOMYCIN (Humatin)	Luminal amebicide; an aminoglycoside effective against *Entamoeba histolytica*; used as alternate the Metronidazole	Nausea, increased gastointestinal motility, abdominal pain, diarrhea; rash; headache, vertigo; vomiting; (ototoxicity and nephrotoxicity is limited due to minimal absorption)	Mild to moderate intestinal amebiasis

78

AMINOGLYCOSIDES and SPECTINOMYCIN:

DRUG	MECHANISM OF ACTION and RESISTANCE	ADVERSE EFFECTS	SPECTRUM
AMIKACIN (Amikin)	Aminoglycoside; see Gentamicin	Neuromuscular blockade, ototoxicity, nephrotoxic, apnea; **Pregnancy category D**	Staphylococci *Acinetobacter* species Enterobacter species *Escherichia coli* *Hemophilus influenzae* *Klebsiella* species *Neisseria* species *Proteus* species *Pseudomonas aeruginosa* *Salmonella* species *Shigella* species *Yersinia pestis*
GENTAMICIN (Garamycin)	Aminoglycosides bind the 30 S subunit of bacterial ribosomes, interfere with the initiation complex, cause misreads of mRNA and inhibits protein synthesis; aminoglycosides are bacteriocidal Mechanisms of resistance: adenylation, acetylation, or phosphorylation of the drug by the bacteria; is usually plasmid mediated resistance; alteration of bacterial cell surface; alteration of ribosomal 30 S subunit Aminoglycosides have poor GI absorption; peak plasma levels within 30-90 minutes after IM injection; 10% plasma protein bound; have a narrow therapeutic window Aminoglycosides are commonly used parenterally for severe gram negative infections	Confusion, fever, lethargy, vomiting, nausea, anemia, leukopenia, thrombocytopenia, rash, urticaria, itching, dizziness, tinnitus, vertigo, ototoxic (hearing loss, deafness), elevated liver enzymes, pain or irritation at injection site, hypotension; **Pregnancy category D**	*Staphylococcus aureus* *Streptococcus faecalis* Enterobacter species *Escherichia coli* *Klebsiella* species *Proteus* species *Pseudomonas aeruginosa* *Salmonella* species *Shigella* species *Yersinia pestis*
KANAMYCIN (Kantrex)	Aminoglycoside; see Gentamicin	Neuromuscular blockade, ototoxicity, nephrotoxicity, apnea, pain or irritation at injection site	Staphylococci Acinetobacter species Enterobacter species *Escherichia coli* *Hemophilus influenzae* *Klebsiella* species *Neisseria* species *Proteus* species *Salmonella* species *Shigella* species *Yersinia pestis*

AMINOGLYCOSIDES and SPECTINOMYCIN:

DRUG	MECHANISM OF ACTION and RESISTANCE	ADVERSE EFFECTS	SPECTRUM
NEOMYCIN (Neo-Tabs)	**Oral aminoglycoside**; only used for suppression of gastrointestinal flora; see Gentamicin	Nausea, vomiting, diarrhea, malabsorption syndrome, *Clostridium difficile* associated colitis, nephrotoxicity, ototoxicity; **Pregnancy category D**	Suppression of Intestinal Bacteria (part of preoperative bowel prep) Hepatic Coma
NETILMICIN (Netromycin)	Aminoglycoside; see Gentamicin	Neuromuscular blockade, ototoxicity, nephrotoxicity, apnea; **Pregnancy category D**	Staphylococci *Streptococcus faecalis* Enterobacter species *Escherichia coli* *Klebsiella* species *Neisseria* species *Proteus* species *Pseudomonas aeruginosa* *Salmonella* species *Shigella* species *Yersinia pestis*
STREPTOMYCIN	Aminoglycoside; see Gentamicin	Fever, neuromuscular blockade, vomiting, nausea, eosinophilia, leukopenia, thrombocytopenia, rash, urticaria, ototoxicity, azotemia, apnea	*Mycobacterium tuberculosis* (given IM route only) *Streptococcus faecalis* *Brucella* species Enterobacter species *Escherichia coli* *Hemophilus influenzae* *Klebsiella* species *Neisseria* species *Proteus* species *Pseudomonas aeruginosa* *Salmonella* species *Shigella* species *Yersinia pestis*

80

AMINOGLYCOSIDES and SPECTINOMYCIN:

DRUG	MECHANISM OF ACTION and RESISTANCE	ADVERSE EFFECTS	SPECTRUM/USE
TOBRAMYCIN (Tobrex)	Aminoglycoside; see Gentamicin	Headache, confusion, fever, lethargy, disorientation, nausea, vomiting, diarrhea, anemia, leukopenia, thrombocytopenia, rash, urticaria, itching, dizziness, tinnitus, vertigo, ototoxicity, nephrotoxicity, liver enzymes elevation, increased bilirubin, apnea, irritation at injection site; **Pregnancy category D**	Staphylococci *Streptococcus faecalis* Enterobacter species *Escherichia coli* *Klebsiella* species *Proteus* species *Pseudomonas aeruginosa* *Salmonella* species *Shigella* species *Yersinia pestis*
SPECTINOMYCIN (Trobicin)	Aminocyclitol antibiotic that is related to the aminoglycosides; binds 30 S ribosomal subunit of bacteria and inhibits bacterial protein synthesis by preventing initiation and causing misreads of mRNA; rapid absorption after intramuscular injection	Urticaria, dizziness, nausea, chills, fever, anemia, decreased creatinine clearance, elevated alkaline phosphatase, BUN and ALT; safety in pregnancy not established	Acute Gonococcal Urethritis Acute Gonococcal Cervicitis Acute Gonococcal Proctitis

81

ANABOLIC STEROIDS:

AGENT	ORGAN SYSTEM EFFECTS	ADVERSE REACTIONS	THERAPEUTIC USE
NANDROLONE DECANOATE (Deca-Durabolin) **NANDROLONE PHENPROPIONATE** (Durabolin)	**Anabolic steroid**; increases muscle mass and strength; enhances performance; weight gain; LESS masculinization effects, MORE anabolic activity	Aggressiveness; gynecomastia; decreased spermatogenesis; decreased testicular size; liver damage; increases cholesterol and LDL, decreases HDL; increases risk of arteriosclerosis; depression; psychosis	Use in some body wasting chronic diseases Athletic performance enhancer (doping in sports) Testosterone also used in sports for anabolic effects
OXANDROLONE	Same as Nandrolone	Same as Nandrolone	Same as Nandrolone
STANOZOLOL (Winstrol)	Anabolic steroid; synthetic derivative of Testosterone	Same as Nandrolone; **pregnancy category X**; Cholestatic jaundice, hepatocellular neoplasm (rare), reversible liver enzyme changes, phallic enlargement, increased frequency of erection, inhibition of testicular function, testicular atrophy, oligospermia, impotence, chronic priapism, epididymitis, clitoral enlargement, menstrual irregularities, changes in libido, gynecomastia, deepening of voice in women, hirsutism and male pattern baldness in women, retention of water and electrolytes, increases LDL and HDL	Hereditary Angioedema Illegal doping in athletes

ANALGESICS, NON-OPIOID:

AGENT	ORGAN SYSTEM EFFECTS	ADVERSE REACTIONS	INDICATIONS
ACETAMINOPHEN (Tylenol)	**Aspirin free;** 60% is conjugated through glucuronide; small amount metabolized to intermediate that requires - SH groups to be detoxified (role in hepatic toxicity in overdose); NOT antiinflammatory; **NOT an NSAID**	Safe drug; has been traced to hepatic failure due to overdose, ties up IC glutathione SH groups of hepatic cells → **hepatocellular necrosis** (treat with **N-acetyl-cysteine**)	Minor Aches Mild Pain Headache Fever (NOT antiinflammatory)
ASPIRIN	**Analgesic; anti-pyretic; antiinflammatory;** mechanism of action is **cyclooxygenase inhibition; acetylation of platelets** and decreases platelet aggregation; NO known cardiovascular effects; GI ulceration due to decreased PG synthesis and salicylic acid is irritating (superficial erosions); **increases bleeding time,** NO effect on prothrombin time; **uricosuric;** potent platelet inhibitor	GI irritation (15%); frank ulcer (1%); Reye's syndrome in children following febrile, viral infection; increases bleeding time; small child poisoning (acidosis)	Antipyretic Analgesic Antiinflammatory
DICLOFENAC (Cataflam, Voltaren)	Nonsteroidal drug with analgesic, antiinflammatory, and antipyretic effects; inhibits prostaglandin synthesis; mean half-life is 2 hours	Gastrointestinal effects, renal and hepatic toxicities; edema, dizziness and tinnitus	Rheumatoid Arthritis Ankylosing Spondylitis Osteoarthritis Mild to Moderate Pain Dysmenorrhea
DIFLUNISAL (Dolobid)	Non-steroidal drug with analgesic, anti-inflammatory and antipyretic effects; peripherally acting non-narcotic; exact mechanism of action is unknown; Diflunisal is a prostaglandin synthetase inhibitor; complete po absorption; peak plasma levels within 2-3 hours; urine excretion; also classified as a non-acetylated salicylate	Nausea, vomiting, dyspepsia, gastrointestinal pain, diarrhea, constipation, rash, headache; associated with gastric and duodenal ulcer; **Pregnancy category C**	Mild to Moderate Pain Osteoarthritis Rheumatoid Arthritis
ETODOLAC (Lodine)	Given po, bid; may give false positive for urine bilirubin and/or urine ketones	GI upset, dyspepsia in 10%; GI bleeding, ulceration, and perforation can occur with chronic use; **Preganancy category C**	Osteoarthritis Management of pain
FENOPROFEN (Nalfon)	Non-steroidal antiinflammatory drug with antiinflammatory, analgesic and antipyretic actions; inhibits prostaglandin synthesis; peak effect occurs within 1-2 hours	Dyspepsia, abdominal pain, diarrhea, flatulence, nausea; associated with gastric and duodenal ulcer; malaise, dizziness; pruritus, rash; blurred vision, tinnitus; **Pregnancy category C**	Osteoarthritis Pain management

83

ANALGESICS, NON-OPIOID:

AGENT	ORGAN SYSTEM EFFECTS	ADVERSE REACTIONS	INDICATIONS
IBUPROFEN (Motrin, Advil)	Non-steroidal antiinflammatory drug with analgesic and antipyretic properties; inhibits prostaglandin synthesis	Nausea, epigastric pain, heartburn; associated with gastric and duodenal ulcer; dizziness, rash	Antipyretic Osteoarthritis Rheumatoid arthritis Mild to moderate pain Primary dysmenorrhea
KETOPROFEN (Oruvail, Orudis)	Non-steroidal antiinflammatory drug with analgesic and antipyretic properties; rapid po absorption with peak plasma levels within 0.5-2 hours	Dyspepsia, nausea, abdominal pain, diarrhea, constipation, flatulence, headache; tinnitus; associated with gastric and duodenal ulcer; **Pregnancy category B**	Rheumatoid Arthritis Osteoarthritis Primary Dysmenorrhea
KETOROLAC (Toradol)	Non-steroidal antiinflammatory drug with analgesic and antipyretic properties; inhibits prostaglandin synthesis; **efficacy comparable to opioid analgesics**; 99% plasma protein bound; peak plasma level IM within 50 minutes and po within 45 minutes; only NSAID available po, IM, and IV; dose adjustments must be made in elderly and in those with renal impairment	Nausea (12%), dyspepsia (12%), gastrointestinal pain (!3%); headache (17%); edema, pruritus, diarrhea, drowsiness, dizziness; associated with gastric and duodenal ulcer; **Pregnancy category C**	Short term management of pain (less than 5 days) NOT for chronic conditions Ocular Itching (topical)
MECLOFENAMATE	Similar to other NSAIDs; po peak level within 3-6 hours; half-life is 2 hours	Similar to Ibuprofen	Analgesic Dysmenorrhea Rheumatoid Arthritis
MEFENAMIC ACID (Ponstel)	Nonsteroidal antiinflammatory, analgesic and antipyretic agent; peak plasma level within 2-4 hours	Diarrhea, nausea, vomiting, gastrointestinal symptoms, abdominal pain; associated with gastric and duodenal ulcer; **Pregnancy category C**	Moderate pain Primary Dysmenorrhea (use restricted to less than one week)
NAPROXEN (Naprosyn) (Anaprox) (Aleve)	Non-steroidal antiinflammatory drug with analgesic and antipyretic activities; rapid and complete gastrointestinal absorption; peak plasma levels within 2-4 hours	Constipation, heartburn, abdominal pain, nausea; headache, dizziness, drowsiness; skin eruptions, ecchymoses; tinnitus; edema, dyspnea; associated with gastric and duodenal ulcer; **Pregnancy category B**	Rheumatoid Arthritis Osteoarthritis Juvenile Arthritis Ankylosing Spondylitis Tendinitis Bursitis Acute Gout Mild to Moderate Pain Primary Dysmenorrhea

ANALGESICS, NON-OPIOID:

AGENT	ORGAN SYSTEM EFFECTS	ADVERSE REACTIONS	INDICATIONS
TRAMADOL (Ultram)	**Centrally acting synthetic analgesic agent;** Tramadol and its metabolite bind to μ-opioid receptors and weakly inhibit reuptake of norepinephrine and serotonin; analgesic potency is between Codeine alone and combination Codeine/Aspirin and is comparable to combination Propoxyphene/Acetaminophen; 20% plasma protein bound; well metabolized following oral dosage; urine excretion, 30% unchanged	Malaise, vasodilation, anxiety, confusion, euphoria, nervousness, sleep disorder, abdominal pain, anorexia, flatulence, rash, urinary retention or frequency; seizures; may have additive effects with CNS depressants; **Pregnancy category C**	Moderate to Moderately Severe Pain Management

85

ANALGESICS, OPIOID:

DRUG	ORGAN SYSTEM EFFECTS	PHARMACOKINETICS	ADVERSE REACTIONS	THERAPEUTIC USE
ALFENTANIL (Alfenta)	Very potent opioid; analgesic; induction agent for anesthesia; about 10 times potency of morphine	Immediate onset of action IV; half-life is 1-2 hours	Respiratory depression; skeletal muscle rigidity; hypotension; **Pregnancy category C**	Analgesic Adjunct Anesthetic Agent
BUPRENORPHINE (Buprenex)	Opioid analgesic 25-50 times more potent than morphine for analgesia and respiratory depression; high affinity binding to μ-opioid receptors in CNS; classified as agonist-antagonist	IM, IV; onset of action within 15 minutes of IM shot, lasts 6 hours; IV onset of action is shorter	Sedation; nausea, dizziness, vertigo; sweating; hypotension; headache; hypoventilation; **Pregnancy category C**	Moderate to Severe Pain
BUTORPHANOL (Stadol)	Synthetic opioid agonist-antagonist; Butorphanol and its metabolites are agonists at K-opioid receptors and mixed agonist-antagonists at μ-opioid receptors; analgesic; central depression of respiration and cough; stimulates emesis center, miosis and sedation; low addiction liability; classified as agonist-antagonist	IM, IV, metered aqueous nasal spray; onset within minutes IV, 10-15 minutes IM, and within 15 minutes via nasal spray; peak activity within 30-60 minutes IV and IM and within 1-2 hours after nasal spray	Asthenia, lethargy, headache; vasodilation, palpitation; dry mouth; confusion; **Pregnancy category C**	Postoperative Analgesia Migraine Headache Pain Preanesthetic Agent Balanced Anesthesia Labor
CODEINE 3-methyl-morphine	**Analgesic and anti-tussive**; very potent increased release of histamine; combined with aspirin and acetaminophen in preparations	High oral bioavailability; some biotransformation to morphine	Constipation; **Pregnancy category C**	Analgesic Antitussive
DEZOCINE (Dalgan)	Synthetic opioid agonist-antagonist; strong opioid analgesic with potency, onset, and duration of action similiar to that of morphine; produces similiar respiratory depression as does morphine when given at analgesic dose but Dezocine has ceiling effect at higher doses; low addiction liability	IM, IV; rapid onset in 30 minutes; duration of action is 2-4 hours	Nausea, vomiting; sedation; injection site reaction; **Pregnancy category C**	Post Op Analgesia Chronic Pain
FENTANYL (Sublimaze) (Duragesic)	One of the MOST potent opioids; analgesic **neuroleptanalgesic** (Fentanyl + Droperidol); **neuroleptanesthetid**(Fentanyl + Droperidol + N2O); transdermal patch (Duragesic) available	IV; transdermal patch has peak plasma levels within 24-72 hours of application	Nausea, vomiting, constipation, dry mouth, somnolence, confusion, asthenia, sweating; **Pregnancy category C**	Transdermal patch is indicated for Chronic Pain; IV form is anesthetic and analgesic

86

ANALGESICS, OPIOID:

DRUG	ORGAN SYSTEM EFFECTS	PHARMACOKINETICS	ADVERSE REACTIONS	THERAPEUTIC USE
HYDROCODONE (in Vicodin)	Opioid analgesic and antitussive with actions similar to those of Codeine	po; well absorbed	Lightheadedness, dizziness, sedation, nausea, vomiting; respiratory depression; **Pregnancy category C**	Moderate to moderately severe pain Anti-tussive
HYDROMORPHONE (Dilaudid)	Centrally acting narcotic analgesic and antitussive; no intrinsic limit to analgesic effect; like Morphine, adequate doses will relieve even the most severe pain	MOST water soluble of opioids; IV, IM, po; onset within 15 minutes, duration of action 5 hours	Dose limiting effects include: respiratory depression, nausea and vomiting; abuse potential; **Pregnancy category C**	Moderate to severe pain
LEVORPHANOL	Highly potent synthetic analgesic similar to Morphine; about 5 times potency of Morphine	Duration of action 4-8 hours; onset of action within 30 minutes	Nausea, vomiting, dizziness; respiratory depression, hypotension, urinary retention; may be habit forming	Indicated whenever narcotic analgesia is needed
LEVOMETHADYL (Orlaam)	Opioid agonist at the μ-receptor; produces analgesia and sedation	Long duration of action; may be given every 2-3 days; well absorbed orally	Sedation, respiratory depression; decreased cardiovascular function	Treatment of Opioid Addiction
MEPERIDINE (Demerol)	Synthetic opioid; phenylpiperdine compound; **anti-muscarinic**; potent analgesic commonly used in obstetrics during active labor (intrapartum); respiratory depression; poor antitussive activity; weakly constipating	High oral bioavailability; injectable; metabolized to **normeperidine**; half-life is 15-20 hours	High potential for abuse by medical personnel; less severe side effects than Morphine due to antimuscarinic activity; may cause tachycardia; CNS stimulation and seizures due to normeperidine; respiratory depresion	Obstetric analgesic of choice; also used for management of other types of pain
METHADONE (Dolophine)	Analgesic; **long duration**; once achieve steady state, can maintain levels with 1 dose/day; advantage for non-compliant patients	LONG duration; good oral bioavailability; HIGH protein binding, > 90%; longer but milder withdrawal than morphine	Less sedation and euphoria than morphine; NOT commonly abused	Morphine addiction treatment Methadone Maintenance

ANALGESICS, OPIOID:

DRUG	ORGAN SYSTEM EFFECTS	PHARMACOKINETICS	ADVERSE REACTIONS	THERAPEUTIC USE
MORPHINE	**Sedation (k receptor)**, general CNS depression; mental clouding; **euphoria** (may relate to being free of pain, may see dysphoria if no initial pain); non-pain sensations NOT affected; **decreases respiration; stimulates CTZ; orthostatic hypotension;** few cardiac effects; smooth m. contraction, biliary contraction (gall stones, exacerbates pain); GI muscle spasm, decreases peristalsis → **constipation;** miosis (pinpoint pupils); ↑ **histamine** (itching, allergic rxns); **decreases body temp; hyperglycemia; antitussive**	Water soluble; 15-20% oral bioavailability; injected dose; tolerance and dependence; NO tolerance to miosis or histamine release; biotrans to morphine-3-glucuronide (inactive); **morphine-6-glucuronide** (active); eliminated by kidney	Nausea, vomiting; decreases respiratory rate; orthostatic hypotension; skeletal m. rigidity at high dose constipation; increases histamine, itching; hypothermia; bradycardia at near toxic doses; respiratory arrest in overdose at medulla; abuse/dependence/withdrawal; **Pregnancy category C**	Analgesia for sharp, focal, surgical type pain; sedation; commonly used agent in PCA pumps (patient controlled analgesia)
NALBUPHINE (Nubain)	Synthetic narcotic agonist-antagonist; potent analgesic equivalent to Morphine; analgesic effect mediated through κ-receptors (kappa)	Onset of action within 2-3 minutes of IV dose and less than 15 minutes of IM dose; duration of action is 3-6 hours	Sedation; sweaty/clammy; nausea/vomiting; dizziness and vertigo; dry mouth; headache;	Moderate to severe pain Balanced anesthesia Preoperative pain Postoperative pain Obstetric analgesia
OXYCODONE (in Percocet, Percodan)	Semi-synthetic narcotic analgesic with actions similar to Morphine; therapeutic use for analgesia and sedation; generally combined in preparations with aspirin or acetaminophen	Good oral bioavailability	Lightheadedness, dizziness, sedation, nausea, vomiting; respiratory depression at higher dose; **Pregnancy category C**	Moderate to severe pain
OXYMORPHONE (Numorphan)	Semi-synthetic narcotic potent analgesic; about 10 times potency of morphine; reversible with Naloxone	Onset of action within 5-10 minutes; duration of action is 3-6 hours; IM, IV, rectal suppository	Drowsiness, nausea, vomiting, miosis, itching, dysphoria, light-headedness, and headache	Moderate to severe pain
PENTAZOCINE (Talwin)	Opioid analgesic about 1/3 potency of morphine; classified as mixed agonist-antagonist; analgesia through κ-receptor	Onset of action withing 15-20 minutes when given IM, within 2-3 minutes of IV dose	Nausea, dizziness, light-headedness, vomiting, euphoria; respiratory depression; psychotomimetic effects	Moderate to severe pain
PROPOXYPHENE (In Darvon, Darvocet))	WEAK analgesic; low milligram potency; respiratory deaths at high dose	Administered po; half-life 6-12 hours	HIGHLY abused; respiratory deaths at high doses	Analgesic
REMIFENTANIL (Ultiva)	Potent opioid for μ-receptor; related to Fentanyl group	Onset is very rapid	Respiratory depression, bradycardia, skeletal muscle rigidity; reversed by Naloxone	Analgesic

ANALGESICS, OPIOID:

DRUG	ORGAN SYSTEM EFFECTS	PHARMACOKINETICS	ADVERSE REACTIONS	THERAPEUTIC USE
SUFENTANIL (Sufenta)	Potent opioid analgesic **10 times** more potent than fentanyl; **625 times** more potent than morphine!	IV, epidural	Respiratory depression, skeletal muscle rigidity, especially chest wall rigidity; bradycardia, hypertension; hypotension, somnolence; pruritus; nausea, vomiting; **Pregnancy category C**	Balanced anesthesia Epidural in labor

EQUIANALGESIC DOSES PO (mg)		POTENCY vs. MORPHINE
7.5	Hydromorphone (Dilaudid)	8
20	Methadone	3
30	Oxycodone (Percocet)	2
60	Morphine	--
130	Propoxyphene (Darvocet)	0.5
200	Codeine	0.3

EQUIANALGESIC DOSES IM (mg)		POTENCY vs. MORPHINE
0.02	Sufentanyl	500
0.1	Fentanyl	100
1.5	Hydromorphone (Dilaudid)	8
2.0	Butorphanol (Stadol)	5
10	Morphine	--
10	Nalbuphine (Nubain)	1
10	Dezocine (Dalgan)	1
75	Meperidine (Demerol)	0.1

ANALGESICS, TOPICAL:

DRUG	ORGAN SYSTEM EFFEFECTS	PRECAUTIONS	THERAPEUTIC USE
CAPSAICIN (Zostrix)	Exact mechanism is not known; May leave skin and joints insensitive to pain by depleting substance P	Avoid contact with eyes, mucous membranes Avoid inhaling residue	Temporary relief of rheumatoid and osteoarthritis Relief of neuralgias from shingles or diabetic neuropathy
TROLAMINE SALICYLATE (Myoflex)	Topical pain reliever; mechanism unknown	For enteral use only; may cause local irritation; precaution same as Capsaicin	Topical for relief of pain of arthritis, strains, sprains and simple backache

ANDROGEN HORMONE INHIBITORS and ANTI-ANDROGENS:

DRUG	ORGAN SYSTEM EFFFECTS	KINETICS	ADVERSE EFFECTS	THERAPEUTIC USE
FINASTERIDE (Proscar)	Competitive inhibitor of 5α-reductase; produces rapid decrease in serum dihydrotestoerone	90% plasma protein bound; crosses blood brain barrier; oral dosage	Impotence, decreased libido, decreased ejaculate volume; breast tenderness and enlargement; **Pregnancy category X**	Symptomatic Benign Prostatic Hyperplasia
FLUTAMIDE (Eulexin)	Androgen antagonist; blocks testosterone negative feedback on pituitary; increases circulating testosterone, estradiol and lutinizing hormone; blocks testosterone receptors	Rapid and near complete oral absorption	Hot flashes, loss of libido, impotence, diarrhea, nausea, vomiting, gynecomastia; **Pregnancy category D**	Metastatic Prostatic Carcinoma (Stage D2)
GOSERELIN (Zoladex)	Synthetic decapeptide analog of lutenizing hormone releasing hormone (LHRH) which inhibits pituitary gonadotropin (FSH, LH) secretion; initial effect is increased LH, FSH and testosterone; chronic effects are decreased LH, FSH, and testosterone to levels seen in castrated males; in women chronic effects are decreased FSH and LH with reduction of estradiol to levels seen in postmenopausal women	Implant subcutaneously with release over 28 days	Males: hot flashes, sexual dysfunction, lethargy, rash, anorexia, insomnia, nausea Females: hot flashes, amenorrhea, vaginitis, decreased libido, depression, acne, breast atrophy, injection site reactions; **Pregnancy category X**	Prostate Cancer Endometriosis
HISTRELIN (Synarel)	Same as Leuprolide	Subcutaneously administered	Skin reactions, hot flashes, diarrhea, increased heart rate; **Pregnancy category X**	Central Precocious Puberty (in children)
LEUPROLIDE (Lupron)	Initial effect is increased LH, FSH, and testosterone, then eventually decreases these hormone levels	Subcutaneous and IM doses; half-life is 3 hours	Ishcemia, edema, constipation, gynecomastia, dizziness, hot flashes, impotence	Prostatic Carcinoma Endometriosis
NAFARELIN (Synarel)	Same as Leuprolide	Nasal spray; protein binding is 80%; 10-40 minutes to maximal serum levels	Chest pain, rash, hot flashes, insomnia, nasal irritation, acne	Endometriosis Precocious Puberty (in children)
SPIRONOLACTONE (Aldactone)	Blocks aldosterone; blocks androgen receptors as well	po dose	Lethergy, ataxia, diarrhea, irregular menses, gynecomastia	Hirsutism in women (takes weeks to months to see effects on unwanted hair)

91

ANDROGENS:

DRUG	ORGAN SYSTEM EFFECTS	PHARMACOKINETICS	ADVERSE REACTIONS	THERAPEUTIC USE
DANAZOL (Danocrine)	Synthetic steroid derived from ethisterone; suppresses the pituitary-ovarian axis; decreases FSH and LH; in treatment of endometriosis, Danazol causes atrophy in normal and ectopic endometrial tissue; in treatment of fibrocystic breast disease, causes reduction in nodularity, pain and tenderness	Plasma half-life is 4.5 hours; mostly excreted in urine, but some in feces	Weight gain, edema, acne, oily skin, hirsutism, decreased breast size, amenorrhea; **Pregnancy category X**	Endometriosis Fibrocystic Breast Disease Hereditary Angioedema
FLUOXYMESTERONE	Same as Testosterone	po; half-life is about 9 hours	Same as Testosterone	Male Hypogonadism Estrogen Sensitive Breast Cancer (females)
METHYL TESTOSTERONE	Same as Testosterone	Methyl results in less 1st pass effect; 8-12 hour duration	See Testosterone	
OXYMETHOLONE (Anadrol-50)	Potent anabolic and androgenic drug; anabolic steroids are synthetic derivatives of testosterone; improves nitrogen balance if sufficient calories and protein are taken; increases production of erythropoietin in patients with anemia due to bone marrow failure	Oral dose	Cholestatic jaundice; phallic enlargement, increased frequency of erection, inhibits testicular function, testicular atrophy, oligospermia, impotence, chronic priapism; clitoral enlargment, menstrual irregularities; gynecomastia in men; voice deepening in women; hirsutism and male pattern baldness in women; acne; edema and electrolyte retention; **Pregnancy category X**	Anemia secondary to deficient red cell production
TESTOLACTONE (Teslac)	Produces antineoplastic effects via inhibition of steroid aromatase activity and reduction in estrone synthesis; anti-estrogenic effects in treatment of breast cancer; no *in vivo* androgenic effects	Oral dosage; well absorbed from GI tract; metabolized to several products by the liver	Maculopapular erythema, increased blood pressure, paresthesia, aches and extremity edema, glossitis, anorexia, nausea, vomiting; **Pregnancy category C**	Palliative treatment for advanced Breast Cancer

ANDROGENS:

DRUG	ORGAN SYSTEM EFFECTS	PHARMACOKINETICS	ADVERSE REACTIONS	THERAPEUTIC USE
TESTOSTERONE	**Increased growth and development of male sex characteristics**; body hair, testicle and penile development, deepening of voice, spermatogenesis; increased muscle and bone growth; increased sebaceous gland secretion; male pattern baldness; increased erythropoietin; dihydrotestosterone (DHT) is MORE active form of testosterone	Binds receptor in cytoplasm; reduced to **dihydrotestosterone (DHT)** by 5-α-reductase; DHT-testosterone-R complex goes to nucleus; stimulates chromosomal activity; increases synthesis of mRNA; increases protein synthesis; endogenous testosterone lasts 10-20 minutes	Female hirsutism; masculinization; male feminization with chronic use; **gynecomastia** in males; **acne; liver dysfunction:** cholestatic jaundice, hepatocellular carcinoma; **hypercalcemia; water and sodium retention; teratogenic;** NOT used in prostatic cancer; **Pregnancy category X**	Replacement therapy for Male Hypogonadism Anemia of Renal Dysfunction Breast cancer Endometriosis Abused for Anabolic Effects in Athletes
TESTOSTERONE CYPIONATE (Depo-Testosterone)	Same as Testosterone	**Depot form of** testosterone; 1-2 week duration	See Testosterone	See Testosterone
TESTOSTERONE PROPIONATE	Same as Testosterone	Less metabolism; less 1st pass effect; 8-10 hour duration	See Testosterone	See Testosterone

93

ANESTHETICS, GENERAL:

DRUG	SYSTEMIC EFFECTS	MAC	ADVERSE REACTIONS	THERAPEUTIC USE
ENFLURANE (Ethrane)	Same as Halothane	MAC = 1.70%; sufficient oil/gas coefficient	**Arrhythmia; convulsion** (associated with electron cloud density near ether oxygen); **renal toxicity;** malignant hyperpyrexia	Inhalational Anesthetic Stage 3 Anesthesia
FENTANYL (Sublimaze)	**IV narcotic;** pain management; also decreases the amount of general anesthetic required to achieve Stage 3 anesthesia	IV administration		Anesthetic Analgesic Transdermal Patch for Chronic Pain
HALOTHANE Fluothane	**Complete anesthetic;** alters ionic fluxes in CNS; changes membrane stiffness causing ion channels to close; **respiratory depression; cholinergic stimulation,** decreases HR and contractility, vasodilation thus decreasing cardiac work	MAC = 0.77%; HIGH oil/gas coefficient	Arrhythmia; **halothane hepatitis; bromide sedation** (hangover); malignant hyperpyrexia	Inhalational Anesthetic Stage 3 Anesthesia
ISOFLURANE (Forane)	Same as Halothane	MAC = 1.15%; sufficient oil/gas coefficient	Arrhythmia; malignant hyperpyrexia; **most expensive general anesthetic**	Inhalational Anesthetic Stage 3 Anesthesia
KETAMINE	IV barbiturate used to get patients into Stage 3 anesthesia quickly	IV		Dissociative Anesthetic Anesthesia Induction Agent
MEPERIDINE (Demerol)	Synthetic opioid; phenylpiperidine compound; **anti-muscarinic;** potent analgesic in obstetrics; respiratory depression; POOR anti-tussive; weakly constipating	High oral bioavailability; injectable; metabolized to **normeperidine**	ABUSED by medical personnel; less severe than morphine due to anti-muscarinic activity; tachycardia; CNS stimulation and seizures due to normeperidine	Obstetric Analgesic (Often given with Phenergan) Post Operative Analgesic

94

ANESTHETICS, GENERAL:

DRUG	EFFECTS	MAC	ADVERSE REACTIONS	THERAPEUTIC USE
NITROUS OXIDE (Inorganic gas)	**Incomplete anesthetic** (no receptor site); **alters ionic fluxes in CNS only**; change membrane stiffness, causing ion channels to close; **respiratory depression** (direct effect); **cholinergic stimulation**: decreases HR, decreases contractility, causes vasodilation thus decreases cardiac work; <u>nitrous oxide is unique</u>: slight sympathetic effects, slight increase in HR, contractility and vasoconstriction	**Rapid onset**; CANNOT achieve stage 3 anesthesia; diffusible through all membranes; MAC = 110% (very high); LOW oil/gas coefficient	Arrhythmia; **gas pocket swelling**; NO malignant hyperpyrexia	Induction Anesthetic Stage 1 Anesthesia Suitable for Dental Procedures Adjunct for Other General Anesthetics and Fentanyl
PROPOFOL (Diprivan)	Sedative-hypnotic; not chemically related to other intravenous anesthetic agents; oil at room temperature; IV administration; major advantage is rapid induction and recovery		No impairment of hepatic or renal function; causes severe respiratory depression, apnea	Similar use as Thiopental Must combine with opioids or NO2 for complete anesthesia
THIOPENTAL (Pentothal)	**IV barbiturates**; helps patient past overpressure, irritating administration, problems of slow induction of anesthetic, and into Stage 3 anesthesia as quickly and problem free as possible	IV administration		Induction Agent (Bypass stage 1 and 2)

ABBREVIATION: MAC - minimum alveolar concentration so that 50% of patients fail to respond to surgical incision; 99% of people remain immobile when given 1.3 times the MAC of an anesthetic; units of % atmosphere

95

ANESTHETICS, LOCAL:

DRUG	MECHANISM OF ACTION/EFFECTS	ADVANTAGES/ DISADVANTAGES	ADVERSE REACTIONS	THERAPEUTIC USE
BENZOCAINE	**Permanently charged ester;** ethyl aminobenzoate	**LACKS terminal hydrophilic amine, LOW water solubility;** prolonged duration		Topical Anesthetic Used on Gums
BUPIVACAINE (Marcaine, Sensoricaine)	Similar to Lidocaine, but more potent and longer duration of action than Lidocaine	Long duration of action	More cardiotoxic than Lidocaine	Widely used local anesthetic Epidural anesthetic
COCAINE *Erythroxylon coca* plant	Ester; sodium influx inhibition; **intrinsic vasoconstrictor; blocks reuptake of NE**	Vasoconstrictor	True CNS stimulant; causes euphoria, major drug of abuse; associated with sudden death syndrome	Surface Anesthetic
DIBUCAINE	Amide similar to Lidocaine	**Powerful, long duration,** can use to avoid general anesthesia	Same as Lidocaine	Spinal Anesthetic
ETIDOCAINE	Amide similar to Lidocaine; long duration of action	**HIGHEST** lipid solubility among local anesthetics; **long acting**	Same as Lidocaine	Infiltration or Field Block Anesthesia
LIDOCAINE	Amide; sodium influx inhibitor; local anesthetic effect is dose, site and administration dependent; **crosses BBB with** systemic absorption	More potent, longer duration, less vasodilation, standard for local anesthetics; **decreased chance of arrhythmia**	Systemic absorption: CNS stimulation then CNS depression; excitement; apprehension, confusion, disorientation, tremors, convulsion; high dose effects: gen vasodilation, hypo-tension, direct depression of excitability, contractility; death	Local Anesthetic (most widely used) Prophylactic Antiarrhythmic
MEPIVACAINE	Amide similar actions as Lidocaine	NO vasodilation so need little or no EPI	**NOT used in obstetric anesthesia** due to prolonged metabolism in fetus and neonate, increases chance of toxicity	Peripheral Nerve Block Anesthetic Agent
PROCAINE	Synthetic ester similar to Lidocaine; **short acting**	Causes vasodilation so MUST add EPI, not good as surface anesthetic	Same as Lidocaine	Subcutaneous Infiltration Anesthetic Agent
TETRACAINE	Ester that is similar to Lidocaine	**Long acting,** can use to avoid general anesthetic	Same as Lidocaine	Spinal Anesthetic

GENERAL: Local anesthetics with lower pKa's exhibit faster onset than drugs with higher pKa.
Ester local anesthetics are metabolized by pseudocholinesterase in plasma, amide local anesthetics in the liver.

96

ANOREXIANTS:

DRUG	ORGAN SYSTEM EFFFECTS	ADVERSE EFFECTS	THERAPEUTIC USE
AMPHETAMINE SULFATE	Amphetamines are non-catecholamine sympathomimetic amines with CNS stimulant activity; elevates blood pressure; weak bronchodilator and respiratory stimulant action; drugs in this class used in obesity are referred to as *anorectic* or *anorexigenic* agents	Palpitations, tachycardia, elevates blood pressure; CNS overstimulation, restlessness, dizziness, insomnia, euphoria, dyskinesia, dysphoria, tremor, headache, exacerbation of motor and phonic tics and Tourette's syndrome; dry mouth, diarrhea, constipation, anorexia, weight loss; **Pregnancy category C**; high abuse potential	Attention Deficit Disorder with Hyperactivity Exogenous Obesity Narcolepsy
BENZPHETAMINE (Didrex)	See profile of Amphetamine	See Amphetamine; **Pregnancy category X**; lower abuse potential than Amphetamine	Exogenous Obesity (short term management)
DIETHYLPROPION	Anorexiant		
FENFLURAMINE (Pondimin)	Anorectic drug in the class of sympathomimetic amines; differs from prototype drug of this class Amphetamine as Fenfluramine is more CNS depressant than stimulant; causes profound reduction in brain serotonin	Drowsiness, diarrhea, dry mouth most common; dizziness, confusion, incoordination, headache, elevated mood, depression, anxiety, nervousness, tension, insomnia, weakness/fatigue, agitation, constipation, abdominal pain, nausea, palpitation, changes in blood pressure; **Pregnancy category C**	Exogenous Obesity (short term management)
MAZINDOL (Sanorex)	An isoindole with action similar to prototype anorectic agent, Amphetamine; CNS stimulant	See Amphetamine profile; should not be used during breast feeding; lower abuse potential than Amphetamine	Exogenous Obesity (short term management)
METHAMPHETAMINE (Desoxyn)	Sympathomimetic amine with CNS stimulant activity; elevates blood pressure; weak bronchodilator and respiratory stimulant; so-called *anorectic* or *anorexigenic* agent	Elevates blood pressure, tachycardia, palpitation; dizziness, dysphoria, CNS overstimulation, euphoria, tremor, restlessness, headache, diarrhea, constipation, dry mouth; **Pregnancy category C**; High abuse potential	Attention Deficit Disorder with Hyperactivity Exogenous Obesity
PHENDIMETRAZINE	Anorexiant		
PHENTERMINE (Ionamin, Fastin)	Sympathomimetic amine with activity profile similar to Amphetamine; Phentermine Resin form available	Palpitation, tachycardia, elevates blood pressure; CNS overstimulation, restlessness, dizziness, insomnia, euphoria, dysphoria, tremor, headache, dry mouth; safe use in pregnancy not established	Exogenous Obesity (short term management)

NOTE: The natural history of obesity is observed over years, while clinical drug trials with anorectic agents are typically weeks in duration.
A combination of fenfluramine and phentermine, known as Fen/Phen, was a popular and effective anorexiant until its recall by its manufacturer in September 1997.

97

ANTACIDS:

DRUG	MECHANISM OF ACTION	KINETICS	ADVERSE EFFECTS	THERAPEUTIC USE
ALUMINUM HYDROXIDE	Antacid and osmotic laxative; slower onset than magnesium hydroxide	Insoluble	Constipating	Antacid Gastritis Peptic Ulcer Gastroesophageal Reflux Disease (GERD)
CALCIUM CARBONATE	Antacid with RAPID onset	Insoluble	Acid rebound	Antacid Gastritis Peptic Ulcer GERD
MAGALDRATE (Riopan)	Combination of magnesium and aluminum oxides	Suspension available		Antacid Gastritis Peptic Ulcer GERD
MAGNESIUM HYDROXIDE	Antacid and osmotic laxative	Insoluble	Laxative	Antacid Gastritis Peptic Ulcer GERD
SODIUM BICARBONATE	Increases stomach pH; systemically absorbed	Soluble	Increases blood pH; **acid rebound**	Antacid (usually self prescribed)

NOTE: The combination of aluminum hydroxide and magnesium hydroxide (Maalox) is widely used.
The constipating effect of aluminum are counteracted by the laxative effects of magnesium.

98

ANTHELMINTICS:

DRUG	MECHANISM OF ACTION	KINETICS	ADVERSE EFFECTS	INDICATIONS
MEBENDAZOLE (Vermox)	Blocks microtubule polymerization; decreases glucose uptake by worm; broad spectrum anthelmintic; used when Pyrantel pamoate fails	2 doses over 2 weeks	**Teratogenic;** abdominal pain; headache; dizziness; **Pregnancy category C**	*Enterobius vermicularis* (if pyrantel pamoate fails); ascaris, trichuris, necator
NICLOSAMIDE (Niclocide)	Blocks anaerobic metabolism of worm by inhibiting oxidative phosphyorylation in mitochondria of cestodes	NOT absorbed	Nausea, vomiting, abdominal discomfort, anorexia, drowsiness, dizziness, headache, skin rash; no known major toxicities; **Pregnancy category B**	Cestodes (tapeworms) *Taenia saginata* (beef tapeworm) *Diphyllobothrium latum* (fish tapeworm) *Hymenolepis nana* (dwarf tapeworm)
OXAMNIQUINE (Vansil)	Alkylates worm DNA; cure rate varies from 90-100%; resistance has been reported in Brazil and Kenya	IM and po (preferred); well absorbed po; peak plasma levels within 3 hours; excreted in urine	Dizziness, somnolence, nausea, vomiting, fever, eosinophilia, liver enzymes elevations, EEG changes, hallucination, seizure have been reported; may cause orange urine; **Pregnancy category C**	Alternative agent for *Schistosoma mansoni*
PRAZIQUANTEL (Biltricide)	Increases calcium ion influx into worm, causes tetanic paralysis and distorts tegmentum of worm; broad spectrum of activity against treamtodes (flukes) and cestodes (tapeworms)	80% po absorption; extensive hepatic first pass hydroxylation	Dizziness, headache, malaise, abdominal pain, nausea; **Pregnancy category B**	*Schistosoma haematobium, mansoni, japonicum* *Clonorchis* and *Opisthorchis* (Chinese liver flukes) *Cysticercosis*
PYRANTEL PAMOATE (Antiminth)	Depolarizing neuronal blocker; paralyzes the worm; anticholinesterase	Poor gastrointestinal absorption; 2 doses over 2 weeks	Anorexia, nausea, headache, dizziness, drowsiness, rash; transient liver enzyme elevations	*Enterobius vermicularis* Ascariasis Uncinariasis (hookworm)
THIABENDAZOLE (Mintezol)	Exact mechanism of action is not known; theoretical action is inhibition of fumarate reductase in helminths	Well absorbed po; peak plasma levels within 1 hour	Dizziness, drowsiness, giddiness, anorexia, nausea, vomiting, diarrhea, fever, epigastric pain, flushing, chills, pruritus, lethargy, rash, headache; Stevens Johson syndrome has been reported; **Pregnancy category C**	*Strongyloides stercoralis* (threadworm) Ancylostoma braziliense *Toxocara canis* and *cati*

ANTIACNE AGENTS:

AGENT	ORGAN SYSTEM EFFECTS	SUPPLIED AS	ADVERSE REACTIONS	THERAPEUTIC USE
BENZOYL PEROXIDE	Antibacterial action against *Propionibacterium acnes*	Topical gel, wash, bars, pads	Allergic contact dermatitis and dryness; **Pregnancy category C**	Topical treatment of Acne Vulgaris
CLINDAMYCIN (Cleocin T)	Antibacterial action against *Propionibacterium acnes*	Topical solution, gel, lotion	Skin dryness; **Pregnancy category B**; diarrhea, bloody diarrhea and colitis have been reported with topical use	Topical treatment of Acne Vulgaris
ERYTHROMYCIN (T-Stat, Erycette)	Reduces inflammatory lesions of acne vulgaris	Solution and pads	Dryness, tenderness, pruritus, desquamation, erythema, oiliness, burning sensation; **Pregnancy category C**	Topical treatment of Acne Vulgaris
ISOTRETINOIN (Accutane)	Retinoid that inhibits sebaceous gland function and keratinization; mechanism of action unknown	Food or milk ↑ po absorption; metabolized to 4-oxo-isotretinoin; $t_{1/2}$ = 25 hours	**Pregnancy category X**, MUST confirm negative pregnancy test before starting therapy; <u>Serum lipid effects</u>: increased serum triglyceride in 25%, decreased HDL in 15%, increased cholesterol in 7%; avoid vitamin A supplementation	**Severe recalcitrant nodular acne** not responsive to conventional therapy; informed consent is recommended prior to starting therapy; Unlabled uses include: keratosis and leukoplakia
MECLOCYCLINE (Meclan)	Mechanism not known, but assumed to have localized effects	Topical cream	Skin irritation; **Pregnancy category B**	Topical treatment of Acne Vulgaris
TRETINOIN (Retin-A)	Mechanism not known, but may decrease follicular epithelial cell cohesiveness, decreasing microcomedo formation	Topical liquid, cream, gel	Skin erythema, edema, blistering, crusting; **Pregnancy category C**; gel forms are flammable!	Topical treatment of Acne Vulgaris Unlabeled uses include: skin wrinkles, aged skin, liver spots, skin cancer and other dermatoses

ANTIALCOHOLIC:

DRUG	ORGAN SYSTEM EFFFECTS	KINETICS	ADVERSE EFFECTS	THERAPEUTIC USE
DISULFIRAM (Antabuse)	Taken alone, Disulfiram has no apparent pharmacologic effects; taken with alcohol causes a toxic reaction seen as cutaneous sensation of heat, flushing, vasodilation, hypotension, palpitation, increased heart rate, dizziness, vomiting, unconsciousness and collapse; magnitude of symptoms dependent on dose of Disulfiram and amount of alcohol taken; this reaction a.k.a. **acetaldehyde syndrome; NOT a cure for alcoholism**	80% GI absorption; peak plasma levels in 1-2 hours; lipid soluble	Contraindicated in patients with severe myocardial disease or coronary occlusion, psychosis or previous hypersensitivity	Management of selected chronic alcoholic patients

ANTIALLERGICS:

DRUG	ORGAN SYSTEM EFFFECTS	SUPPLIED AS	ADVERSE EFFECTS	THERAPEUTIC USE
CROMOLYN SODIUM	Inhibits release of histamine and other immediate hypersensitivity mediators from mast cells; may stabilize mast cell membranes	Capsule, nebulizer, inhaler, nasal solution, ophthalmic solution	**Pregnancy category B**	Allergic Rhinitis Asthma Mastocytosis Prevention of Exercise-Induced Bronchospasm Food and Skin Allergy
LEVOCABASTINE (Livostin)	H1 receptor antagonist	Ophthalmic solution	**Pregnancy category C**	Ophthalmic Antiallergic Allergic Conjunctivitis
LODOXAMIDE (Alomide)	Mast cell stabilizer; inhibits Type I immediate hypersensitivity reactions; inhibits increase in cutaneous vascular permeability associated with IgE and antigen mediated reactions; also inhibits mast cell release of slow reacting substance of anaphylaxis (SRS-A); inhibits eosinophil chemotaxis; thought to stabilize mast cell membranes	Cphthalmic solution	Transient burning or stinging upon instillation; **Pregnancy category B**	Vernal Keratoconjunctivitis Vernal Conjunctivitis Vernal Keratitis

102

ANTIANGINALS:

DRUG	ORGAN SYSTEM EFFECTS	PHARMACOKINETICS	ADVERSE REACTIONS	THERAPEUTIC USE
AMYL NITRATE	Inhalational nitrate which relieves pain of angina within 1-3 minutes	Inhalation	See Nitroglycerin	Acute Anginal Episodes
ISOSORBIDE NITRATE	LONG acting nitrate; decreases frequency of attacks, prophylactic; long term studies show NO major effect on mortality	Oral, sublingual; several hour duration	Cross tolerance to nitroglycerin	Maintenance therapy for Angina
ISOSORBIDE MONONITRATE (Dilatrate SR)	Organic nitrate whose principal action is relaxation of vascular smooth muscle; decreases left ventricular end-diastolic pressure and pulmonary capillary wedge pressure (preload)	Highly variable bioavailability (10-90%) with high first pass metabolism by liver	Headache, lightheadedness, hypotension, syncope, tolerance	Angina pectoris
NITROGLYCERIN (Glycerol trinitrate)	Prototype nitrite anginal agent; **selective vasodilator**, venous (decreases preload), less effective in arteriole dilation; smooth m. relaxant; EDRF → NO → GC → ↑ cGMP → vasodilation; acute use for angina; continuous use with abrupt withdrawal of agent causes **rebound angina**; see pseudotolerance	QUICK tolerance; sublingual, IV and transdermal dosage; NOT oral; metabolize to dinitrites (inactive) → urine; RAPID onset, SHORT duration (20 mins); light sensitive	Headache; decreases BP, reflex tachycardia; severe hypotension; tolerance limits use (give Hydralazine or ACE inhibitors to reverse this); increases plasma volume	Acute Angina
ATENOLOL	Same as Propranolol (except ß1 > ß2 blocker)			Antianginal
METOPROLOL	Same as Propranolol (except ß1 > ß blocker)			Antianginal
NALDOLOL	See Propranolol			Antianginal
PROPRANOLOL (non-selective ß blocker)	Prototype beta adrenergic antagonist antianginal agent; decreases frequency of anginal attacks; increases exercise tolerance; **decreases HR** (CW = HR x BP); **decreases BP** (slight); **antiarrhythmic** (only agents proven to decrease subsequent MI and mortality)	Oral dose	Irritability, mood swings, depression, tiredness, impotence	Antianginal
BEPRIDIL (Vascor)	Calcium channel blocker antianginal agent with poorly characterized antiarrhythmic and antihypertensive properties	Peak plasma levels within 2-3 hours; 70% urine and 22% fecal excretion	Dizziness, gastrointestinal symptoms, ventricular arrhythmia, syncope; headache, drowsiness; **Pregnancy category C**	Chronic Stable Angina (Effort Associated Angina)
DILTIAZEM benzothiazepine	Calcium channel blocker; see prototype agent, Verapamil	Oral dose	Low incidence of side effects; Pedal edema, dizziness, headahce, rash are reported	Variant Angina Effort Angina

103

ANTIANGINALS:

DRUG	ORGAN SYSTEM EFFECTS	PHARMACOKINETICS	ADVERSE REACTIONS	THERAPEUTIC USE
NICARDIPINE (Cardene)	Dihydropyridine antianginal and antihypertensive agent; calcium channel blocker; see Verapamil	Peak plasma level within ½ - 2 hours; >95% plasma protein bound; extensively metabolized in liver; 60% urine and 35% fecal excretion	Pedal edema, dizziness, headache, asthenia, flushing, increased angina, palpitation, nausea, dyspepsia, dry mouth; **Pregnancy category C**	Stable Angina Hypertension
NIFEDIPINE (Procardia)	General vasodilator; **dihydropyridine** calcium channel blocker; good arterial vasodilator; see Verapamil	Oral dose	Dizziness, lightheadedness, flushing, headache, weakness, nausea, heartburn, muscle cramps, tremor, peripheral edema, nervousness, palpitation; **Pregnancy category C**	Vasospastic Angina Chronic Stable Angina Hypertension
VERAPAMIL (Calan)	*Prototype calcium channel blocker antianginal agent;* modulates influx of ionic calcium across cell membranes of arterial smooth muscle; antihypertensive effects mediated by decreased systemic vascular resistance; dilates main coronary arteries and arterioles; reduces cardiac afterload; prolongs refractory period at the AV node	90% oral absorption; high first pass effect, bioavailability is 20-35%; peak plasma levels within 1-2 hours; 90% plasma protein bound; 75% urine and 16% fecal excretion	Constipation, dizziness, nausea, hypotension, headache, edema, fatigue; **Pregnancy category C**	Essential Hypertension Classic Angina of Effort Atrial Tachycardia

Abbreviations: EDRF - endothelium dependent relaxing factor
CW - cardiac work

104

ANTIANXIETY AGENTS:

DRUG	ORGAN SYSTEM EFFECTS	PHARMACOKINETICS	ADVERSE REACTIONS	THERAPEUTIC USE
ALPRAZOLAM (Xanax)	See Diazepam for benzodiazepine effects and mechanism of action	Short acting (3-20 hrs); BZs have good oral absorption; **Phase I oxidation** (multiple active metabolites); **Phase II conjugation** (NO active metabolites)	Sedation; ataxia; lethargy; anterograde amnesia; tolerance; dependence; Rare: syncope; hypotension; skin rash; menstrual irregularities; resp arrest; low dose dependency: slight withdrawal; anxiety symptoms; high dose abuse: severe withdrawal with convulsion and hypothermia; contraindications: BZ, alcohol and barbiturates; **Pregnancy category D**	Anxiety Disorder
CHLORDIAZEPOXIDE (Librium)	Effective in management of generalized anxiety disorder and symptoms of alcohol withdrawal	Long acting (more than 20 hrs)	Drowsiness, confusion, ataxia; safety in pregnancy and lactation not established	Anxiety Disorder Alcohol withdrawal
CLONAZEPAM (Klonopin)	Exhibits several properties characteristic of benzodiazepines	Max blood level within 1-2 hours; excreted in urine	Very sedating and tolerance develops to antiepileptic effects thus limits utility; ataxia, drowsiness, dysarthria; safety in pregnancy is unknown	Anxiety Antiepileptic Anticonvulsant
CLORAZEPATE (Tranxene)	Benzodiazepine used as central nervous system depressant; see Alprazolam	Long acting; **prodrug**; converted by gastric acid	Drowsiness, dizziness, nervousness, blurred vision, dry mouth, confusion; use not advised in pregnancy and lactation	Anxiety disorders Partial Seizure adjunct
DIAZEPAM (Valium)	*Prototype benzodiazepine* that enhances inhibitory action of GABA; **absolute requirement for GABA**; anti-anxiety at low dose; sedative-hypnotic at moderate dose; skeletal m. relaxant at high dose; anti-convulsant at high IV/IM doses; **disinhibitory effect** (suppression of behavior inhibitors such as punishment)	Long acting (more than 20 hrs)	Blurred vision, diplopia, hypotension, amnesia, slurred speech, tremor, urinary incontinence, constipation; risk of congenital malformations with use in 1st trimester of pregnancy; should be avoided in pregnancy	Alcohol withdrawal Convulsions Skeletal m. relaxant Anesthesia adjunct
HALAZEPAM	Benzodiazepine; see Diazepam		See Diazepam	Antianxiety
LORAZEPAM (Ativan)	Benzodiazepine antianxiety and sedative activity; anxiolytic used as preanesthesia medication to produce sedation, perioperative amnesia	Short acting (3-20 hrs) IM, IV, po	Sedation, dizziness, weakness, ataxia; **Pregnancy category D**	Preanesthesia medication Anxiolytic

105

ANTIANXIETY AGENTS:

DRUG	ORGAN SYSTEM EFFECTS	PHARMACOKINETICS	ADVERSE REACTIONS	THERAPEUTIC USE
OXAZEPAM (Serax)	Benzodiazepine effective in generalized anxiety disorder, alcohol withdrawal and insomnia; anticonvulsant	Short acting (3-20 hrs)	Drowsiness, rash, nausea, dizziness, syncope, hypotension, tachycardia, edema, nightmares, lethargy, slurred speech and paradoxical reactions such as excitement and confusion; risk of congenital malformation with use in 1st trimester; **should be avoided in pregnancy and lactation**	Anxiety disorders Alcohol withdrawal
PRAZEPAM (Centrax)	Effective in treament of generalized anxiety disorder	Long acting; **prodrug;** must be oxidized in liver	Fatigue, dizziness, weakness, drowsiness, lightheadedness, ataxia	Antianxiety
BUSPIRONE (Buspar)	**Decreases 5-HT activity**; especially at 5-HT$_{1A}$ R; pre-synaptic agonist; post-synaptic partial agonist/blocker; **anti-anxiety only**; NOT anti-convulsant; NOT sedative-hypnotic; NOT skeletal muscle relaxant	Non-benzodiazepine; Low dependency and low tolerance	Dizziness, nausea, headache, nervousness, lightheadedness, excitement; **Pregnancy category B**	Antianxiety LSD overdose
CHLORMEZANONE (Trancopal)	Nonhypnotic antianxiety agent that improves emotional state by allaying mild anxiety: non-benzodiazepine	Onset usually within 15-30 minutes; duration up to 6 hours	Drowsiness, drug rash, dizziness, flushing, nausea, depression, edema, inability to void, tremor, confusion, headache; safety in pregnancy not established	Mild anxiety and tension
DOXEPIN (Sinequan)	Tricyclic antidepressant; see Desipramine	See Desipramine	Dry mouth, blurred vision, constipation, urinary retention; drowsiness, nausea, vomiting, diarrhea; safety in pregnancy not established	Anxiety Depression
HYDROXYZINE (Vistaril)	Mild anti-anxiety; Antihistiminic; Sedative; Antiemetic given IM to decrease vomiting after induction of anesthesia; Non-benzodiazepine antianxiety agent	4-6 hrs duration of action	Potentiates CNS depressant effects of benzodiazepine and barbiturates	Antiemetic Antihistamine Antianxiety

106

ANTIANXIETY AGENTS:

DRUG	ORGAN SYSTEM EFFECTS	PHARMACOKINETICS	ADVERSE REACTIONS	THERAPEUTIC USE
MEPROBAMATE (Miltown, Equanil)	Non-benzodiazepine that is similar to barbiturates; CNS depressant; daytime sedative; used to reduce anxiety and tension	Good gastrointestinal absorption; urine excretion; crosses placenta	Tolerance, dependency, and abuse are reported; may have additive effects with other CNS depressants; may cause drowsiness, ataxia, dizziness, slurred speech, headache, vertigo, weakness, paresthesia, euphoria, paradoxical excitement; nausea, vomiting, diarrhea; risk of congenital malformation with use in 1st trimester; **should be avoided in pregnancy** and lactation	Anxiolytic

107

ANTIARRHYTHMICS:

DRUG	GROUP	ORGAN SYSTEM EFFECTS	DOSE/DYNAMICS	ADVERSE REACTIONS	THERAPEUTIC USE
DISOPYRAMIDE (Norpace)	IA	Similar action as Procainamide	Oral dosing every 6 hours	Dry mouth, urinary hesitancy, constipation; blurred vision, dry nose, eyes, throat, nausea, abdominal pain; dizziness, fatigue, malaise; **Pregnancy category C**	Ventricular Arrhythmia
QUINIDINE (Quinidex)	IA	Class Ia antiarrhythmic agent; depresses depolarization; prolongs repolarization; slows conduction; prolongs refractory period; Na^+ depressant drug; decreases the slope of phase 4 (decreases automaticity)	Oral; NOT used IV (causes hypotension)	50% show nausea, vomiting, GI disturbance; **tinnitus**; headache; blurred vision (**cinchonism**); 2° thrombocytopenic purpura; **Pregnancy category C**	Premature atrial and ventricular contractions; Atrial tachycardia; AV junctional rhythm; Atrial flutter; Atrial fibrillation; Ventricular tachycardia
PROCAINAMIDE (Procan SR)	IA	Class Ia antiarrhythmic agent; same as Quinidine; increases refractory period of the atria, bundle of His-Purkinje, and ventricles; NO anticholinergic effects; limited use; antiarrhythmic agents have not been shown to increase survival in patients with ventricular arrhythmia	Oral	Anorexia, nausea, vomiting, bitter taste, diarrhea; positive ANA titer with or without a **lupus erythematosus like syndrome (up to 30%)**; secondary thrombocytopenic purpura; **Pregnancy category C**	Ventricular arrhythmias
LIDOCAINE	IB	Class Ib antiarrhythmic agent; **Short acting**; slightly depresses depolarization; **shortens repolarization; slows conduction**; action is greater in ischemic or diseased hearts; selectively **decreases impulse conduction; prevents re-entry; decreases slope of phase 4**; greater effects on ventricle than atria; little effects on nodal conduction; **does NOT promote purkinje automaticity**; LITTLE effect on atrial flutter	IV not oral; short acting; HIGH first pass effect	Vasodilation and cardiac depression in overdose	Post MI Ventricular Dysrhythmia Digitalis Induced Arrhythmia
MEXILETINE (Mexitil)	IB	Sodium channel blockade; slight depression of depolarization; shortens repolarization; slows conduction	Oral dosing every 8 hours with food or antacid	Dizziness, lightheadedness, tremor, nervousness, changed sleep habits, paresthesias; **Pregnancy category C**	Ventricular Arrhythmia

108

ANTIARRHYTHMICS:

DRUG	GROUP	ORGAN SYSTEM EFFECTS	DOSE/DYNAMICS	ADVERSE REACTIONS	THERAPEUTIC USE
TOCAINIDE (Tonocard)	IB	Class Ib antiarrhythmic agent; primary amine analog of Lidocaine	**ORAL;** NO first pass effect in liver	Tremor, blurred vision, lethargy, nausea, vomiting, rash, fever; **agranulocytosis;** proarrhythmic effects; pulmonary fibrosis; **Pregnancy category C**	Ventricular arrhythmias
FLECAINIDE (Tambocor)	IC	Sodium channel blockade; depolarization markedly depressed; slight effect on repolarization; slows conduction	Oral dosing every 12 hours	Dizziness, vision disturbances, dyspnea, headache, nausea, fatigue, palpitation; **Pregnancy category C**	Paroxysmal Supreventricular Tachycardia (PSVT) Ventricular Tachycardia
MORICIZINE (Ethmozine)	IC	Sodium channel blockade; potent local anesthetic activity and myocardial membrane stabilizing effects	Oral dosing every 8 hours; peak plasma levels within 0.5-2 hours	Dizziness, nausea, headache, dyspnea, fatigue; **Pregnancy category B**	Ventricular Arrhythmia
PROPAFENONE (Rythmol)	IC	Sodium channel blockade; same as Flecainide	Oral dosing every 8 hours; peak plasma level within 3.5 hours	Unusual taste, dizziness, first degree AV block, headache, constipation, intraventricular conduction delay, nausea, vomiting, blurred vision, dry mouth; positive ANA titers; **Pregnancy category C**	Ventricular Arrhythmia
PROPRANOLOL (Inderal, Inderide)	II	Class II antiarrhythmic agent; classic ß blocker, decreases automaticity; delays conduction; counteracts increases catecholamines released post myocardial infarction and in heart failure; **membrane stabilizing activity (MSA)** aids in antiarrhythmic effects; high lipid solubility with high penetration into CNS	Good oral absorption, high first pass effect, **highest** lipid solubility of the beta blockers	Nausea, vomiting, anorexia, gastric pain, flatulence, dizziness, vertigo, fatigue, insomnia, depression, hallucinations, visual disturbances, mild diarrhea or constipation, rash, pruritus; **Pregnancy category C**	Hypertension Cardiac arrhythmias Supraventricular arrhythmia Ventricular arrhythmia Tachyarrhythmia (of digitalis) Myocardial infarction Hypertrophic subaortic stenosis
ESMOLOL (Brevibloc)	II	Class II antiarrhythmic agent; VERY SHORT acting ß blocker	IV; low lipid solubility	Hypotension, dizziness, diaphoresis, bronchospasm, wheezing, nasal congestion, nausea, infusion site reactions; **Pregnancy category C**	Rapid control of ventricular rate in atrial fibrillation or atrial flutter

109

ANTIARRHYTHMICS:

DRUG	GROUP	ORGAN SYSTEM EFFECTS	DOSE/DYNAMICS	ADVERSE REACTIONS	THERAPEUTIC USE
AMIODARONE (Cordarone)	III	Class III antiarrhythmic agent; Sodium channel blocker, β adrenergic blocker, weak calcium channel blocker, also blocks potassium channels; prolongs repolarization; **stops re-entry pathways;** last resort antiarrhythmic; only used in severe dysrthymia	Oral absorption is slow and variable; peak plasma concentration 3-7 hrs after dose	Mortality, pulmonary toxcity, arrhythmia, liver injury, **pregnancy category D;** deposited in ALL tissues, corneal deposition (impairs vision), photosensitivity, thyroid abnormalities; skin discoloration; photodermatitis in 25%; pulmonary fibrosis in 25%; causes *torsade de pointes*	Recurrent Ventricular Fibrillation Recurrent Hemodynamically Unstable Ventricular Tachycardia
BRETYLIUM (Bretylol)	III	Class III antiarrhythmic agent; quaternary amine that prolongs repolarization; adrenergic neuronal blocker; LAST resort anti-arrhythmic **(potent on ventricles);** **increases ERP in His/purkinje system;** little effects on atrial muscle; **STOPS ventricular fibrillation;** emergency use	Poor oral absorption; IM, IV use	Transient hypertension with tachycardia, followed by postural hypotension; dizziness, lightheadedness and syncope are reported	Ventricular Fibrillation (v-fib)
IBUTILIDE (Corvert)	III	Prolongs action potential duration in cardiac myocytes and increases both atrial and ventricular refractoriness	80% urine excretion	Arrhythmia, syncope, renal failure, nausea; **Pregnancy category C**	Atrial Fibrillation Atrial Flutter
SOTALOL (Betapace)	III	Class III antiarrhythmic agent; β adrenergic blocker; sodium and potassium channel blocker; prolongs Q-T interval	Complete oral absorption; urine excretion	Tiredness, lassitude, impotence, depression, headache	Class III Antiarrhythmic
DILTIAZEM (Cardizem)	III	Calcium channel blocker; main activity is on slow-response fibers; suppresses automaticity and delays conduction	Well absorbed orally; 70-80% protein bound; high first pass effect	Headache, dizziness, bradycardia, first degree AV block, edema; **Pregnancy category C**	Atrial Flutter Atrial Fibrillation PSVT
VERAPAMIL (Calan)	III	Class IV antiarrhythmic; calcium channel blocker; increases atrial and AV nodal effective refractory period; slows sinus rate		Hypotension, dizziness, lightheadedness, headache, nausea; **Pregnancy category C**	Essential Hypertension Supraventricular tachyarrhythmia
ADENOSINE (Adenocard)	IV	Purkinje receptor antagonist; slows conduction time through the AV node; interrupts re-entry pathways; does NOT convert atrial flutter or fibrillation or ventricular tachycaria to sinus rhythm	Rapid IV bolus	Facial flushing, dyspnea, chest pressure, nausea, headache, lightheadedness; **Pregnancy category C**	Paroxysmal Supraventricular Tachycardia (PSVT)

110

ANTIARTHRITIC:

DRUG	ORGAN SYSTEM EFFECTS	KINETICS	ADVERSE EFFECTS	THERAPEUTIC USE
AUROTHIOGLUCOSE (Solganal)	Gold containing antiarthritic agent; mechanism not well understood; reported to decrease synovial inflammation and retard cartilage and bone destruction; storage of gold in tissues depends on the organ and gold concentration; major areas of deposit: bone marrow, liver, skin, bone	IM injection; peak plasma levels within 4-6 hours; 95% plasma albumin bound; 70% of gold excreted in urine, 30% in feces	Dermatitis is most common reaction including pruritus and erythema; stomatitis is next most common reaction; nephrotoxic leading to mild nephrotic syndrome or glomerulonephritis if diagnosed early; **Pregnancy category C**	Rheumatoid Arthritis

111

ANTIASTHMATICS:

DRUG	ORGAN SYSTEM EFFECTS	KINETICS	ADVERSE EFFECTS	THERAPEUTIC USE
CROMOLYN SODIUM	Inhibits release of histamine and other immediate hypersensitivity mediators from mast cells; thought to stabilize mast cell membranes; may also inhibit PAF (platelet activating factor)	Capsule, nebulizer, inhaler, nasal solution, ophthalmic solution	**Pregnancy category B**	Seasonal Allergy Asthma
NEDOCROMIL SODIUM (Tilade)	**Inhaled antiinflammatory,** effect depends on topical application to lungs; NOT bronchodilator	Inhalation aerosol; unknown whether excreted in breast milk	Unpleasant taste **Pregnancy category B**	Maintenance therapy for mild to moderate **bronchial asthma**
THEOPHYLLINE (Respbid, Slo-Bid, Theo-Dur)	Chemical structure is methylxanthine; classified as a bronchodilator; mechanism is antagonism of adenosine receptors	POOR water solubility; good ORAL absorption; available as capsule, elixir, sustained release tablets and syrup preparations	CNS: restlessness, anxiety, insomnia, tremor, seizure, increases respiratory rate CV: ↑ HR, ↑ CO, ↑ O₂ use; vasodilation (except meningeal blood vessels, which constrict) GI: increases acid and pepsin Renal: increases loss of Na, K, Cl, and H2O **Pregnancy category C**	Relief of symptoms of Asthma and reversible bronchospasm associated with Chronic Bronchitis and Emphysema
ZAFIRLUKAST (Accolate)	**Synthetic, selective leukotriene receptor antagonist (LTRA);** is a selective and competitive inhibitor of leukotriene D₄ and E₄ (components of slow reacting substance of anaphylaxis (SRSA); decreases airway responsiveness and bronchoconstriction caused by antigen challenge; decreases need for beta agonist rescues; has NO effect on bronchospasm in acute asthmatic attacks	Oral dose twice daily; should be taken 1-2 hours prior to meals; peak plasma level within 3 hours; cytochrome P450 metabolized; 90% feces and 10% urine excretion; >99% plasma protein bound; Erythromycin and Theophyllin *decrease* plasma levels of Zafirkulast; Aspirin *increases* plasma levels of Zafirlukast; NO significant effect on Ethinyl Estradiol plasma levels or oral contraceptive efficacy; excreted in breast milk	Headache, increased respiratory infection, nausea, vomiting, diarrhea, asthenia, dizziness, myalgia, fever, reversible hepatic transaminase elevation; **Pregnancy category B**	Prophylaxis and Treatment of Chronic Asthma in children 12 years and older

ANTICHOLINERGICS:

DRUG	ORGAN SYSTEM EFFECTS	PHARMACOKINETICS	ADVERSE REACTIONS	THERAPEUTIC USE
ATROPINE alkaloid	**Antimuscarinic;** decreases salivation, decreases bronchiolar secretion, decreases sweating, pupillary dilation, non-accommodation, increases HR, decreases GI motility **(antispasmodic)**, decreases gastric acid secretion, CNS stimulation	Rapid and almost complete GI absorption; peak plasma concentration 1 hr after dose; majority is urine excreted	**Dry mouth** (classic), atropine fever due to decreased sweating, vision disturbance (mydriasis and cycloplegia), heart palpitation, CNS excitation at high doses	Organophosphate poisoning: artificial respiration, atropine and pralidoxime (Protopam); Preanesthesia to dry respiratory tract; **cycloplegia** for eye exam
BENZTROPINE (Cogentin)	Antimuscarinic; a tropanol derivative; effective in decreasing extrapyramidal reactions induced by antipsychotic agents such as Haloperidol	Oral dose at bedtime	Similar to Atropine	Parkinson's disease Drug-induced extrapyramidal reactions
DICYCLOMINE tertiary amine	Decreases GI smooth m. spasms via antimuscarinic and musculotropic antispasmodic effects	Rapid oral absorption; peak plasma level 60-90 min after dose	Dry mouth, dizziness, blurred vision	Antispasmodic
HOMATROPINE	**Mydriasis and cycloplegia** (paralysis of accommodation) lasting 1-3 days	Similar to Atropine	Similar to Atropine	Induces mydriasis in ophthalmology
IPRATROPIUM (Atrovent)	Bronchodilation without inhibiting mucociliary escalator	Aerosol administration	Dry mouth with improper aerosol administration	Bronchodilator used in COPD
PROPANTHELINE quaternary ammonium	**Ganglionic blocker** (non-selective); cholinergic blocker, decreases gastric secretions	Polar molecule that does not cross BBB well	Ganglionic blocker adverse effects similar to atropine	Antiulcer Anticholinergic Antispasmotic
SCOPOLAMINE (Transderm Scop)	Anti-motion sickness agent, given through **transdermal patch** (CNS action but mechanism not clear, probably related to sedation); antimuscarinic activity	Transdermal absorption; dose 4 hours prior to activity, lasts 42 hours	Less side effects than atropine; dry mouth (66%), blurred vision (14%), bizarre hallucination (rare)	Motion sickness; prep for anesthesia to dry respiratory tract, sedative effects
TROPICAMIDE	**Mydriasis** lasting 6 hours and **cycloplegia** lasting 2 hours with maximal effects 20-35 min after application	Topical application with rapid onset and short duration of action	Rarely causes side effects due to short duration of action	Induces mydriasis in ophthalmology; cycloplegia for eye exam

NOTE: cycloplegia - paralysis of accommodation (shape of lens is fixed allowing refractive studies)

113

ANTICOAGULANTS:

DRUG	ORGAN SYSTEM EFFECTS	PHARMACOKINETICS/ DYNAMICS	ADVERSE REACTIONS	THERAPEUTIC USE
DICUMAROL	Inhibits **gamma-carboxylation** of clotting **factors II, VII, IX, and X** (all vitamin K dependent); PT is 1.4-2.0 x's normal; does NOT work in vitro	24-36 hours to onset; in vivo ONLY; incomplete, slow absorption; DMMS: hydroxylated then conjugated → **urine excretion;** 1-8 days to return to normal	Hypoprothrombinemia → hemorrhage (give whole fresh blood or **phytonadione (vit K1)** to restore gamma-carboxylation of II, VII, IX, and X); diarrhea; urticaria; alopecia (reversible)	Oral anticoagulant Prevention and Treatment of Deep Venous Thrombosis and Pulmonary Emboli
ENOXAPARIN (Lovenox)	Low molecular weight heparin with antithrombotic properties; has anti-Factor Xa and antithrombin (anti-Factor IIa) activity; decreased total deep vein thrombosis (DVT) by 80% in hip replacement surgery trials	Subcutaneous administration, NOT intramuscular; usually no need for daily PTT monitoring in patients with normal presurgical coagulation values	Hemorrhage, thrombocytopenia, local irritation; **pregnancy category B;** overdosage may be reversible with Protamine sulfate	Prevention of Deep Venous Thrombosis Thrombosis in Hip Replacement Surgery
DALTEPARIN (Fragmin)	Low molecular weight heparin with antithrombotic properties; inhibits factor Xa without significant effect on the PTT	Given subcutaneously only	Hemorrhage (incidence depends on dosage and patient population); thrombocytopenia; injection site pain **Pregnancy category B**	Deep Venous Thrombosis Prophylaxis
HEPARIN	**Accelerates antithrombin III binding to** clotting factors **Xa and IIa;** strong negative charge; PTT is 1.5-2.0 x's normal	Immediate onset; **IV dose** or subcutaneous dose; works in vitro and in vivo; **95% plasma protein binding;** converted to uroheparin (slightly active) by heparinase	**Hemorrhage;** fever, urticaria, anaphylaxis, osteoporosis; **alopecia** (reversible); **heparin-induced thrombocytopenia** → platelet aggregation; **Pregnancy category C**	Prevention and Treatment of Deep Venous Thrombosis and Pulmonary Emboli Anticoagulant for lab and blood bank specimens and during extra-corporeal circulation
WARFARIN SODIUM	Similar agent, but preferred over Dicumarol	24-36 hours to onset; BETTER absorption than dicumarol; injectable form available; HIGH (99%) plasma protein binding; **displaced by salicylates, chloral hydrate** → **hemorrhage;** 1-8 days to return to original coagulation state	Usually direct effect of overdosage resulting in hypoprothrombinemia manifested by ecchymoses and/or hemorrhage; uncommon effects include alopecia, urticaria, dermatitis, nausea, diarrhea, necrosis; **Pregnancy category X**	Oral anticoagulant Prevention and Treatment of Deep Venous Thrombosis and Pulmonary Emboli

Notes: PTT - 20-35 seconds is normal
        PT - 11-13 seconds is normal

Decreased vitamin K absorption (due to antibiotics) OR agents that displace anticoagulants from serum albumin (Salicylates, Chloral Hydrate) OR agents that inhibit the DMMS (Cimetidine, Disulfiram and Ketoconazole) will increase anticoagulant effects

114

ANTIDEPRESSANTS:

DRUG	MECHANISM OF ACTION/EFFECTS	PHARMACOKINETICS	ADVERSE REACTIONS	CLINICAL USE
AMITRIPTYLINE (Elavil)	Tricyclic antidepressant; elevates mood by decreasing sensitivity of post-synaptic NE and 5-HT receptors; anticholinergic; **blocks reuptake of NE and 5-HT** (results in down regulation of post-synaptic ß2 receptors); **α2 antagonist;** decreases sensitivity of post-synaptic ß receptors; sedation (through anti-histaminic activity), decreases anxiety; Desipramine may be stimulatory, effective for lethargy in depression; decreases REM; **elevation of mood;** anticholinergic; increases HR; antiarrhythmic (at low dose)	Rapid oral absorption, peak plasma levels within 2-4 hrs; undergoes first pass effect; extensive hepatic metabolism; metabolized to Nortriptyline	Antimuscarinic effects: dry mouth, blurred vision, constipation, tachycardia or palpitation, dizziness, urinary retention; **Pregnancy category C**	Depression
AMOXAPINE (Asendin)	Tricyclic antidepressant with less anticholinergic effects than Desipramine; unique in having neuroleptic effects (structural relationship to antipsychotic drug, Loxapine)	Biotransformed to active hydroxylated products in liver	Extrapyramidal reactions; **Pregnancy category C**	Depression
DESIPRAMINE (Norpramin)	Tricyclic antidepressant; Desipramine is active metabolite of imipramine; see Amitriptyline	Absorbed well p.o.; 2-6 weeks to onset of antidepressant; 70-90+% protein binding; biotransformed by microsomal system (N-demethylation, hydroxylation); elimination through kidney; some enterohepatic circulation; conjugated with glucuronic acid in liver	Contraindications: CNS depressants (morphine, anti-histamines, alcohol), **sympathomimetic amines** (HTN crisis), **MAOI** (hyperpyrexia, convulsion, coma, death) and **anticholinergics** Adverse: seizures; arrhythmic at high dose; palpitation, tachycardia, orthostatic hypotension; twitching, confusion, anxiety; safety in pregnancy not established Rare: leukopenia, skin rash, agranulocytosis, photosensitivity and cholestatic jaundice	Depression
DOXEPIN (Sinequan)	Tricyclic antidepressant; See Desipramine	Same as Desipramine	Same as Desipramine; safety in pregnancy not established	Depression

ANTIDEPRESSANTS:

DRUG	MECHANISM OF ACTION/EFFECTS	PHARMACOKINETICS	ADVERSE REACTIONS	CLINICAL USE
FLUOXETINE (Prozac) 1st member of this class introduced 1988	**Selective serotonin reuptake inhibitor (SSRI)**; little or no anticholinergic effects, sedation, or cardiac toxicity in overdose (better for suicidal patients); widely used anti-depressant; no more suicidal tendency than any other TCAs	Phenylpropylamine derivative; 2° amine; almost 100% oral absorption; peak blood levels 4-8 hrs after dose; high plasma protein binding	Dizziness, CNS stimulation, insomnia, anxiety, restlessness, GI upset, dry mouth, tremors, anorgasmia in women, ejaculatory delay in men; **Pregnancy category B**	Depression
IMIPRAMINE (Tofranil)	Tricyclic antidepressant; see Amitriptyline	Similar to Amitriptyline; metabolized to Desipramine	See Amitriptyline; safety in pregnancy not established	Depression
MAPROTILINE (Ludiomil)	Tricyclic antidepressant with less anticholinergic effects, less sedation	Similar to other tricyclic antidepressants	Antimuscarinic side effects, causes sedation; **Pregnancy category B**	Depression
NORTRIPTYLINE (Pamelor)	Tricyclic antidepressant; Nortriptyline is active metabolite of Amitriptyline	See Amitriptyline	LEAST likely to cause orthostatic hypotension; safety in pregnancy not established	Depression
PAROXETINE (Paxil)	Selective serotonin reuptake inhibitor (SSRI); potentiates serotonergic activity in CNS by inhibiting serotonin neuronal reuptake; not related to other selective serotonin reuptake inhibitors or other antidepressants; has little affinity for other pharmacologic receptors	Complete po absorption; 95% plasma protein bound; urine and fecal excretion	Asthenia, nausea, dry mouth, constipation, diarrhea, somnolence, dizziness, insomnia, ejaculatory disturbance; **Pregnancy category C**	Depression Panic Disorder Obsessive Compulsive Disorder
PHENELZINE (Nardil)	Monoamine oxidase inhibitor; **down regulates ß2 post-synaptic receptors**	Oral dosage; onset of action within 2-4 weeks	Contraindicated with sympathomimetic amines (taken together may cause hypertensive crisis); tyramine containing foods (wine, cheese); orthostatic hypotension, hepatocellular necrosis; **Pregnancy category C**	Depression
PROTRIPTYLIN (Vivactil)	Tricyclic antidepressant; same as Desipramine; protriptylin may be stimulatory, effective for lethargy in depression	Same as Amitriptyline	Same as Amitriptyline; safety in pregnancy not established	Depression

ANTIDEPRESSANTS:

DRUG	MECHANISM OF ACTION/EFFECTS	PHARMACOKINETICS	ADVERSE REACTIONS	CLINICAL USE
SERTRALINE (Zoloft)	Selective serotonin reuptake inhibitor (SSRI)	Same as Fluoxetine	Same as Fluoxetine; **Pregnancy category B**	Depression
TRANYLCYPROMINE (Parnate)	Monoamine oxidase inhibitor; **down regulates ß2 post-synaptic receptors**	See Phenelzine	Same as Phenelzine; safety in pregnancy not established	Depression
TRAZODONE (Desyrel)	Weak activity in blocking reuptake of serotonin and norepinephrine; Less anticholingeric effects; less sedation; little or no cardiac toxicity in overdose (better for suicidal patients)	Oral dosage; peak plasma level within 1-2 hours; biphasic elimination	Lightheadedness, orthostatic hypotension, confusion; **priapism** (many cases have required corrective surgery or caused permanent loss of erectile function); **Pregnancy category C**	Depression
TRIMIPRAMINE (Surmontil) (TCA)	Tricyclic antidepressant; same as Imipramine	See Amitriptyline	See Amitriptyline **Pregnancy category C**	Depression
VENLAFAXINE (Effexor)	Antidepressant not related to tricyclic or other antidepressants; mechanism associated with potentiation of neurotransmitter activity in CNS; inhibits serotonin and norepinephrine reuptake and weakly inhibits dopamine reuptake	Well absorbed po; extensive liver metabolism	Nausea, somnolence, insomnia, dizziness, nervousness, dry mouth, anxiety, abnormal ejaculation, impotence, headache, asthenia, sweating; **Pregnancy category C**	Depression

NOTES:

EPR - extrapyramidal reactions (dystonia, akathesia {restlessness}, parkinson-like syndrome)
Depression is also treatable with **electroconvulsive therapy (ECT)**, which also down regulates the ß2 post-synaptic receptors in CNS.
Tyramine is an indirect NE agonist.

117

ANTIDIARRHEALS:

DRUG	ORGAN SYSTEM EFFFECTS	KINETICS	ADVERSE EFFECTS	THERAPEUTIC USE
ATTAPULGITE (Kaopectate)	Taken at first sign of diarrhea and after each subsequent bowel movement	Available in liquid, capsule, and tablet form		Diarrhea Abdominal Cramps
BISMUTH SUBSALICYLATE (Pepto-Bismol)	Over the counter stomach remedy proven effective for upper and lower GI symptoms; also has some antibacterial action	Available in liquid, tablet and caplet form	Excessive dosage may cause constipation Warning: may cause Reye syndrome in children with flu or chicken pox	Diarrhea Heartburn Indigestion Nausea Upset Stomach
DIPHENOXYLATE (Lomotil)	Chemically related to narcotic analgesics; Lomotil is combination preparation of Diphenoxylate, an antidiarrheal, and Atropine, an anticholinergic to discourage abuse by overdosage	Liquid and tablets are available	Paresthesia, euphoria, depression, confusion, sedation, dizziness, restlessness, headache, nausea, vomiting, anorexia, abdominal discomfort; has potential for abuse and dependence; **Pregnancy category C**	Diarrhea
LOPERAMIDE (Imodium)	Slows intestinal motility and water and electrolyte movement through the bowel	Liquid and tablets are available	Constipation, CNS depression, nausea	Acute Nonspecific Diarrhea Traveler's Diarrhea

118

ANTIEMETICS:

DRUG	ORGAN SYSTEM EFFECTS	KINETICS	ADVERSE EFFECTS	THERAPEUTIC USE
BENZQUINAMIDE (Emete-Con)	Antiemetic, antihistaminic, and mild anticholinergic and sedative activity		Drowsiness, dry mouth, dizziness, anorexia; not recommended in pregnancy	Antiemetic for nausea and vomiting associated with surgery and anesthesia
CHLORPROMAZINE (Thorazine)	Blocks chemotactic trigger zone (CTZ) to prevent vomiting; also is psychotropic; also sedative; activity on all areas of CNS; strong antiadrenergic and mild anticholinergic activity; slight ganglionic blocker; slight antihistaminic and antiserotonin action	Po, per rectum	Tardive dyskinesia; neuroleptic malignant syndrome (NMS); safety in pregnancy not established; drowsiness, jaundice, blood disorders including agranulocytosis; hypotension; ECG changes; pseudo-Parkinsonism	Nausea and vomiting Psychotic disorders Preoperative restlessness Acute intermittent porphyria Tetanus (adjunct) Mania Intractable hiccups Explosive hyperexcitable behavior in children
CYCLIZINE (Marezine)	H1 receptor antagonist, common use as antiemetic	Taken ½ hour prior to travel; po dose	Sedation, dry mouth	Antiemetic Motion Sickness
DIMENHYDRINATE (Dramamine)	Exact mechanism not known, but thought to have depressant effect on hyperstimulated labyrinthe function	Taken ½ - 1 hour prior to travel; po dose	Sedation, dry mouth	Antiemetic Antivertigo
DIPHENHYDRAMINE (Benadryl)	**H1 blocker**; but also is antimuscarinic; metabolized by DMMS (some tolerance to sedative effects)	Po, IM; ½ hour onset; 4-6 hour duration	**Sedation**; dry mouth; constipation; contraindication with alcohol; CNS depression; convulsion in children	Antiemetic Acute Hypersensitivity Reactions Sedative (good OTC drug for insomnia) Motion sickness
DRONABINOL (Marinol)	Cannabinoid,delta-9-tetrahydrocannabinol (delta-9-THC) is active extract from *Cannabis sativa* or marijuana; orally active cannabinoid with complex CNS effects including central sympathomimetic activity; appetite stimulant effect in AIDS related weight loss; has antiemetic activity	90-95% po absorption; first pass liver metabolism; 10-20% reaches circulation	Asthenia, palpitations, tachycardia, facial flushing, abdominal pain, nausea, vomiting, anxiety, dizziness, euphoria, paranoid reaction, somnolence; **Pregnancy category C**	Anorexia associated with AIDS Antiemetic in cancer chemotherapy

119

ANTIEMETICS:

DRUG	ORGAN SYSTEM EFFFECTS	KINETICS	ADVERSE EFFECTS	THERAPEUTIC USE
GRANISETRON (Kytrel)	Antiemetic that is **selective 5-HT3 receptor antagonist** without affinity for other serotonin receptors	Injection	Headache, asthenia, somnolence, diarrhea; **Pregnancy category B**	Nausea and Vomiting Associated with Emetogenic Chemotherapy
HYDROXYZINE (Atarax)	Not a cortical depressant; may suppress regions of subcortical areas of CNS; bronchodilator activity, antihistaminic and analgesic effects; potentiates CNS depressants such as narcotics, non-narcotic analgesics and barbiturates	Po, syrup and capsules	Dry mouth, drowsiness, tremor; should be avoided in pregnancy and lactation	Pruritus associated with skin rashes Sedative premedication Antianxiety
METOCLOPRAMIDE (Reglan)	Stimulates upper GI motility; its activity is inhibited by anticholinergic agents; increases gastric contraction, relaxes pyloric sphincter; accelerates gastric emptying and intestinal transit time; increases lower esophageal sphincter resting tone; little effect on colon or gall bladder motility	Rapid and complete GI absorption	Restlessness, drowsiness, fatigue and lassitude in 10%; acute dystonic reactions in 0.2%; **Pregnancy category B;** excreted in human breast milk	Gastroesophageal reflux Diabetic gastroparesis Antiemetic in chemotherapy Post operative antiemetic Small bowel intubation Radiological examination
ONDANSETRON (Zofran)	Selective serotonin 5-HT3 receptor blocking agent; not a dopamine receptor antagonist; no effect on esophageal motility, gastric motility, lower esophageal sphincter pressure, or small intestinal transit time	Extensively metabolized; IV and po	Constipation, rash, transient blurred vision, **Pregnancy category B**	Antiemetic in courses of emetogenic cancer chemotherapy Postoperative antiemetic
PERPHENAZINE (Trilafon)	Blocks chemotactic trigger zone (CTZ); also has some antipsychotic effects	Po and injectable dosages	Extrapyramidal reactions, tardive dyskinesia; dry mouth, nausea, vomiting, diarrhea, anorexia, constipation	Antipsychotic Antiemetic
PROCHLORPERAZINE (Compazine)	Blocks dopamine receptors of the chemotactic trigger zone (CTZ); mild sedative, antiemetic, alters temperature regulation, alters skeletal muscle tone, endocrine alterations, potentiates analgesics; alpha adrenergic blocker, inhibits bioamine uptake and adrenergic potentiation, cholinergic blocking effects; serotonin and histamine receptor blocking properties	Po, syrup, suppository, and injectable dosages	Tardive dyskinesia, neuroleptic malignant syndrome (NMS); safety in pregnancy not established; drowsiness, dizziness, amenorrhea, blurred vision, skin reactions, hypotension; dystonias	Severe nausea and vomiting Psychotic disorders

120

ANTIEMETICS:

DRUG	ORGAN SYSTEM EFFFECTS	KINETICS	ADVERSE EFFECTS	THERAPEUTIC USE
PROMETHAZINE (Phenergan)	Blocks dopamine receptors at the chemoreceptor trigger zone (CTZ); also has antihistaminic, sedative, antimotion sickness, and anticholinergic activity; does not block histamine release, but is competitive histamine antagonist	4-6 hour duration of action; po, injectable and suppository dosages	Drowsiness, dizziness, tinnitus, incoordination, fatigue, blurred vision, euphoria, tremors, changes in blood pressure and heart rate	Antiemetic Allergic reactions to blood or plasma Anaphylaxis as adjunct agent Motion sickness Preop, postop, and obstetric (labor) sedation Analgesic adjunct (postoperative)
SCOPOLAMINE (Transderm Scop)	Anti-motion sickness agent, given through **transdermal patch** (CNS action but mechanism not clear, probably related to sedation)	Dose 4 hours prior to activity, lasts 42 hours	Less side effects than atropine; dry mouth (66%), blurred vision (14%), bizarre hallucination (rare)	**Motion sickness;** prep for anesthesia to dry respiratory tract, sedative effects
THIETHYLPERAZINE (Torecan)	Phenothiazine with exact mechanism of action unknown; probable action on chemotactic trigger zone (CTZ) and vomiting center via dopamine receptors	Po and injectable dosages	Extrapyramidal reactions such as dystonia, torticollis, oculogyric crises, akathisia and gait disturbances; dry mouth, blurred vision, tinnitus; **contraindicated in pregnancy**	Nausea and Vomiting
TRIMETHOBENZAMIDE (Tigan)	Work at the chemotactic trigger zone (CTZ) by blocking dopamine receptors	Capsules Suppositories Injectable	Blood dyscrasia, blurred vision, convulsion, diarrhea, dizziness, drowsiness, headache; safety in pregnancy and lactation not established	Antiemetic

121

ANTIENURETIC:

DRUG	ORGAN SYSTEM EFFFECTS	KINETICS	ADVERSE EFFECTS	THERAPEUTIC USE
DESMOPRESSIN ACETATE (DDAVP)	Antidiuretic analog of posterior pituitary hormone that affects renal water conservation; synthetic analog of 8-arginine vasopressin; increases plasma clotting factor VIII in patients with hemophilia and von Willebrand's disease Type I	Clotting effects within 30 minutes, maximum effect within 90 minutes to 2 hours; available in tablets, injectable and spray forms	Transient headache, nausea, abdominal cramping, vulval pain; **Pregnancy category B**	Injection for : Hemophilia A von Willebrand's Disease (Type I) Central Cranial Diabetes Insipidus Pirmary Nocturnal Enuresis

122

ANTIEPILEPTICS and ANTICONVULSANTS:

DRUG	ORGAN SYSTEM EFFECTS	ADVERSE REACTIONS	INDICATIONS
CARBAMAZEPINE (Tegretol)	Appears to work on seizure focus; decreases Na$^+$ influx thus decreases repetitive firing from seizure focus; NO effect on post tetanic potentiation	Dizziness, unsteadiness, nausea, vomiting; xerostomia; diarrhea; jaundice; **aplastic anemia** (rare); **Pregnancy category C**	Complex Partial Seizures Generalized Tonic-Clonic Seizures Mixed Seizures
CLONAZEPAM (Klonopin)	Secondary agent in epilepsy treatment; also has antianxiety activity	Sedation is side effect and tolerance develops to antiepileptic effects thus limiting utility of this agent; ataxia, drowsiness, dysarthria; **safety in pregnancy is unknown**	Lennox-Gestaut Syndrome (Petit Mal variant) Akinetic and Myoclonic Seizures Abscence Seizures Antianxiety
CLORAZEPATE (Tranxene)	Has the characteristics of benzodiazepines; has depressant effect on the central nervous system; effective for partial seizures; metabolized in the liver and urine excreted	Drowsiness, dizziness, gastrointestinal complaints, nervousness, blurred vision, dry mouth, headache, confusion, insomnia, irritability, tremor; **increased risk of congenital malformation with use in 1st trimester**	Anxiety disorders Adjunctive agent in Partial Seizures
DIAZEPAM (Valium)	Benzodiazepine with mild sedative effects along with anticonvulsant and skeletal muscle relaxant properties; acts on limbic system, thalamus, hypothalamus producing a calming effect; not used daily for treatment of any epileptic condition; use reserved for status epilepticus	Sedation, lightheadedness, ataxia, lethargy; **increased risk of congenital malformations with use in 1st trimester**	Status Epilepticus Anxiety Disorders Acute Alcohol Withdrawal Preoperative Sedation Skeletal Muscle Relaxant Preoperative Premedication
DIVALPROEX (Depakote)	Antiepileptic which becomes valproate in the gastrointestinal tract; activity related to increased brain levels of GABA (gamma-amino butyric acid); also may decrease sodium influx and prevent repetitive firing of seizure focus; primary metabolism in liver; 90% plasma protein bound	Nausea, vomiting, indigestion, diarrhea, abdominal cramps, constipation, both anorexia and increased appetite are reported, sedation, alopecia, skin rash, photosensitivity, weakness, thrombocytopenia, liver enzyme changes, irregular menses, secondary amenorrhea, breast enlargement, galactorrhea; Stevens Johnson syndrome; **Teratogenic**	Simple and Complex Abscence Seizures Generalized Tonic Clonic and Partial Seizures in presence of Abscence Seizures
ETHOTOIN (Peganone)	Antiepileptic without CNS depressant effect; stabilizes seizure threshold; prevents spread of seizure activity (does not abolish primary focus of seizure discharge); may block sodium influx into neurons (like Phenytoin)	Ataxia, gum hypertrophy, nausea, vomiting, nystagmus, diplopia, fever, dizziness, diarrhea, headache, insomnia, fatigue, numbness, rash, isolated cases of lymphadenopathy and lupus reported; **Pregnancy category C**	Tonic-Clonic (Grand mal) Seizures Complex Partial (Psychomotor) Seizures

123

ANTIEPILEPTICS and ANTICONVULSANTS:

DRUG	ORGAN SYSTEM EFFECTS	ADVERSE REACTIONS	INDICATIONS
ETHOSUXIMIDE (Zarontin)	May block calcium ion influx in thalamus; blocks T-type calcium ion channels	Dizziness; drowsiness; ataxia: sedation; **renal, hepatic and bone marrow toxicity**	**Absence Seizures**
FELBAMATE (Felbatol)	Antiepileptic agents with weak inhibitory effect on GABA receptor binding and benzodiazepine receptor binding	Anorexia, vomiting, insomnia, nausea, dizziness, somnolence, headache; **aplastic anemia; Pregnancy category C**	Partial Seizures (with and without generalization) Lennoz-Gastaut syndrome in children
GABAPENTIN (Neurontin)	Related to neurotransmitter GABA; inhibits seizure through unknown mechanism	Somnolence, dizziness, ataxia, fatigue, nystagmus, alopecia; **Pregnancy category C**	Partial Seizures Chronic Pain Control Adjunct
MEPHENYTOIN (Mesantoin)	Antiepileptic agent that inhibits seizures and has effects similar to the barbiturates; causes behavioral and EEG changes similar to those of barbiturates	Blood dyscrasias; drowsiness, ataxia, diplopia, nystagmus, dysarthria, fatigue, nervousness, nausea, vomiting, dizziness, hepatitis, jaundice, nephrosis are reported; effects in pregnancy and nursing are not known	Tonic Clonic and Partial Seizures
MEPHOBARBITAL (Mebaral)	**Enhances GABA; suppresses excitatory action of glutamic acid;** some conversion to phenobarbital	Overdose and abuse potential; somnolence, agitation, confusion, hyperkinesia, ataxia, CNS depression, hallucinations, insomnia, anxiety, dizziness, apnea, bradycardia, hypotension, nausea, vomiting, constipation, headache; **Pregnancy category D**	Tonic Clonic Seizures Simple Partial Seizures Sedative
METHSUXIMIDE (Celontin)	Anticonvulsant that suppresses paroxysmal spike and wave activity associated with loss of consciousness common in absence (petit mal) seizures; may block calcium ion influx into neurons (like Ethosuximide)	Blood dyscrasias, nausea, vomiting, anorexia, diarrhea, weight loss, abdominal pain, constipation; drowsiness, ataxia, dizziness, irritability, headache, blurred vision, photophobia, hiccups, insomnia, effects in pregnancy and nursing are not known; Stevens-Johnson syndrome (reported)	Absence (Petit Mal) Seizures

ANTIEPILEPTICS and ANTICONVULSANTS:

DRUG	ORGAN SYSTEM EFFECTS	ADVERSE REACTIONS	INDICATIONS
PHENACEMIDE (Phenurone)	A monoureide that resembles many older hypnotics; well absorbed from GI tract; very toxic drug; last resort antipileptic only	Liver and bone marrow toxicity; psychic changes in up to 20%, GI distress, skin rash, drowsiness, headache, insomnia, dizziness, parestheisa, blood dyscrasia, hepatitis; **Pregnancy category D**	Refractory Severe Epilepsy Mixed forms of Complex Partial Seizures
PHENOBARBITAL (Luminal)	Enhances GABA; suppresses excitatory action of glutamic acid	Sedation; paradoxical excitement in elderly and children; exfoliative dermatitis; megaloblastic anemia; abuse potential; **Pregnancy category D**	Tonic-Clonic Seizures Simple Partial Seizures
PHENYTOIN (Dilantin)	**Decreases post tetanic potentiation;** decreases Na$^+$ influx during depolarization, decreases Ca^{++} influx (essential for NT release), decreases K$^+$ efflux (slows repolarization, increases refractory period); **blocks reuptake of GABA;** advantage: little or NO sedation (good for children)	Dizziness; drowsiness; ataxia; tremors; epigastric pain; **gingival hyperplasia;** hirsutism; hepatitis; **Stevens Johnson syndrome** (rare); congenital malformation must be considered if used during pregnancy	Generalized Tonic-Clonic Seizures Complex Partial Seizures Pre and Post Neurosurgery Seizure Prophylaxis Status Epilepticus
PRIMIDONE (Mysoline)	Non-barbiturate anticonvulsant that **decreases post tetanic potentiation (PTP)** in neuronal circuits of CNS; decreases spread of seizure focus; some conversion to phenobarbital; may decrease sodium entrance into neurons (like Phenytoin)	Drowsiness; sedation; dizziness; ataxia; **contraindicated in acute intermittent porphyria;** exfoliative dermatitis, megaloblastic anemia (rare); **contraindicated with Phenobarbital;** effects in pregnancy and nursing are not known	Tonic-Clonic Seizures Partial Seizures

125

ANTIEPILEPTICS and ANTICONVULSANTS:

DRUG	ORGAN SYSTEM EFFECTS	ADVERSE REACTIONS	THERAPEUTIC USE
TRIMETHADIONE (Tridione)	Antiepileptic agent with sedative and respiratory depression effects; rapidly absorbed from GI tract; liver metabolized to active metabolite, dimethadione; drug has limited usage due to adverse reactions	Nausea, vomiting, abdominal pain, gastric distress, drowsiness, fatigue, malaise, insomina, vertigo, headache, paresthesia, irritability, bleeding gums, epistaxis, vaginal bleeding, neutropenia, skin rash, hiccups, anorexia, weight loss, alopecia, blood pressure changes, photophobia; **risk of congenital malformation** if used during first trimester	Absence Seizures
VALPROIC ACID (Depakene)	Blocks sodium ion influx into neurons and decreases repetitive firing of neurons; also inhibits GABA transaminase and succinic semialdehyde DH (enzymes that breakdown GABA), thus increases GABA; blocks reuptake of GABA; metabolite is δ-4-valproic acid which inhibits biotransformation of phenobarbital, phenytoin, carbamazepine	Dizziness; drowsiness; ataxia; sedation; diarrhea, abdominal cramps, constipation, anorexia or increased appetite, tremor, hallucination, skin rash, photosensitivity; irregular menses, secondary amenorrhea, breast enlargement galactorrhea; acute pancreatitis; hepatotoxicity; alopecia; **Pregnancy category D**	Absence Seizures Partial Seizure if patient has accompanying Absence Seizures

126

ANTIFLATULENTS:

DRUG	ORGAN SYSTEM EFFFECTS	KINETICS	ADVERSE EFFECTS	THERAPEUTIC USE
SIMETHICONE (Mylicon, Mylanta GAS Relief)	Antiflatulent agent which relieves painful symptoms of gastrointestinal gas caused by swallowed air or dyspepsia; works by changing surface tension of trapped gas which allows them to coalesce and be passed as eructation or flatulence	po tablets and liquid forms	No signigicant side effects reported	Gas pain and other symptoms associated with indigestion, dyspepsia, and reflux in the digestive tract

ANTIFUNGALS:

DRUG	ORGAN SYSTEM EFFECTS	KINETICS	ADVERSE EFFECTS	THERAPEUTIC USE
AMPHOTERICIN B (Fungizon)	**Binds ergosterol**; polyene macrolide; has *in vitro* activity against a variety of fungi; fungicidal or fungistatic depending on concentration achieved in tissue; has no effect on bacteria, rickettsiea or viruses	POOR oral absorption; will NOT cross blood brain barrier; t½ = 24 hours; 90% plasma protein bound; po, topical, IV, intrathecal administration; extremely slow renal excretion (over weeks to months)	Fever, malaise, weight loss, hypotension, tachypnea, anorexia, nausea, vomiting, diarrhea, dyspepsia, epigastric pain, anemia, injection site pain, agranulocytosis, hearing loss, tinnitus; renal and liver toxic; **Pregnancy category B**	Aspergillosis Cryptococcosis North American Blastomycosis Systemic candidiasis Coccidioidomycosis Histoplasmosis Zygomycosis (mucromycosis)
FLUCONAZOLE (Diflucan)	Synthetic triazole antifungal agent; selective inhibitor of fungal cytochrome P450; active against *Cryptococcus neoformans*, *Candida* species, *Aspergillus* species, *Coccidioides immitis*; action by inhibiting erosterol synthesis	po tablets, IV; renal excretion	Drug interactions with oral hypoglycemics, Coumarin type anticoagulants, phenytoin, cyclosporine, Rifampin, Theophylline; nausea, headache, skin rash, vomiting, abdominal pain, diarrhea, hepatotoxic; **Pregnancy category C**	Oropharyngeal and Esophageal Candidiasis Cryptooccal meningitis Fungal prophylaxis
FLUCYTOSINE (Ancobon)	Its active product, 5'-fluorodeoxyuridylic acid **inhibits thymidylate synthetase**; triphosphate-5-fluorouracil gets **incorporated into fungal RNA**; Amphotericin B and Flucytosine are synergists	**Prodrug:** flucytosine is converted to 5-fluorouracil which is then converted to 5'-fluoro-deoxyuridylic acid; AND flucytosine is converted to triphosphate-5-fluorouracil; good oral absorption; urine excretion (80% unchanged)	Rash, pruritus, photosensitivity, nausea, vomiting, abdominal pain, diarrhea, anorexia, dry mouth, renal toxic, aplastic anemia, thrombocytopenia; paresthesia, confusion; hepatotoxicity; **Pregnancy category C**	Candida Septicemia Endocarditis Urinary infection Cryptooccus Meningitis Pulmonary infection
GRISEOFULVIN (Fulvicin)	Binds to keratin in skin, nail, and hair; **blocks fungal mitosis** (binds microtubules and disrupts spindles)	**ORAL dose:** delayed onset	Oral thrush, nausea, vomiting, epigastric pain, diarrhea, headache, fatigue, insomnia, nephrosis, leukipenia, hepatotoxicity, GI bleeding and menstrual abnormalities are reported; **should NOT be used in pregnancy**	Oral antifungal agent used to dermatophytic infections only Tinea pedis Tinea cruris Tinea barbae Tinea capitis Tinea unguium NOT used for systemic infection

128

ANTIFUGALS:

DRUG	ORGAN SYSTEM EFFFECTS	KINETICS	ADVERSE EFFECTS	THERAPEUTIC USE
ITRACONAZOLE (Sporanox)	This triazole compound inhibits the cytochrome **P450** dependent synthesis of ergosterol, a vital fungal membrane component	Itraconazole and its metabolite, hydroxyitraconazole inhibit the cytochrome P450 system; not removed by dialysis; dosing po with food (increases bioavailability)	Nausea, vomiting, diarrhea, edema, fatigue, headache, HTN, rash, pruritus; **Contraindicated with Astemizole, Terfenadine and Cisapride,** may cause ventricular tachycardia and *torsades de pointes*; **Pregnancy category C**	Blastomycosis, Histoplasmosis, and Aspergillosis in patients intolerant of or refractory to amphotericin B
KETOCONAZOLE (Nizoral)	Imidazole that **blocks ergosterol synthesis**; Ketoconazole may be used for ALL fungal infections, but is a second line agent	Requires acidic medium for absorption; antacids, anti-cholinergics, and H2 blockers decrease absorption; used systemically if cannot use Amphotericin B or Amphotericin B with Flucytosine is not effective	Anti-androgenic effects: decreases testosterone synthesis, may cause gynecomastia; hepatotoxic; **safety in pregnancy is not known;** serious cardiac effects may occur if taken with Terfenadine (see Seldane) or Erythromycin	Blastomycosis Histoplasmosis Aspergillosis
MICONAZOLE (Micatin)	Synthetic imidazole derivative with effects similar to Ketoconazole	IV administration is highly toxic and thus reserved for only severe systemic fungal infections that fail Amphotericin B therapy	IV use may cause nausea, vomiting, anemia, anaphyloid reactive, phlebitis and hyponatremia	2nd line agent for systemic fungal infection
NYSTATIN (Mycostatin)	Oral or topical antifungal that binds ergosterol causing cell swelling and lysis	Available in suspension, tablets, pastilles, cream, ointment, powder, and vaginal tablets; not used intravenously	Virtually nontoxic and non-sensitizing; well tolerated by all age groups	Cutaneous and Mucocutaneous Mycotic Infections caused by *Candida albicans* and other Candida species

129

ANTIGLAUCOMA AGENTS:

AGENT	ORGAN SYSTEM EFFECTS	ADVERSE REACTIONS	THERAPEUTIC USE
ACETAZOLAMIDE (Diamox)	Inhibits carbonic anhydrase; controls fluid secretion in some types of glaucoma; a bacteriostatic sulfonamide; decreases intraocular pressure; diuretic action in conditions of fluid retention such as heart failure; available po and IV	Paresthesia, hearing dysfunction or tinnitus, loss of appetite, taste changes, GI upset; **Pregnancy category C**	Chronic Simple (Open Angle) Glaucoma Secondary Glaucoma Acute Mountain Sickness Adjunct for Edeme in Heart Failure Epilepsy
BETAXOLOL (Betoptic)	Beta-1-adrenergic blocker without significant membrane stabilizing activity and no intrinsic sympathomimetic action; given po will decrease cardiac output in healthy patients and those with impaired cardiac function; given topically in ophthalmic solution, Betaxolol reduces both elevated and normal intraocular pressures, with or without glaucoma	Local eye irritation, blurred vision, foreign body sensation, dry eye, ocular pain; systemic effects: bradycardia, dyspnea, bronchospasm, insomnia, dizziness, vertigo, headache, depression; safety in nursing mothers is not established (oral or ophthalmic); **Pregnancy category C**	Ocular Hypertension Chronic Open-Angle Glaucoma
BRIMONIDINE (Alphagan)	Alpha-2 adrenergic receptor agonist; peak ocular hypotensive effects within 2 hours; reduces aqueous humor production; increases uveoscleral outflow	Oral dryness, ocular hyperemia, burning, stinging, headache, blurring, foreign body sensation, fatigue, drowsiness, allergic reaction, ocular pruritus	Intraocular Pressure Elevation Open-angle Glaucoma Ocular Hypertension
CARBACHOL (Isopho Carbachol)	Direct-acting miotic agent that has parasympathetic (cholinergic) activity same as acetylcholine; onset of action within seconds when given as intraocular dose, within 10-20 minutes when used topically	Transient stinging, burning, tearing, corneal clouding, retinal detachment, ciliary and conjunctival injection, ciliary spasm, temporary decrease in visual acuity; **Pregnancy category C**	Intraocular Pressure Elevation in Glaucoma; Induces Miosis during surgery
CARTEOLOL (Ocupress)	Nonselective, beta-adrenergic blocker with intrinsic sympathomimetic activity; long acting beta blocker; no significant membrane stabilizing activity	Asthenia, muscle cramping; **Pregnancy category C**	Glaucoma
DEMECARIUM (Humoriol)	Indirect acting cholinesterase inhibitor; topical application to the eye produces miosis and muscle contraction	Iris cysts, burning, lacrimation, lid muscle twitching, conjunctival and ciliary redness, browache, headache, myopia with visual blurring; **Pregnancy category X**	Open-angle Glaucoma
DIPIVEFRIN (Propine)	A prodrug of epinephrine; hydrolysis of this drug yields epinephrine which decreases aqueous production and increases outflow	Burning, stinging, conjunctival injection; systemic effects may include tachycardia, arrhythmia, hypertension; **Pregnancy category B**	Chronic Open-angle Glaucoma
DORZOLAMIDE (Trusopt)	Carbonic anhydrase inhibitor for topical ophthalmic use; when applied topically, this agent reaches systemic circulation	Ocular burning, stinging, bitter taste, blurred vision, tearing, dryness, photophobia; **Pregnancy category C**	Elevated Intraocular Pressure Open-angle Glaucoma

130

ANTIGLAUCOMA AGENTS:

AGENT	ORGAN SYSTEM EFFECTS	ADVERSE REACTIONS	THERAPEUTIC USE
ECHOTHIOPHATE (Phospholine Iodide)	Indirect acting cholinesterase inhibitor; topical application to the eye produces miosis and muscle contraction	Iris cysts, burning, lacrimation, lid muscle twitching, conjunctival and ciliary redness, browache, headache, myopia with visual blurring; **Pregnancy category C**	Open-angle Glaucoma
LATANOPROST (Xalatan)	Prostaglandin $F_{2\alpha}$ analog thought to reduce intraocular pressure by increasing flow of aqueous humor; absorption occurs through the cornea; hydrolysis of this prodrug forms the active metabolite	Blurred vision, burning, stinging, conjunctival hyperemia, foreign body sensation, itching, dry eye, tearing, eye pain, lid crusting, lid edema, lid erythema, photophobia; **Pregnancy category C**	Elevated Intraocular Pressure
LEVOBUNOLOL (AKBeta, Betagan Liquifilm))	Nonselective beta adrenergic blocker used in glaucoma; action is thought to be reduction of aqueous production	Transient irritation, burning, tearing, conjunctival hyperemia, edema, blepharitis, blurred vision, browache, photophobia; **Pregnancy category C**	Chronic Open-angle Glaucoma
METIPRANOLOL (OptiPranolol)	Nonselective beta adrenergic blocker used in glaucoma; action is thought to be reduction of aqueous production	Transient irritation, burning, tearing, conjunctival hyperemia, edema, blepharitis, blurred vision, browache, photophobia; **Pregnancy category C**	Chronic Open-angle Glaucoma
PHYSOSTIGMINE (Eserine)	Indirect acting cholinesterase inhibitor; topical application to the eye produces miosis and muscle contraction	Iris cysts, burning, lacrimation, lid muscle twitching, conjunctival and ciliary redness, browache, headache, myopia with visual blurring; **Pregnancy category C**	Open-angle Glaucoma
PILOCARPINE (Pilocar)	Cholinergic parasympathomimetic agent with muscarinic action; stimulates sweat, salivary, lacrimal, gastric, pancreatic, and intestinal glands; ophthalmic use causes miosis, spasm of accomodation, and decrease in intraocular pressure	Local eye irritation, blurred vision, lacrimation; **Pregnancy category C**	Glaucoma
TIMOLOL (Timoptic)	Non-selective beta-adrenergic receptor blocker; topical application in the eye reduces elevated as well as normal intraocular pressures	Ocular irritation, conjunctivitis, blepharitis, keratitis, decreased corneal sensation, diplopia, ptosis; **Pregnancy category C**	Ocular Hypertension Open Angle Glaucoma

131

ANTIGOUT AGENTS:

DRUG	ORGAN SYSTEM EFFECTS	ADVERSE REACTIONS	THERAPEUTIC USE
ALLOPURINOL (Zyloprim)	**Xanthine oxidase inhibitor;** decreases uric acid; hypoxanthine and xanthine shunt back, and are more soluble than uric acid	Safe drug; some drug interactions; skin rash (exfoliative dermatitis); kidney failure (rare); **Pregnancy category C**	Hyperuricemia Gout
COLCHICINE alkaloid	**Resolves acute gouty arthritis; NOT** anti-inflammatory; NOT cyclooxygenase inhibitor; NO effect on uric acid or its handling; 1 tablet per day is prophylactic	Diarrhea, headache, dizziness, nausea, vomiting; **teratogenic** effects; contraindicated in pregnancy	Acute Gouty Arthritis Gout Prophylaxis
PROBENECID (Benemid)	**Uricosuric** (blocks uric acid reabsorption) and renal tubular blocking agent; inhibits tubular secretion of penicillin and increases plasma levels of penicillin; inhibits renal transport of several other compounds; **NOT** antiinflammatory	Headache, dizziness, may precipitate acute gouty arthritis, hepatic necrosis, nausea, vomiting, anorexia, sore gums, nephrotic syndrome, urticaria, pruritus, aplastic anemia, dermatitis, alopecia, flushing; crosses placenta and appears in umbilical cord blood; safety in pregnancy not established	Hyperuricemia Gout Gouty Arthritis Adjuvant to many penicillin antibiotics
SULFINPYRAZONE (Anturane)	Uricosuric agent which potentiates urine excretion of uric acid; reduces blood urate levels in patients with chronic tophaceous gout and acute intermittent gout, and promotes resorption of tophi	Upper GI disturbances, blood dyscrasiea; safety in pregnancy and lactation not established	Chronic Gouty Arthritis Intermittent Gouty Arthritis

132

ANTIHISTAMINES, SYSTEMIC:

DRUG	MECHANISM OF ACTION	KINETICS	ADVERSE EFFECTS	USES
ASTEMIZOLE (Hismanal)	Long acting histamine H1 receptor antagonist; best used as prophylactic antihistamine and not as an "as needed" agent	Does NOT cross BBB 2-3 day duration	**Contraindicated with Erythromycin and Ketoconazole** because may lead to QT prolongation and ventricular arrhythmias including torsades de pointes; drowsiness, fatigue, increased appetite, weight increase, dry mouth; **Pregnancy category C**	Seasonal Allergic Rhinitis Chronic Idiopathic Urticaria
AZATADINE (Optimine)	Competitive H1 receptor antagonist; moderate antihistaminic activity; moderate sedation; moderate anticholinergic activity	bid dosage	Sedation, rash, palpitation, bradycardia, tachycardia, dizziness, epigastric distress; **Pregnancy category B**	Seasonal Allergy
BROMPHENIRAMINE (Dimetane)	H1 receptor antagonist; high antihistaminic activity; low sedation; moderate anticholinergic effects	tid/qid dosage	See Diphenhydramine; **Pregnancy category C**	Seasonal Allergy
CETIRIZINE (Zyrtec)	Orally active selective H1 receptor antagonist; primary action on peripheral H1 receptors; does not prolong the QTc interval on ECG	Human metabolite of Hydroxyzine; peak plasma levels within 1 hour; 93% plasma protein binding	Somnolence, fatigue, dry mouth, pharyngitis, dizziness, diarrhea, nausea, vomiting; **Pregnancy category B**; no interactions with Theophylline, Azithromycin, Pseudoephedrine, Ketoconazole or Erythromycin	Seasonal Allergic Rhinitis Perennial Allergic Rhinitis Chronic Urticaria
CHLORPHENIRAMINE (Chlor-Trimenton)	Alkylamine that is competitive, reversible H1 blocker; alkylamine; same as effects as Diphenhydramine	See Diphendyramine and Dimenhydrinate	See Diphenhydramine; **Pregnancy category B**	Acute Type I Hypersensitivity
CLEMASTINE (Tavist)	Competitive H1 receptor antagonist; high anticholinergic and antiemetic effects	bid dosage	See Diphenhydramine; **Pregnancy category B**	Seasonal Allergy
CYCLIZINE (Marezine)	Piperazine that is competitive, reversible H1 blocker; same as Diphenhydramine	See Diphenhydramine and Dimenhydrinate	See Diphenhydramine; **Pregnancy category B**	Acute Type I Hypersensitivity Sedation Motion Sickness
CYPROHEPTADINE (Periactin)	Piperidine that is competitive, reversible H1 blocker; same as Diphenhydramine; moderate antihistaminic and antiemetic action	tid dosage	See Diphenhydramine; **Pregnancy category B**	Seasonal Allergy

133

ANTIHISTAMINES, SYSTEMIC:

DRUG	MECHANISM OF ACTION	KINETICS	ADVERSE EFFECTS	USES
DEXCHLOR-PHANIRAMINE (Polaramine)	Alkylamine that is competitive, reversible H1 blocker with high antihistaminic activity; moderate antiemetic activity	tid/qid dosage	See Diphenhydramine; **Pregnancy category B**	Seasonal Allergy
DIMENHYDRINATE (Dramamine)	Aminoalkylether that is competitive, reversible H1 blocker; no significant H2 effects; no effect on synthesis, release or metabolism of histamine	Good GI absorption; effects begin within 30 minutes, peak 1-2 hrs after dose	See Diphenhydramine; **Pregnancy category B**	Motion Sickness Sedation Acute Type I Hypersensitivity Antimuscarinic
DIPHENHYDRAMINE (Benadryl)	Aminoalkylether that is competitive, reversible H1 blocker; anti-muscarinic; local anesthetic; aminoalkylether	ORAL; 30 min to onset; 4-6 hour duration; metabolized by DMMS	Sedation; may see agitation, nervousness, delirium, tremors, incoordination, hallucinations, convulsions; anorexia, diarrhea or constipation, epigastric pain; **Pregnancy category B**	Acute Type I Hypersensitivity Sedation Antimuscarinic Motion Sickness
FEXOFENADINE (Allegra)	Selective peripheral histamine H1 receptor antagonist, a metabolite of Terfenadine; **NO interaction with Erythromycin or Ketoconazole**	Max plasma levels within 2.5 hours; 60-70% plasma protein bound	Dysmenorrhea, drowsiness, dyspepsia, fatigue; **Pregnancy category C**; does NOT prolong QTc interval on electrocardiogram (see Terfenadine)	Seasonal Allergic Rhinitis
PHENINDAMINE (Nolahist)	Piperadine that is a competitive, reversible H1 blocker; moderate antihistaminic and anticholinergic effects	tid/qid dosage	See Diphendyramine	Seasonal Allergy
TRIPELENNAMINE (PBZ)	Ethylenediamine that is a competitive, reversible H1 blocker; moderate antihistaminic and sedative activity	tid/qid dosage	See Diphenhydramine	Seasonal Allergy
LORATADINE (Claritin)	Long acting tricyclic antihistamine with selective peripheral histamine H1 receptor antagonistic activity	Does NOT cross BBB; 12-15 hour duration	Changes in blood pressure, palpitations, tachycardia, hyperkinesia, paresthesia, dizziness, migraine, tremor, vertigo, dysphonia, GI discomfort, nausea, vomiting, flatulence, anxiety, agitation, insomnia, menorrhagia, dysmenorrhea; **Pregnancy category B**	Seasonal Allergic Rhinitis

134

ANTIHISTAMINES, SYSTEMIC:

DRUG	MECHANISM OF ACTION	KINETICS	ADVERSE EFFECTS	USES
MECLIZINE (Antivert)	Piperazine that is competitive, reversible H1 blocker; same as Diphenhydramine	taken every 4-6 hours	Drowsiness, dry mouth; **Pregnancy category B**	Motion Sickness Vertigo
PROMETHAZINE (Phenergan)	Phenothiazine that is competitive, reversible H1 blocker	Oral, IV, IM	Drowsiness, dizziness, tinnitus, incoordination, fatigue, blurred vision, euphoria, tremors, changes in blood pressure and heart rate; **Pregnancy category C**	Motion Sickness Nausea, Vomiting Sedation Potentiates Opiate Analgesia
PYRILAMINE *(Various)*	H1 histamine receptor antagonist; structural class is ethylenediamine	tid/qid dosage	See Diphenhydramine	Seasonal Allergic Rhinitis
TERFENADINE (Seldane)	Non-sedating H1 blocker	Does NOT cross BBB; duration of action is 8-12 hours; onset of action within 1-2 hours	**Contraindicated** with **Erythromycin** and **Ketoconazole** because may lead to QT prolongation and ventricular arrhythmias including torsades de pointes; **Pregnancy category C**	Seasonal Allergic Rhinitis Sneezing Rhinorrhea Pruritus Lacrimation

135

ANTIHISTAMINES, TOPICAL:

AGENT	ORGAN SYSTEM EFFECTS	PHARMACOKINETICS	ADVERSE REACTIONS	THERAPEUTIC USE
AZELASTINE (Astelin)	H1 receptor antagonist	Intranasal dosage; systemic bioavailability is 40%; peak plasma levels within 2-3 hours	Bitter taste, headache, somnolence, nasal burning, pharyngitis, dry mouth, sneezing, rhinitis, dizziness; **Pregnancy category C**	Allergic Rhinitis
DIPHENHYDRAMINE (Benadryl Cream)	Aminoalkylether that is competitive, reversible **H1 blocker**; antimuscarinic; local anesthetic (like quinidine); aminoalkylether	1% and 2% cream available for topical application	Systemic absorption may cause sedation; agitation, nervousness, delirium, tremor, incoordination, hallucinations, convulsions; anorexia, nausea, vomiting, diarrhea or constipation, epigastric pain	Acute Type I allergy Local Anesthetic

136

ANTIHYPERTENSIVES:

DRUG	ORGAN SYSTEM EFFECTS	PHARMACOKINETICS	ADVERSE REACTIONS	THERAPEUTIC USE
BENAZEPRIL (Lotensin)	ACE inhibitor; see Captopril	Daily or twice daily oral dosage	Headache, dizziness, fatigue, GI upset, cough, angioedema, orthostatic hypotension, hyperkalemia; **Pregnancy category C (1st trimester) and D (2nd and 3rd trimester)**	Hypertension
CAPTOPRIL (Capoten)	**ACE** inhibitor; decreases PAR; decreases BP; slight to no change in CO; metabolized to inactive product; **inhibits metabolism of bradykinin (a vasodilator)**	Moderate oral bioavailability (35-75%); rate of absorption ↓ by food (captopril especially); 15 minutes to onset; **ALL long acting (up to 24 hours)**; elimination 40-50% in urine, 50-60% in feces	Hypotension (1st dose phenomena, just stop diuretic); transient increased BUN and creatinine; CNS: headache, dizziness, nausea and vomiting; GI: diarrhea, abdominal pain, **dysgeusia** (decreased taste acuity, captopril ONLY); **cough**	Hypertension Heart Failure
CLONIDINE (Catapres)	Central acting selective α2 agonist; same as methyldopa; **decreases HR; increases plasma volume**; NOT used IV because may stimulate peripheral α1 receptors causing hypertension	GOOD oral bioavailability; oral and **transdermal** use; 30-60 minutes to onset; 12-24 hour duration	Same as methyldopa; **constipation**; dermatologic reactions; NO lupus-like syndrome; NO positive Coombs	Hypertension (used with diuretic)
DIAZOXIDE (Hyperstat)	Direct acting arterial vasodilator; structurally related to thiazide diuretics, but NO diuretic activity	**Used IV for acute HTN crisis**, 1-2 mins to onset, 3-8 hour duration; used p.o. for chronic hypoglycemia	Hypokalemia; hyperuricemia; **hyperglycemia**	Hypertension (IV); Hypoglycemia (p.o.)
DILTIAZEM (Cardizem SR) benzothiazepine	**Calcium channel blocker vasodilator**; block voltage dependent calcium channels in cardiac tissue and arterial and venous vascular smooth m.; dilates coronary a. and arterioles; inhibit coronary a. spasm; decreases contractility; **slows AV conduction, increases ERP, decreases SAN automaticity**; metabolized to **desacetyl-diltiazem** (active)	Ca^{++} **channel blockers**: LOW bioavailability, HIGH 1st pass effect; ALL used orally for HTN; rapid onset (20-45 mins) $t\frac{1}{2}$ = 2-4 hours; HIGH plasma protein binding; ALL eliminated through kidney; available in SR	**Calcium channel blockers**: peripheral edema; hypotension; palpitations; dizziness, headache; constipation, nausea, abdominal cramping	Hypertension Angina Arrhythmia

137

ANTIHYPERTENSIVES:

DRUG	ORGAN SYSTEM EFFECTS	PHARMACOKINETICS	ADVERSE REACTIONS	THERAPEUTIC USE
DOXAZOSIN (Cardura)	Selective alpha-1 adrenergic blocker	Daily oral dosing	Syncope, dizziness, somnolence, fatigue, malaise, edema, rhinitis, abnormal vision, tinnitus, epistaxis, orthostatic hypotension, sexual dysfunction, polyuria, urinary incontinence, ataxia, leukopenia, neutropenia, arrhythmia; **Pregnancy category C**	Hypertension
ENALAPRIL (Vasotec)	ACE inhibitor; metabolized to **enalaprilat** (active); more potent than captopril	1 hour to onset; **prodrug**; longer acting than captopril	Less side effects than Captopril	Hypertension Heart Failure
FELODIPINE (Plendil)	Dihydropyridine calcium channel blocker vasodilator; slight increase in cardiac output	2 hours to onset; t½ = 11-16 hours; 99% plasma protein bound	Decreased cardiac contractility and cardiac output; cardiac slowing and heart block may precipitate heart failure	Vasopastic Angina
FOSINAPRIL (Monopril)	ACE inhibitor; metabolized to **fosinoprilat** (active)	1 hour to onset; **prodrug**	Headache, cough, dizziness, GI upset, hyperkalemia, orthostatic hypotension, angioneurotic edema; **Pregnancy category C (1st trimester) and D (2nd and 3rd trimester)**	Hypertension Heart Failure
GUANABENZ (Wytensin)	Central acting selective α2 agonist; same as methyldopa; **decreases HR; decreases plasma renin activity (PRA)**	60 minutes to onset; 6-12 hour duration	NO edema	Hypertension
GUANADREL (Hylorel)	Adrenergic neuronal blocking agent; similar mechanism to Guanethidine	Good GI absorption; does not readily enter CNS	Similar side effect profile as Guanethidine, but less diarrhea, hypotension and impaired ejaculation	Hypertension
GUANETHIDINE (Ismelin)	Displaces norepinephrine from terminal neuronal storage vesicles thereby decreasing its availability for neuronal release	Incomplete GI absorption; 40% metabolized to inactive metabolites; urine excretion	Orthostatic hypotension, dizziness, weakness, lassitude, syncope, bradycardia, diarrhea, inhibition of ejaculation, fluid retention, edema	Hypertension
GUANFACINE (Tenex)	Central acting selective α2 agonist; **decreases plasma renin activity**	30 minutes to onset; 12-24 hour duration	Dry mouth, sedation, asthenia, dizziness, NO edema; **Pregnancy category B**	Hypertension

138

ANTIHYPERTENSIVES:

DRUG	ORGAN SYSTEM EFFECTS	PHARMACOKINETICS	ADVERSE REACTIONS	THERAPEUTIC USE
HYDRALAZINE (Apresoline)	**Direct acting arterial vasodilator; EDRF (nitric oxide free radical)** is proposed mechanism; sodium and water retention	Oral bioavailability 30-50% (need high mg dose); HIGH plasma protein binding (90%); biotransformed by **acetylation**; plasma levels are widely variable	High drug-drug interaction; **fluid retention**; Common: headache; nausea and vomiting; dizziness; **tachycardia;** Less common: anginal pain, nasal congestion, **lupus-like syndrome**	Hypertension (used with diuretic)
ISRADIPINE (DynaCirc)	Dihydropyridine calcium channel blocker vasodilator; slight increase in cardiac output	2 hours to onset	Decreased cardiac contractility and cardiac output; cardiac slowing and heart block may precipitate heart failure	Vasospastic Angina
LABETOLOL (Trandate)	Non-selective ß blocker, selective α1 blocker; **decreases TPR; decreases HR; decreases renin** activity; **increases plasma volume** → use with diuretic; action is similar to Propranolol + Prazosin	High first pass effect, only 25% bioavailability	**Fluid retention**	Hypertension (used with diuretic)
LOSARTAN (Cozaar)	Highly selective **angiotensin II receptor antagonist;** directly inhibits binding of angiotensin II to AT1 receptor; affinity much greater for AT1 than AT2 receptor; no significant effect on heart rate	Once a day tablets	Dizziness, insomnia, muscle cramps, leg pain, upper respiratory effects, GI upset; **Pregnancy category C (1st trimester) and D (2nd and 3rd trimesters)**	Hypertension
LISINOPRIL (Privinil, Zestril)	ACE inhibitor; metabolized to **lisinoprilat**	1 hour to onset	Dizziness, headache, fatigue, diarrhea, cough, nausea, hyperkalemia, orthostatic hypotension, renal impairment, angioedema; **Pregnancy category C (1st trimester) and D (2nd and 3rd trimesters)**	Hypertension
MECAMYLAMINE (Inversine)	Ganglionic blocking agent that reduces ganglionic transmission in both sympathetic and parasympathetic autonomic nervous systems	Onset within 1.5-2 hours; duration 6-12 hours	Ileus, constipation, nausea, vomiting, anorexia, glossitis, dry mouth, orthostatic dizziness, postural hypotension, convulsions, mental aberration, tremor, paresthesias, pulmonary edema and fibrosis, urinary retention, impotence, decreased libido, blurred vision, dilated pupils, weakness, fatigue, sedation; **Pregnancy category C**	Essential Hypertension

139

ANTIHYPERTENSIVES:

DRUG	ORGAN SYSTEM EFFECTS	PHARMACOKINETICS	ADVERSE REACTIONS	THERAPEUTIC USE
METHYLDOPA (Aldomet) prodrug	**Central acting selective α2 agonist**; act at solitary tract nucleus to decreases activity of vasomotor center which decreases sympathetic tone and increases vagal tone; **decreaes PVR; increases plasma volume** → use with diuretic	LOW oral bioavailability; ORAL dosage; IV use in emergency; MUST metabolize to **methyl-norepinephrine**; 120 minutes to onset; 12-24 hour duration; **prodrug**	<u>CNS:</u> sedation, dizziness, headache; <u>CVS:</u> **bradycardia, edema;** xerostomia; <u>Other:</u> drug fever, lupus-like syndrome; **pos Coombs test**	Hypertension (used with diuretic)
METOPROLOL (Lopressor)	Selective ß1 > ß2 blocker; ↓ **renin release;** no intrinsic sympathomimetic activity (ISA); weak membrane stabilizing activity (MSA)	Rapid and complete GI absorption; high first pass effect; urine excretion	LESS likely to cause bronchoconstriction than Propranolol	Essential Hypertension Angina; post-MI
METYROSINE (Demser)	α-methylated derivative of tyrosine; competitive inhibitor of tyrosine hydroxylase; decreases formation of endogenous epinephrine and norepinephrine	30% GI absorption; metabolized to Methyldopa; urine excretion	Sedation, extrapyramidal symptoms, anxiety, depression, nausea, vomiting, diarrhea, abdominal pain, nasal stuffiness; **Pregnancy category C**	Hypertension
MINOXIDIL (Loniten) prodrug	Direct acting arterial vasodilator; MORE potent than hydralazine	**Prodrug,** HIGH oral bio-availability; NO significant plasma protein binding (10-15%); inactivated through conjugation	**Fluid retention; hypertrichosis** (increased hair growth); tachycardia; ECG changes; pericardial effusions; pericarditis	Hypertension (used with diuretic)
MOEXIPRIL (Univasc)	ACE inhibitor; see Captopril	Daily or twice daily oral dosage	Cough, dizziness, diarrhea, flu syndrome fatigue, pharyngitis, flushing, rash, myalgia; **Pregnancy category C (1st trimester) and D (2nd and 3rd trimesters)**	Hypertension
NICARDIPINE (Cardene)	Dihydropyridine calcium channel blocker vasodilator; slight increase in cardiac output	t½ = 2-4 hours	See Diltiazem	Vasospastic Angina
NIFEDIPINE (Procardia)	Dihydropyridine calcium channel blocker vasodilator; slight increase in cardiac output; available in sustained release (SR)	t½ = 2-4 hours	See Diltiazem	Vasospastic Angina
NITROGLYCERIN	Direct acting arterial AND venous vasodilator; used IV for controlled hypotension	**IV dose for Hypertensive Crisis**	Throbbing headache, facial flushing, dizziness are common; postural hypotension; nausea, vomiting when given po	Hypertensive Crisis Angina pectoris Congestive Heart Failure (CHF)

140

ANTIHYPERTENSIVES:

DRUG	ORGAN SYSTEM EFFECTS	PHARMACOKINETICS	ADVERSE REACTIONS	THERAPEUTIC USE
NITROPRUSSIDE	Direct acting arterial **AND venous vasodilator**; used IV for Hypertensive crisis; generates nitric oxide free radical	Rapid onset (15-30 sec), short duration (5 mins); converted to cyanide by erythrocytes; CN metabolized by liver **rhodanase** to SCN; light sensitive	**Cyanide toxicity** in overdose and in malnourished patients	Hypertensive Crisis (IV)
PRAZOSIN (Minipress)	Peripheral acting **α1 > α2 blocker**; decreases arterial resistance; decreases venous tone; mild tachycardia; hypotension (orthostatic); **1st dose phenomena**	Active metabolite; t½ = 2-3 hours; excretion in **feces** (90%) and urine (10%)	<u>CNS</u>: dizziness, headache, drowsiness, asthenia (muscle weakness) <u>CVS</u>: palpitations <u>Other</u>: nasal stuffiness	Hypertension
PROPRANOLOL (Inderal)	Noncardioselective ß blocker; **decreases renin release**	See β adrenergic blockers	Heart failure, hypotension, bronchospasm, bradycardia, heart block, fatigue, dizziness, depression, GI upset, pharyngitis, agranulocytosis; **Pregnancy category C**	Hypertension
QUINAPRIL (Accupril)	**ACE inhibitor**; decreases PAR; decreases BP; slight to no change in cardiac output	Daily or twice daily po dosage	Headache, dizziness, fatigue, cough, GI upset, hyperkalemia, back pain, tachycardia, dry mouth, somnolence, sweating, sinusitis; **Pregnancy category C (1st trimester) and D (2nd and 3rd trimesters)**	Hypertension
RESERPINE (Diupres)	Adrenergic neuronal blocker; irreversibly blocks **Mg^{2+} ATPase on NE storage vesicles**	Days to onset; used in small dose and with other agents	Serious side reactions; high incidence of depression with chronic use; **Pregnancy category C**	Refractory Hypertension
RAMIPRIL (Altace)	ACE inhibitor; see Captopril	Onset of action within 1 hour; rate of absorption decreased by food	Headache, dizziness, fatigue, cough, GI upset, hyperkalemia, back pain, tachycardia, dry mouth, somnolence, sweating, siusitis, impotence, neutropenia; **Pregnancy category C (1st trimester) and D (2nd and 3rd trimesters)**	Hypertension Heart Failure

ANTIHYPERTENSIVES:

DRUG	ORGAN SYSTEM EFFECTS	PHARMACOKINETICS	ADVERSE REACTIONS	THERAPEUTIC USE
TERAZOSIN (Hytrin)	Peripheral acting α1 > α2 blocker; same as prazosin just longer duration	90% oral bioavailability; NO active metabolite; t½ = 9-12 hours; excretion in **feces** (60%) and urine (40%)	Syncope, dizziness, somnolence, asthenia, nausea, nasal congestion, palpitations, orthostatic hypotension, blurred vision, peripheral edema; **Pregnancy category C**	Hypertension
VALSARTAN (Diovan)	Highly selective **angiotensin II receptor antagonist**; directly inhibits binding of angiotensin II to AT1 receptor; affinity much greater for AT1 than AT2 receptor; no significant effect on heart rate	Peak plasma levels within 2-4 hours; food decreases absorption; 85% excreted in feces	Headache, dizziness, dry cough, diarrhea; dry mouth; may cause fetal or neonatal injury when taken during 2nd or 3rd trimesters; **Pregnancy category C (first trimester) and D (second and third trimesters)**	Hypertension
VERAPAMIL (Calan SR) (Isoptin SR)	Diphenylalkylamine; Ca++ channel blocker vasodilator; slows AV conduction; prolongs ERP in AVN; decreases automaticity of SAN; available in SR	Dealkylated to **norverapamil** (active)	Constipation, dizziness, nausea, hypotension, headache, edema, AV block, bradycardia, CHF, fatigue, dyspnea, rash, flushing, elevated liver enzymes, paralytic ileus; **Pregnancy category C**	Hypertension

Abbreviations:

PVR - peripheral vascular resistance
PRA - plasma renin activity
Coombs test - an indicator of hemolytic anemia
EDRF - endothelial derived relaxing factor
ERP - effective refractory period
SR - sustained release
PAR - peripheral arterial resistance

General: **Decreased PVR:**   **Dihydropyridines > Verapamil > Diltiazem**
       Cardiac Effect: **Verapamil > Diltiazem > Dihydropyridines**

Antihypertensive agents that should be used with a diuretic (2° to fluid retention):
   Clonidine
   Hydralazine
   Labetalol
   Methyldopa
   Minoxidil

ANTIINFLAMMATORY AGENTS, BOWEL:

AGENT	ORGAN SYSTEM EFFECTS	PHARMACOKINETICS	ADVERSE REACTIONS	THERAPEUTIC USE
MESALAMINE (Asacol)	Antiinflammatory agent; Sulfasalazine is converted to Sulfapyridine and Mesalamine by bacteria in colon; mechanism of Mesalamine is not known but appears to be topical rather than systemic	Asacol tablets have acrylic based resin to delay release of agent until the terminal ileum and beyond	Diarrhea, exacerbated colitis, dizziness, nausea, joint pain, headache, rash, lethargy, constipation, dry mouth, malaise, lower back discomfort, dyspepsia, vomiting; **Pregnancy category B**	Ulcerative Colitis
OLSALAZINE (Dipentum)	Sodium salt of a salicylate; converted to 5-aminosalicylic acid (5-ASA); antiinflammatory activity in ulcerative colitis	Limited systemic bioavailability; peak plasma levels within 1 hour; >99% plasma protein bound	Diarrhea, abdominal pain, rash, itching, insomnia, dizziness; **Pregnancy category C**	Ulcerative Colitis
SULFASALAZINE (Azulfidine)	Metabolized to 5-aminosalicylic acid (5-ASA) and Sulfapyridine by colonic bacteria	1/3 of given dose is absorbed in small intestine; 2/3 of dose reaches colon and it metabolized	Anorexia, headache, nausea, vomiting, gastric upset, reversible **oligospermia**, rash, pruritus, urticaria, fever, blood dyscrasia, Stevens Johnson syndrome; **Pregnancy category B**	Ulcerative Colitis

143

ANTIINFLAMMATORY AGENTS, SYSTEMIC:

S/E Cox-1
upper GI - dyspepsia & ulceration
lower GI - diarrhea, ulceration, hemorrhage

AGENT	ORGAN SYSTEM EFFECTS	ADVERSE REACTIONS	THERAPEUTIC USE
ASPIRIN ASA	**Analgesic; antipyretic; antiinflammatory;** mechanism of action is cyclooxygenase inhibition; **acetylation of platelets and decreases platelet aggregation;** NO known CV effects; GI ulceration due to decreased PG synthesis and salicylic acid is irritating (superficial erosions); **increases bleeding time,** NO effect on prothrombin time; uricosuric; potent platelet inhibitor	GI irritation (15%); frank ulcer (1%); Reye's syndrome in children following febrile, viral infection; increased bleeding time; small child poisoning (acidosis) - lose K⁺ eventually ↑ respiration Vasodilation peripheral uricosuric	Antipyretic - only in febril pts Analgesic - mild - moderate Antiinflammatory → high dose → rheumatoid Arth. (of skeletal origin)
DICLOFENAC (Voltaren, Cataflam)	Analgesic; antipyretic; antiinflammatory; increases platelet aggregation time, no effect on bleeding time, no clinically evident effect on PT/PTT; **prostaglandin synthetase inhibitor**	Nausea, dyspepsia, diarrhea, **peptic ulceration, GI bleeding;** LFT elevation; hypersensitivity; fluid retention and edema; all NSAIDs have been associated with reduced renal blood flow and renal papillary necrosis in elederly; should be avoided in hepatic porphyria, **Pregnancy category B;** tinnitus in 3-9%	Rheumatoid Arthritis Osteoarthritis Ankylosing Spondylitis Dysmenorrhea
DIFLUNISAL (Dolobid)	Non-steroidal drug with analgesic, antiinflammatory and antipyretic effects; peripherally acting non-narcotic; exact mechanism of action is unknown; Diflunisal is a prostaglandin synthetase inhibitor; complete po absorption; peak plasma levels within 2-3 hours; urine excretion	Nausea, vomiting, dyspepsia, gastrointestinal pain, diarrhea, constipation, rash, headache; associated with gastric and duodenal ulcer; **Pregnancy category C**	Mild to moderate pain Osteoarthritis Rheumatoid arthritis
ETODOLAC (Lodine)	Analgesic; antiinflammatory: inhibits prostaglandin synthesis	Dyspepsia (10%); GI ulceration and bleeding; caution in impaired renal function, heart failure, and hepatic dysfunction; false-positive urine bilirubin and/or ketone; pregnancy category C	Osteoarthritis Pain management
FENOPROFEN (Nalfon)	Non-steroidal anti-inflammatory drug with anti-inflammatory, analgesic and antipyretic actions; inhibits prostaglandin synthesis; peak effect occurs within 1-2 hours	Dyspepsia, abdominal pain, diarrhea, flatulence, nausea; associated with gastric and duodenal ulcer; malaise, dizziness; pruritus; rash; blurred vision, tinnitus; **Pregnancy category C**	Osteoarthritis Rheumatoid Arthritis Pain management
FLURBIPROFEN (Ansaid)	Nonsteroidal antiinflammatory agent with analgesic and antipyretic properties; potent prostaglandin synthesis inhibitor; well absorbed after oral dosage; peak plasma levels within 1.5 hours; >99% plasma protein bound; primary excretion is via urine	Dyspepsia, diarrhea, abdominal pain, nausea, headache, edema, signs and symptoms of urinary tract infection, nervousness, anxiety, rhinitis, rash; **Pregnancy category B**	Rheumatoid Arthritis Osteoarthritis

144

ANTIINFLAMMATORY AGENTS, SYSTEMIC:

AGENT	ORGAN SYSTEM EFFECTS	ADVERSE REACTIONS	THERAPEUTIC USE
IBUPROFEN (Advil, Motrin)	Non-steroidal antiinflammatory drug with analgesic and antipyretic properties; inhibits prostaglandin synthesis; analgesic effect is greater than its antiinflammatory effect	Nausea, epigastric pain, heartburn; associated with gastric and duodenal ulcer; dizziness, rash	Osteoarthritis Rheumatoid arthritis Mild to moderate pain Primary dysmenorrhea
INDOMETHACIN (Indocin)	Nonsteroidal antiinflammatory agent with analgesic and antipyretic action; potent prostaglandin synthesis inhibitor; peak plasma levels within 2 hours; 90% dose absorption by mouth within 4 hours; 99% plasma protein bound	Nausea, dyspepsia, dizziness, diarrhea, abdominal pain, constipation, headache, vertigo, somnolence, depression, fatigue, tinnitus; **not recommended in 3rd trimester of pregnancy or nursing mothers**	Rheumatoid Arthritis Ankylosing Spondylitis Osteoarthritis Acute Painful Shoulder Acute Gouty Arthritis
KETOPROFEN (Orudis, Oruvail)	Nonsteroidal antiinflammatory drug with analgesic and antipyretic properties; inhibits prostaglandin and leukotriene synthesis; rapid and complete absorption; peak plasma levels within 0.5-2 hours; > 99% plasma protein bound; Oruvail is controlled release preparation (not for acute pain relief or control)	Dyspepsia, nausea, abdominal pain, diarrhea, constipation, flatulence, headache, rash, tinnitus, dizziness, increased BUN, risk of GI ulceration and perforation; **Pregnancy category B**	Rheumatoid Arthritis Osteoarthritis
KETOROLAC (Toradol)	Non-steroidal antiinflammatory drug with analgesic and antipyretic properties; inhibits prostaglandin synthesis; efficacy comparable to opioid analgesics; 99% plasma protein bound; peak plasma level IM within 50 minutes and po within 45 minutes; only NSAID available po, IM, and IV; dose adjustments must be made in elderly and in those with renal impairment	Nausea (12%), dyspepsia (12%), gastrointestinal pain (13%); headache (17%); edema, pruritus, diarrhea, drowsiness, dizziness; associated with gastric and duodenal ulcer; **Pregnancy category C**	Short term management of pain (less than 5 days)
MECLOFENAMATE	Non-steroidal antiinflammatory agent; anthranilic acid derivative; also competes for binding at the prostaglandin receptor site	Use limited to less than one week because of possible serious GI toxicity, nephrotoxicity, hemolytic anemia, and bone marrow hypoplasia	Analgesia Dysmenorrhea Osteoarthritis/Rheumatoid Arthritis
NABUMETONE (Relafen)	Antiinflammatory; analgesic; antipyretic; metabolite, 6MNA, is potent inhibitor of prostaglandin synthesis; **prodrug** metabolized by liver to 6-methoxy-2-naphthylacetic acid (6MNA) which is active; po dosing	Diarrhea (14%), dyspepsia (13%), abdominal pain (12%), constipation, flatulence, nausea, positive stool guaiac, pruritus, rash, tinnitus, edema (3-9%), **GI ulceration and bleeding with chronic use; Pregnancy category C**	Osteoarthritis Rheumatoid arthritis

145

ANTIINFLAMMATORY AGENTS, SYSTEMIC:

AGENT	ORGAN SYSTEM EFFECTS	ADVERSE REACTIONS	THERAPEUTIC USE
NAPROXEN (Naprosyn, Anaprox, Aleve)	Non-steroidal antiinflammatory drug with analgesic and antipyretic activities; rapid and complete gastro-intestinal absorption; peak plasma levels within 2-4 hours	Constipation, heartburn, abdominal pain, nausea; headache, dizziness, drowsiness; skin eruptions, ecchymoses; tinnitus; edema, dyspnea; associated with gastric and duodenal ulcer; **Pregnancy category B**	Rheumatoid arthritis Osteoarthritis; Juvenile arthritis Ankylosing spondylitis Tendinitis; Bursitis Acute gout Mild to moderate pain Primary dysmenorrhea
OXAPROZIN (Daypro)	Nonsteroidal antiinflammatory, analgesic, antipyretic agent; analgesic effect is observed after single dose, but antiinflammatory effect is reliable after several doses (takes several days to reach steady state); peak plasma levels within 3-5 hours; 99.9% plasma protein bound; unbound agent is active	Photosensitivity, constipation, diarrhea, dyspepsia, nausea, rash; peptic ulceration and/or GI bleeding; **Pregnancy category C**	Osterarthritis Rheumatoid Arthritis
PIROXICAM (Feldene)	Antiinflammatory, analgesic and antipyretic agent; mechanism of action is not fully known; is known prostaglandin synthesis inhibitor; well absorbed; peak plasma levels within 3-5 hours	Not recommended in pregnancy or nursing mothers as safety is not established; Epigastric distress, nausea, decreased hemoglobin, constipation, abdominal pain, anemia, rash, dizziness, vertigo	Osterarthritis Rheumatoid Arthritis
SALSALATE (Disalcid)	Nonsteroidal antiinflammatory agent with weak prostaglandin synthesis inhibitory effects; insoluble in gastric secretions, well absorbed in small intestine; does NOT inhibit platelet action (versus Aspirin)	Tinnitus, nasuea, hearing impairment, rash, vertigo; **Pregnancy category C**	Rheumatoid Arthritis Osteoarthritis Rheumatic Disorders
SULINDAC (Clinoril)	Non-steroidal, antiinflammatory, analgesic, and antipyretic agent; 90% absorption after oral dosage; peak plasma level within 2 hours; prolonged antiinflammatory action allows for twice daily (bid) dosing	Not recommended in pregnancy or nursing mothers since safety is not established; gastrointestinal pain, dyspepsia, nausea, vomiting, diarrhea, constipation, rash, dizziness, headache	Osteoarthritis Rheumatoid Arthritis Ankylosing Spondylitis Acute Painful Shoulder Acute Gouty Arthritis
TOLMETIN (Tolectin)	Antiinflammatory, analgesic, antipyrectic agent; rapid and complete GI absorption; peak plasma levels within 30-60 minutes	Nausea, dyspepsia, GI distress, abdominal pain, diarrhea, flatulence, vomiting, headache, asthenia, elevated blood pressure, edema, weight gain/loss; GI bleeding and ulceration reported; **Pregnancy category C**	Rheumatoid Arthritis Osteoarthritis Juvenile Arthritis

146

ANTIMALARIALS:

AGENT	DESCRIPTION	KINETICS	ADVERSE EFFECTS	THERAPEUTIC USE
CHLOROQUINE (Aralen)	*Prototype antimalarial*, synthetic 4-aminoquinoline derivative; selectively concentrates in parasitized red blood cells; chemically a weak base which **alkalinizes acid vesicles within the parasite**; other proposed mechanism involves inhibition of heme polymerase; other effects include: slight quinidine-like effect on heart and depresses cardiac function; is antiinflammatory; thought to be immunosuppressant	Oral bioavailability is 90%; peak plasma levels within 6 hours; 55% plasma protein bound; normal red blood cells concentrate this drug at 2x's plasma levels; 25% excreted unchanged in urine	Anorexia, nausea, vomiting, diarrhea, abdominal cramps; generalized loss of hair pigment, blue-black skin and mucocutaneous pigmentation; keratopathy, and retinopathy	Acute attacks of Malaria Prophylactic suppression of: *Plasmodia vivex* *Plasmodia ovale* *Plasmodia malariea* *Plasmodia falciparum* Also used as antiinflammatory for: Rheumatoid arthritis Systemic lupus erythematosus
HYDROXYCHLOROQUINE (Plaquenil)	See Chloroquine which is prototype antimalarial agent	See Chloroquine	See Chloroqine; should be avoided in pregnancy unless benefits clearly outweigh possible hazards	Same as Chloroqine
PRIMAQUINE (Primaquine phosphate)	8-aminoquinoline derivative; effective on tissue stages of malaria only this drug has **no effect on erythrocytic forms of malaria** (in contrast to 4-aminoquinolines); site of action is within the mitochondria of the parasite; thought to interfere with electron transport	Rapid and complete GI absorption; peak plasma levels within 2 hours; only 1% is excreted unchanged; excreted in urine	Intravascular hemolysis aka *Primaquine sensitivity* (more common in people with G-6-PD); nausea, headache, visual disturbance, pruritus	Radical cure or causal Prophylaxis of Malaria caused by: *Plasmodia vivex* *Plasmodia ovale* Often used concomitantly or consecutively with Chloroquine for all Plasmodia species
MEFLOQUINE (Lariam)	Quinoline methanol derivative; see prototype Quinine	Delayed absorption; 98% plasma protein bound; long duration of action, half-life is about 3 weeks	Generally well tolerated; nausea, vomiting, diarrhea, dizziness, myalgia, skin rash, vertigo, tinnitus, visual disturbance	Prophylactic and therapeutic agent for *Plasmodia vivex* and resistant *Plasmodia falciparum* malarial infection

Note: G-6-PD - glucose-6-phosphate dehydrogenase deficiency

ANTIMALARIALS:

AGENT	DESCRIPTION	KINETICS	ADVERSE EFFECTS	THERAPEUTIC USE
QUININE	Quinoline methanol derivative antimalarial which is **effective against the erythrocytic stages of malarial infection**; thought to have similar mechanism of action as Chloroquine; also has analgesic and antipyrectic properties; injections produces local anesthesia; also inhibits cholinesterases and has weak curare-like effects	Rapid and complete GI absorption; peak plasma levels within 1-2 hours; 70% plasma protein bound; liver metabolized; 5% left unchanged and excreted in urine	Chronic use may cause *cinchonism*: tinnitus, headache, neausea, and vision disturbance; skin rash, urticaria, angioneurotic edema, asthmatic attacks	Used as component of multi-agent regimen for uncomplicated attack of Chloroquine-resistant *Plasmodia falciparum* malaria
CHLOROGUANIDE PYRIMETHAMINE TRIMETHOPRIM	Anti-folate agents that are active against erythrocytic and hepatic forms of *Plasmodium* infestations; Chloroguanide introduced in England in 1945; **inhibitors of dihydrofolate reductase (DHF)**	Good GI absorption; peak plasma levels within 2-6 hours; 87% plasma protein bound; develops high concentration in tissues; Pyrimethamine concentrates in breast milk at a sufficient level to provide suppression of malaria in infant	Prolonged use can cause smptoms of folic acid deficiency: bone marrow deppression, megaloblastosis (both are readily reversible by leucovorin or cessation of drug)	Pyrimethamine is used alone for prophylaxis of malaria Combination with sulfonamide, Sulfadoxine is preparation known as **Fansidar** which is effective for Chloroquine resistant *Plasmodia falciparum* malaria
SULFONAMIDE SULFONE	Structural analogs of para-aminobenzoic acid (PABA), an essential precursor for folic acid synthesis; **competitive inhibitors of dihydropterate synthetease**; often used in combination with anti-folate agents (Pyrimethamine + Sulfadoxine = Fansidar)	Good GI absorption (70-100%); food delays absorption but does not affect total amount absorbed; readily penetrates tissues, body fluids, eye and CSF; liver metabolized by acetylation or conjugation; excreted in urine	Nausea, vomiting, diarrhea, hypersensitivity reactions including rash, erythema multiforme, Stevens Johnson syndrome, erythema nodosum, vasculitis, drug fever, serum-sickness like syndrome, leukopenia, agranulocytosis, acute hemolytic anemia, thrombocytopenia	Used in combination with other antimalarials for malarial infection Urinary Tract Infection Prophylaxis against Meningococcal Meningitis
DOXYCYCLINE (Vibramycin)	Tetracycline derivative most frequently used against malaria species	Good GI absorption but decreases with milk, antacids or iron	Allergic reactions including skin rash and drug fever; photosensitivity; epigastric pain, nausea, vomiting; may discolor teeth in children or during 2nd or 3rd trimester of pregnancy	Prophylaxis of malaria due to resistant *Plasmodia falciparum*

148

ANTIMANIACALS:

DRUG	ORGAN SYSTEM EFFECTS	PHARMACOKINETICS	ADVERSE REACTIONS	THERAPEUTIC USE
LITHIUM CARBONATE (Eskalith)	NOT antipsychotic; decreases peak of mania thus avoiding the post mania depression; somehow replaces sodium in key areas of brain (probably limbic system); 60-70% therapeutic success; may normalize manic symptoms within 1-3 weeks	Almost 100% orally absorbed; crosses blood brain barrier; excreted by kidney	Arrhythmia especially in ventricles; alters brain function; nephrotoxic; **narrow therapeutic window;** may cause fetal harm in pregnancy; **teratogen**	Manic Depressive Disorder
LITHIUM CITRATE	Same as Lithium Carbonate	Syrup preparation	Same as Lithium Carbonate	Manic Depressive Disorder
VALPROIC ACID (Depakote)	Antiepileptic drug approved to treat manic depressive disorder (bipolar disorder)	Orally absorbed	Sedation, ataxia, liver dysfunction, alopecia; **Pregnancy category D**	Manic Depressive Disorder Absence Seizures
CARBAMAZEPINE (Tegretol)	Antiepileptic drug approved to treat manic depressive disorder (bipolar disorder)	Orally absorbed	Dry mouth, nausea, jaundice; **Pregnancy category C**	Manic Depressive Disorder Tonic Clonic Seizure Partial Seizures

149

ANTIMICROBIALS, SYSTEMIC:
Macrolides, Chloramphenicol, Clindamycin, and Tetracyclines

DRUG	ORGAN SYSTEM EFFECTS	PHARMACOKINETICS	ADVERSE REACTIONS	SPECTRUM/USE
AZITHROMYCIN (Zithromax)	Macrolide antibiotics reversibly binds to the P site of 50 S subunit of ribosome; inhibits RNA-dependent protein synthesis; bacteriostatic or bacteriocidal depending on drug concentration; macrolides have similar antimicrobial spectrum	Excreted unchanged in bile; food decreases GI absorption; 50% plasma protein bound	Diarrhea, loose stools, vomiting, nausea, abdominal pain, photosensitivity; **Pregnancy category B**	*Staphylococcus aureus* *Streptococcus pyogenes* *Streptococcus pneumoniae* *Streptococcus agalactiae* *Streptococcus viridans* *Haemophilus influenzae* *Haemophilus ducreyi* *Moraxella catarrhalis* *Bordetella pertussis* *Legionella pneumophila* *Clostridium perfringens* *Peptostreptococcus* *Borrelia burgdorferi* *Chlamydia trachomatis* *Mycoplasma pneumoniae* *Ureaplasma urealyticum* *Mycobacteria Avian Complex (MAC)*
CLARITHROMYCIN (Biaxin)	See Azithromycin	Excreted in urine; food delays GI absorption but has no effect on amount of drug absorbed	Diarrhea, nausea, abdominal pain, rash, abnormal taste; **Pregnancy category C**	Pharyngitis/Tonsillitis Acute Maxillary Sinusitis Lower Respiratory Infection due to: *S. pneumoniae* *M. Catarrhalis* *H. influenzae* Pneumonia due to: *S. pneumoniae* *M. pneumoniae* Uncomplicated skin infections Component of treatment regimen for Duodenal Ulcer associated with *H. pylori*

150

ANTIMICROBIALS, SYSTEMIC:
Macrolides, Chloramphenicol, Clindamycin, and Tetracyclines

DRUG	ORGAN SYSTEM EFFECTS	PHARMACOKINETICS	ADVERSE REACTIONS	SPECTRUM/USE
ERYTHROMYCIN *(Various)*	Macrolide antibiotics reversibly bind to the P site of 50 S subunit of ribosome; inhibit RNA-dependent protein synthesis; bacteriostatic or bacteriocidal depending on drug concentration; the macrolides have similar antimicrobial spectrum	Over 70% plasma protein bound; taken on empty stomach	Abdominal pain, GI upset, nausea, vomiting, diarrhea, anorexia (GI effects may be seen with both oral and IV routes); venous irritation and phlebitis when given IV; **Pregnancy category B**	Upper Respiratory Infections due to: *Streptococcus pyogenes* (Group A β-hemolytic streptococcus) *S. pneumoniae* Lower Respiratory Infections due to: *S. pyogenes* *S. pneumoniae* *Mycoplasma pneumoniae* Skin infections Pertussis (whooping cough) Diphtheria *(Corynebacterium diphtheriae)* *Entamoeba histolytica* (oral dose only) Conjunctivitis of the Newborn Primary Syphilis (oral dose only) Legionnaire's Disease *(L. pneumophila)* Rheumatic Fever *Listeria monocytogenes* Unlabeled uses: *Campylobacter jejuni* *Lymphogranuloma venereum* Chancroid *(Hemophilus ducreyi)*
CHLORAMPHENICOL (Chloromycetin)	Binds to 50 S ribosomal subunit and inhibits binding of amino acids to the nascent peptide chain; blocks protein synthesis in bacteria and is bacteriostatic	Rapid GI absorption; 60% plasma protein bound; excreted in urine; readily crosses the placenta into fetus	Nausea, vomiting, glossitis, stomatitis, diarrhea, headache, mild depression, confusion, fever, rash, urticaria, optic and peripheral neuritis; **gray baby syndrome**; serious and fatal blood dyscrasias	Serious infections caused by *Salmonella* species, *H. Influenzae*, Richettsiea, Lymphogranuloma-Psittacosis group, anaerobic organisms especially *Bacteroides fragilis*; drug of choice for *Salmonella typhi*

151

ANTIMICROBIALS, SYSTEMIC:
Macrolides, Chloramphenicol, Clindamycin, and Tetracyclines

DRUG	ORGAN SYSTEM EFFECTS	PHARMACOKINETICS	ADVERSE REACTIONS	SPECTRUM/USE
CLINDAMYCIN (Cleocin)	Clindamycin and Lincomycin together are known as the lincosamides; they bind exclusively to the 50 S subunit of bacterial ribosomes and inhibit protein synthesis; the lincosamides are bacteriostatic	Food has no effect on GI absorption; peak plasma levels within 1-2 hours po	Nausea, vomiting, diarrhea, pseudomembraneous colitis (PMC), neutropenia, leukopenia, a g r a n u l o c y t o s i s , thrombocytopenic purpura, skin rash, liver enzymes abnormalities; **Pregnancy category B**	*Staphyloccous aureus* *S. epidermidis* *Streptococcus pneumonia* *S. pyogenes* *S. viridans* Pneumococci *Corynebacterium diphtheriae* *Bacteroides species* *Propionibacterium* *Actinomyces species* *Peptococcus* *Peptostreptococcus* *Clostridium perfringens*
LINCOMYCIN (Lincocin)	See Clindamycin	Food impairs GI absorption; peak plasma levels within 2-4 hours of po dose	See Clindamycin	*Staphyloccous aureus* *S. epidermidis* *Streptococcus pneumonia* *S. pyogenes* β hemolytic streptococci *S. viridans* *Corynebacterium diphtheriae* *Bacteroides species* *Propionibacterium* *Actinomyces species* *Peptococcus* *Peptostreptococcus* *Clostridium perfringens* Drug of choice for Lyme disease *(Borrelia burgdorferi)*

152

ANTIMICROBIALS, SYSTEMIC:
Macrolides, Chloramphenicol, Clindamycin, and Tetracyclines

DRUG	ORGAN SYSTEM EFFECTS	PHARMACOKINETICS	ADVERSE REACTIONS	SPECTRUM AND USE
DEMECLOCYCLINE (Declomycin)	See Tetracycline	65-91% plasma protein bound	See Tetracycline	See Tetracycline
DOXYCYCLINE (Vibramycin)	See Tetracycline	80-95% plasma protein bound; high lipid solubility; GI absorption not affected by food or dairy products	**Pregnancy category D**; see Tetracycline	See Tetracycline Uncomplicated gonococcal infections Nongonococcal urethritis *(Chlamydia trachomatis)* Lyme disease Prevention of Traveler's Diarrhea (unlabeled use)
MINOCYCLINE (Minocin)	See Tetracycline	70-80% plasma protein bound; high lipid solubility; GI absorption not affected by food or dairy products	See Tetracycline	See Tetracycline Elimination of *Neisseria meningitidis* from nasopharynx of asymptomatic carriers Alternative to sulfonamides for *Nocardiosis* (unlabeled use)
OXYTETRACYCLINE (Terramycin)	See Tetracycline	20-40% plasma protein bound	See Tetracycline	See Tetracycline
TETRACYCLINE (Achromycin)	The tetracyclines are bacteriostatic antimicrobials that bind to the 30 S subunit of microbial ribosomes; they block protein synthesis by blocking charged aminoacyl-tRNA	65% plasma protein bound; food, dairy products, and antacids may affect GI absorption; taken po 1-2 before or after meals; readily cross the placenta into fetus	<u>Tetracyclines may cause:</u> anorexia, nausea, vomiting, diarrhea, epigastric distress, stomatitis, glossitis, rash, increased liver enzymes, hemolytic anemia, *pseudotumor cerebri* (adults), bulging fontanels (infant); do not use during pregnancy, may retard fetal skeleton development and may discolor teeth of newborn if given during the last half of pregnancy; may discolor teeth if used in pediatric patients less than eight years old	Rocky Mountain Spotted Fever Typhus fever Q fever *Mycoplasma pneumoniae* Psittacosis Lymphogranuloma Venereum Granuloma inguinale Chancroid *(Hemophilus ducreyi)* *Yersinia pestis* Tularemia *(Francisella tularensis)* *Vibrio cholera* *Escherichia coli* *Enterobacter aerogenes* *Shigella* species *Acinetobacter calcoaceticus* *Klebsiella* species *Streptococcus pneumoniae* *Chlamydia trachomatis*

153

ANTIMIGRAINE AGENTS:

AGENT	ORGAN SYSTEM EFFECTS	PHARMACOKINETICS	ADVERSE REACTIONS	THERAPEUTIC USE
ERGOTAMINE TARTRATE	Vasoconstrictor; acts at the 5-HT_{1D} receptor; also has α-adrenergic receptor activity	Poor GI absorption, thus given with caffeine to enhance absorption; may be given as oral or inhaled dose	Nausea, vomiting, diarrhea, paresthesia of limbs, cramps; **Pregnancy category X**	Acute Migraine Headache
METHYSERGIDE MALEATE (Sansert)	Blocks peripheral effects of 5-hydroxytryptamine (5-HT) receptors; weak oxytocic effects	Semisynthetic ergot derivative; **1-2 days to onset of action** thus NOT for acute treatment	Contraindications same as for ergotamine; fibrotic changes in various tissues (uncommon) with chronic use; nausea, vomiting, diarrhea, insomnia, nervousness, euphoria, dizziness	Vascular Headache and Migraine Prophylaxis
PROPRANOLOL (Inderal)	Beta-adrenergic blocker of choice for prophylaxis of migraine, efficacy in over 60%; unknown mechanism; does NOT prevent cluster headaches	Given po; gradually increase dose over 3-4 weeks until get therapeutic effect; must gradually wean drug if stopping therapy, abrupt withdrawal may precipitate headache, arrhythmia or angina	Well tolerated; fatigue (common), nausea, diarrhea, insomnia lightheadedness; contraindicated in asthma, COPD, CHF and AV conduction defects	Migraine Prophylaxis
SUMATRIPTAN SUCCINATE (Imitrex)	Acute migraine therapy; selective agonist at the 5-HT_{1D} receptor; does not bind adrenergic, dopaminergic nor muscarinic receptors	Subcutaneous injection bioavailability is 97%; also given po; metabolized by liver; both parent and inactive metabolite excreted in urine	Contraindicated in ischemic heart disease and uncontrolled HTN; NOT to be used with MAO inhibitors; **pregnancy category C**; may cause transient paresthesia, flushing, chest discomfort, ↑BP, dizziness, bad taste in mouth, weakness, myalgia	Abortive treatment of Migraine Headache
TIMOLOL (Blocadren)	Non-selective beta-adrenergic receptor blocker	po dosage	Similar side effect profile as seen with Propranolol; **Pregnancy category C**	Migraine Prophylaxis
VALPROIC ACID (Depakote)	Antiepileptic that is also effective in controlling migraine headaches; decreases sodium ion influx across neurons	po dosage	Nausea, vomiting, indigestion, diarrhea, abdominal cramps, constipation, skin rash, photosensitivity; known **teratogen**	Migraine Headache

154

ANTINEOPLASTICS:

AGENT	MECHANISM OF ACTION	USES	TOXICITY
ALTRETAMINE (Hexalen)	Resembles alkylating agent triethylenemelamine Metabolism is essential for cytotoxicity	Endometrial CA Ovarian CA	Nausea, vomiting Bone marrow depression CNS depression Peripheral neuropathy Visual hallucination Tremor Alopecia
ANASTROZOLE (Arimiden)	Aromatase inhibitor that decreases estradiol concentration	Breast CA	Nausea, vomiting, asthenia, headache, hot flushes, pains, dyspnea, coughing, GI upset
ASPARAGINASE (Elspar) **PEGASPARGASE** (Oncaspar)	Causes intracellular depletion of L-asparagine with subsequent inhibition of protein and nucleic acid synthesis	Acute Lymphocytic Leukemia (ALL)	Nausea, vomiting, liver toxicity manifests as hypoalbuminemia, decreased production of clotting factors; unusual chemotherapeutic because does not cause significant bone marrow of GI toxicity
BICALUFAMIDE (Casodex)	Antiandrogen; competitive antagonist at androgen receptors	Prostate CA	Body pains, hot flashes, nausea, vomiting, constipation, infection
BLEOMYCIN (Blenoxane)	Mixture of glycopeptide antibiotics derived from *Streptomyces verticillus*; has antitumor, antiviral and antibacterial activity; binds DNA causing single and double strand breaks; **Cell-cycle specific**	Testicular cancer Hodgkin's and Non-Hodgkin's Lymphoma Squamous cell carcinomas of head and neck, cervix, esophagus and lung	Interstitial pneumonitis which may progress to pulmonary fibrosis (a dose related toxicity)
BUSULFAN (Myleran)	Alkylating agent; kills stem cells and cells in the G_o phase of cell cycle	Myeloproliferative disorders Chronic Myelogenous Leukemia (CML) Polycythemia Vera (PV) Bone marrow transplant	Irreversible bone marrow suppression; less immune system suppression than other alkylating agents; produces little mucositis or GI disturbance
CARBOPLATIN (Paraplatin)	Platinum analog with mechanism similar to that of cisplatin with less toxic effects	Ovarian CA	Nausea, vomiting Bone marrow depression Peripheral neuropathy (unusual) Hearing loss Transient cortical blindness Hemolytic anemia

155

ANTINEOPLASTICS:

AGENT	MECHANISM OF ACTION	USES	TOXICITY
CARMUSTINE (BiCNU)	A nitrosurea alkylating agent	Brain tumors Multiple Myeloma Hodgkin's Disease Non-Hodgkin's Lymphoma	Nausea, vomiting Leukopenia/Thrombocytopenia Pulmonary fibrosis Nephrotoxic and Hepatotoxic
CHLORAMBUCIL (Leukeran)	Alkylating agent	Chronic Lymphocytic Leukemia (CLL) Malignant Lymphomas	Nausea, vomiting Seizure Bone marrow depression Pulmonary fibrosis Leukemia Sterility Hepatotoxicity
CISPLATIN (CDDP, Platinol-AQ)	Inorganic platinum-containing alkylating agent; causes intrastrand cross linking of DNA; mechanism causing cell death not clear; suppresses mitochondrial respiration and inhibits microtubule assembly	Testicular and Ovarian cancers Head, Neck and Bladder cancers	Renal dysfunction, nausea, vomiting, peripheral neuropathy, high-frequency hearing loss, myelosuppression; renal toxicity can be lessened with vigorous hydration prior to dosage
CLADRIDBINE (CdA) (Leustatin)	Phosphorylated *in vivo* to the active 2-chloro-2'deoxy-D-adenosine monophosphate and to the triphosphate form; these active products inhibit deoxycytodine kinase, deoxynucleotidase and adenosine deaminase enzymes	Hairy Cell Leukemia	Myelosuppression, infection, fever, rashes, nausea, fatigue, headache
CYCLOPHOSPHAMIDE (Cytoxan)	Alkylating agent; prodrug that requires biotransformation by the liver	Non-Hodgkin's lymphoma Acute lymphatic leukemia Chronic Lymphocytic Leukemia Myeloma Breast and Ovarian cancers Neuroblastoma Immunosuppressant (connective tissue disorders)	Hemorrhagic cystitis Alopecia Sterility Bone marrow depression

156

ANTINEOPLASTICS:

AGENT	MECHANISM OF ACTION	USES	TOXICITY
CYTARABINE (ARA-C) (Cytosar-U)	Antimetabolite **prodrug** DNA polymerase inhibitor S-phase specific (some G1 phase activity) t½ = 10 min used IV	Acute Leukemias	Profound bone marrow suppression and GI toxicity; high dose may cause elevated liver enzymes and cerebellar toxicity with ataxia
DACARBAZINE (DTIC-Dome)	Alkylating agent that requires hepatic microsomal demethylation for activation; **Cell-cycle nonspecific**	Hodgkin's Disease Soft Tissue Sarcoma Melanoma	Severe nausea, vomiting, moderate myelosuppression, flu-like syndrome, fulminant hepatic veno-occlusive disease
DACTINOMYCIN (Actinomycin D, Cosmegen)	Chromopeptide that forms complex with DNA binding to and intercalating between guanine-cytosine segments, blocking DNA-dependent RNA synthesis; greatest effect in early S phase of cell cycle; also causes single stranded DNA breaks	Wilms' Tumor Ewing's Sarcoma Rhabdomyosarcoma Testicular Carcinoma Gestational Choriocarcinoma Lymphoma Kaposi's Sarcoma	Myelossuppression is most frequent, GI toxicity including stomatitis, nausea, vomiting and diarrhea; can enhance radiation injury; extravasation can cause significant tissue necrosis
DAUNORUBICIN (Cerubidine)	Antibiotic derived from *Streptomyces coeruleorubidus*; precise mechanism not known; may intercalate into DNA	Acute Nonlymphocytic Leukemia (myelogenous, erythroid, and monocytic), Acute Lymphocytic Leukemia	Nausea, vomiting, alopecia, **bone marrow suppression**, mucositis are most common **Cardiotoxicity**
DIETHYLSTILBESTROL (Stilphostrol)	Antiestrogen; a.k.a. DES	Receptor positive Breast CA	Nausea, vomiting Gynecomastia (males) Loss of libido Hepatotoxic Edema Altered menses
DOCETAXEL (Taxotere)	Antineoplasic of the taxoid family; made from Pacific yew tree (See Paclitaxel); binds to cell free tubulin which inhibits the usual stabilization of microtubule bundles which ultimately interferes with cell mitosis	Breast CA	Neutropenia, leukopenia, thrombocytopenia, anemia, nausea, diarrhea, vomiting, stomatitis, myalgia, nail changes, fever, alopecia, infusion site reactions; Pregnancy category D

157

ANTINEOPLASTICS:

AGENT	MECHANISM OF ACTION	USES	TOXICITY
DOXORUBICIN (Adriamycin)	Antibiotic derived from *Streptomyces peucetius*; acts by DNA intercalation, impairs DNA repair, chelates divalent cations, interferes with cell membrane function, and triggers topoisomerase II-dependent DNA fragmentation	Acute Leukemias Lymphoma Breast and Ovarian CA Sarcoma	Bone marrow suppression and mucositis are major side effects; nausea, vomiting, alopecia occur in majority of patients; extravasation can cause severe tissue injury; dose-limiting side effect is cardiac toxicity; **red urine discolorization**
ESTRADIOL	Antiestrogen	Advanced breast cancer in receptor-positive postmenopausal females and in men with advanced prostate carcinoma	GI upset, phlebitis, hypercalcemia flare, gynecomastia in men
ESTRAMUSTINE (Emcyt)	Alkylating agent Weak estrogen	Carcinoma of the Prostate	Nausea, vomiting, diarrhea Pulmonary fibrosis Decreased glucose tolerance Hypertension
ETOPOSIDE (VP-16) (VePesid)	Plant alkaloid synthetic derivative of American mandrage plant (*Podophyllum peltatum*); arrests cells in late S phase or early G_2 phase; stabilizes topoisomerase II cleavable enzyme-DNA complex resulting in double-stranded DNA breaks	Testicular Cancers Small Cell Lung Cancers Lymphoma Leukemia Kaposi's Sarcoma	Dose related myelosuppression, mild nausea, vomiting, reversible alopecia, stomatitis; acute hypersensitivity is described characterized by fever, chills, bronchospasm, flushing, & hypotension
FLOXURIDINE (5-FUdR) (Adrucil)	Antimetabolites pyrimidine derivative antineoplastic Inhibits thymidylate synthetase Interferes with DNA production	Colon CA with liver metastasis	Nausea, vomiting, diarrhea Oral and GI ulceration Bone marrow depression Alopecia Dermatitis
FLUDARABINE PHOSPHATE (Fludara)	Flourinated nucleotide analog of Vidarabine; undergoes intracellular conversion to active triphosphate, 2-fluoro-ara-ATP which inhibits DNA polymerase alpha ribonucleotide reductase and DNA primase which ultimately inhibits DNA synthesis	Chronic Lymphocytic Leukemia	Myelosuppression, fever, chills, infection

158

ANTINEOPLASTICS:

AGENT	MECHANISM OF ACTION	USES	TOXICITY
FLUOROURACIL (5-FU)	Pyrimidine derivative antimetabolite; Thymidylate synthetase inhibitor that interferes with DNA production; active metabolite 5-fluorodeoxyuridine monophsophate (FdUMP)	Carcinoma of Head and Neck, Colon, Rectum, Breast, Stomach, and Pancreas; Topical application effective for Multiple actinic or Solar keratoses	Bone marrow suppression, mucositis, diarrhea, gastrointestinal ulceration and bleeding
FLUTAMIDE (Eulexin)	Antiandrogen that binds dihydrotestosterone receptors on the nuclear membrane Suppresses nuclear androgen binding	Advanced Prostate CA	Nausea, vomiting Gynecomastia Hepatotoxicity
GEMCITABINE (Gemzar)	S-phase inhibitor; ribonucleotide reductase inhibitor; activated *in vivo* to di and triphosphates which inhibit DNA synthesis	Adenocarcinoma of the Pancreas	Myelosuppression, hepatotoxicity, nephrotoxiity, nausea, vomiting, pains, rashes, dyspnea
HYDROXYUREA (Hydrea)	A substituted derivative of urea Reduces ribonucleotides to deoxyribonucleotides Inhibits DNA synthesis	Myeloproliferative disorders Acute Myelogenous Leukemia Melanoma	Nausea, vomiting Bone marrow depression Stomatitis Dysuria Alopecia Pulmonary infiltrate
IDARUBICIN (Idamycin)	Synthetic analog of Daunorubicin Lipid soluble agent Increased cell uptake, decreased cardiac toxicity Inhibits DNA synthesis via DNA intercalation Interacts with topoisomerase II	Acute Lymphocytic Leukemia	Nausea, vomiting, extravasation injury, bone marrow depression, alopecia, myocardial toxicity, infection, abdominal cramps, diarrhea
IFOSFAMIDE (Ifex)	Prodrug that is metabolized by hepatic microsomal enzymes to active product 4-hydroxyifosfamide which is an alkylating agent	Testicular CA	Nausea, vomiting, hematuria, hemorrhagic cystitis, metabolic acidosis, CNS effects, alopecia, infection, myelosuppression
INTERFERON ALFA-2a (Roferon-A)	Antitumor activity; may have antiproliferative action against tumor cells and host immune response modulatory effect; protein made via recombinant DNA technology	Hairy Cell Leukemia AIDS related Kaposi's Sarcoma	Fever, chills, myalgia/arthralgia, fatigue, headache, bone marrow depression, anorexia, neutropenia, nephrotoxic, edema; Pregnancy category C

159

ANTINEOPLASTICS:

AGENT	MECHANISM OF ACTION	USES	TOXICITY
INTERFERON ALFA-2b (Intron A)	Binds specific cell membrane receptors; inhibits viral replication, suppresses cell proliferation, enhances macrophage phagocytosis and augments cytotoxicity of lymphocytes; protein made via recombinant DNA technology	Hairy Cell Leukemia Kaposi's Sarcoma Chronic Hepatitis B Chronic Hepatitis Non-A, Non B/C Condyloma accuminata	Flu-like symmptoms, fever, headache, chills, myalgia, fatigue, dizziness, paresthesia, depression, anxiety, confusion, irritability, decreased libido, nausea, vomitng, diarrhea
INTERFERON ALFA-N3 (Alferon N)	Antineoplastic; used topically	Condyloma accuminata	Local irritation
INTERFERON BETA-1b Betaseron)	Antiviral and immunoregulatory effects	Multiple Sclerosis	Injection site reaction, headache, fever, flu-like syndrome, pain, asthenia, chills, infection, abdominal pain, chest pain, malaise, edema, nausea, vomiting, diarrhea; Pregnancy category C
IRINOTECAN (Camptosar)	Topoisomerase I inhibitor; causes DNA strand damage	Colon CA Rectal CA	Nausea, vomiting, anorexia, hematologic suppression, asthenia, abdominal cramping, pains, weight loss, alopecia, insomnia, cough, dyspnea
LETROZOLE (Femara)	Aromatase inhibitor; decreases concentration of estrogens	Breast CA	Nausea, vomiting, muscle pain, headache, cough, dyspnea
LEUPROLIDE (Lupron)	LH-RH agonist; inhibits GHRH and gonadotropin secretion	Prostate CA	EKG changes, edema, pains, headache, testicular atrophy, hot flashes, sweats
LOMUSTINE (CCNU) (CeeNu)	Alkylating agent; highly reactive compound that forms covalent bonds with electron rich site on nucleic acid, phosphate, amino acids and proteins; causes DNA misreads, single and double stranded DNA breaks and DNA crosslinking; cell ceath occurs through interference with DNA replication and mitosis; **cell cycle nonspecific**	Non-Hodgkin's Lymphoma Brain cancers Small Cell Lung Carcinoma Gastrointestinal cancers Hodgkin's Disease	Myelosuppression, dose related luekopenia and thrombocytopenia; GI toxicity including nausea, vomiting, mucositis, diarrhea; alopecia; impairs spermatogenesis, causes menstrual irregularity, possible irreversible sterility; pulmonary fibrosis; teratogenic in first trimester of pregnancy; increases incidence of Acute myelogenous leukemia, non-Hodgkin's lymphoma and other secondary tumors

160

ANTINEOPLASTICS:

AGENT	MECHANISM OF ACTION	USES	TOXICITY
MECHLORETHAMINE (Mustargen)	See Lomustine; the first clinically tested **alkylating agents**; causes DNA interstrand cross linking and DNA-protein cross linkages; most commonly used as **component of MOPP regimen** (mustargen, vincristine, procarbazine and prednisone) used in Hodgkin's disease	Hodgkin's disease Mycosis Fungoides (topical application) Polycythemia vera Lymphosarcoma Chronic Myelocytic Leukemia Chronic Lymphocytic Leukemia Bronchogenic Carcinoma	See Lomustine
MEGESTROL (Megace)	Progestin; unknown mechanism of action	Breast CA Endometrial CA	Weight gain, increased appetite, nausea, vomiting, breakthrough bleeding, dyspepsia, dys[nea
MELPHALAN (Alkeran)	Alkylating agent Nitrogen mustard	Multiple Myeloma Lymphoma Breast and Ovarian CA	Nausea, hypersensitivity reactions, bone marrow depression; pulmonary fibrosis; amenorrhea; sterility; leukemia
MERCAPTOPURINE (6-MP) (Purinethol)	Purine derivative antimetabolite that is converted to a monophosphate form that blocks *de novo* purine synthesis through inhibition of inosine mono-phosphate synthesis; also inhibits conversion of inosine monophosphate to adenine and guanine; causes DNA strand breaks; Rapid resistance develops	Remission maintenance in Acute Lymphatic Leukemia Acute Myelogenous Leukemia	Myelosuppression, nausea, vomiting, diarrhea, mucositis; reversible cholestatic jaundice; crystaluria; co-administration of **Allopurinol** treats excessive uric acid production due to rapid dissolution of neoplastic cells with liberation of nucleic acid purines which are oxidized to uric acid

METHOTREXATE	**Folate antagonist** antimetabolite
	Activity in **cell cycle S phase**
	Inhibits dihydrofolate reductase
	
	Rapid resistance:
	   increased folate reductase
	   altered enzyme
	   decreased uptake of drug
		Acute Lymphatic Leukemia, Choriocarcinoma, Non-Hodgkin's Lymphoma, Mycosis Fungoides, Sarcoma of bone, Cancers of head, neck, breast, lung; Carcinoma, lymphoma, or leukemia involving the meninges	Myelosuppression, nausea, vomiting, abdominal pain, ulceration and severe mucositis; hepatic fibrosis may occur with chronic maintenance therapy; acute renal failure can occur due to precipitation of agent in renal tubules

161

ANTINEOPLASTICS:

AGENT	MECHANISM OF ACTION	USES	TOXICITY
MITOMYCIN (Mutamycin)	Inhibits DNA synthesis; RNA synthesis and protein synthesis are decreased at high concentration	Gastric Adenocarcinoma Pancreatic Adenocarcinoma	Bone marrow suppression, nephrotoxicity
MITOXANTRONE (Norantrone)	Specific mechanism of action unknonw; inhibits DNA synthesis	Acute Leukemias	GI bleeding, nausea, vomiting, diarrhea, sepsis, fever, alopecia
NILUTAMIDE (Nilandron)	Antiandrogen; blocks androgen receptors	Metastatic Prostate CA	Hot flashes, nausea, dyspnea
PACLITAXEL (Taxol)	Derived from bark of the Pacific yew tree, *Taxus brevifolia*; structure is complex 15-membered taxane ring; antitumor activity by promotion of microtubule assembly from tubulin dimers and microtubule stabilization by preventing depolymerization, leads to bundles of disorganized microtubules; **Cell cycle nonspecific**	Cisplatin resistant Ovarian cancer Metastatic Breast Cancer Malignant Melanoma Acute Myelogenous Leukemia	Dose dependent neutropenia occurring 7-10 days after dosing; hypersensitivity reactions including urticaria, bronchospasm, and hypotension; toxicity is reduced by premedication with corticosteroids, antihistamines, and H_2 receptor antagonists
PLICAMYCIN (Mithracin)	Cytotoxic antibiotic often used as cancer chemotherapeutic agent; **blocks calcium resorption from bone via direct toxic effect on osteoclasts**	Testicular Tumors	Hepatic and renal toxicity, nausea, vomiting and thrombocytopenia
PROCARBAZINE (Matulane)	Methylhydrazine alkylating agent	Hodgkin's Disease Intracranial Tumors	Nausea, vomitng CNS depression Disulfiram reaction Bone marrow depression Peripheral neuropathy
STREPTOZOCIN (Zanosar)	Antineoplastic agent with affinity for pancreatic islet beta cells	Pancreatic Islet Cell Tumors Carcinoid	Nausea, vomiting Nephrotoxic/Hepatotoxic Eosinophilia Nephrogenic Diabetes Insipidus

162

ANTINEOPLASTICS:

AGENT	MECHANISM OF ACTION	USES	TOXICITY
TAMOXIFEN (Nolvadex)	Oral antiestrogen which blocks the activity of estrogen via competitive inhibition of estradiol binding to estrogen receptors; associated with increased risk of endometrial carcinoma; endometrial sampling (biopsy) recomended periodically during Tamoxifen therapy	Receptor positive breast cancer in postmenopausal females	Infrequent side effects include mild nausea, fluid retention, thrombocytopenia, skin rash, vaginal bleeding
TENIPOSIDE (Vumon)	Semisynthetic derivative of podophyllotoxin; cell cycle G_2 phase specific; inhibits DNA synthesis	Acute Lymphoblastic Leukemia (refractory)	Myelosuppression, leukopenia, thrombocytopenia, anemia, nausea, vomiting, anorexia, diarrhea, stomatitis, alopecia
TESTOLACTONE (Teslac)	Inhibits steroid aromatase activity and decreases estrone synthesis	Breast CA in postmenopausal women	Glossitis, nausea, vomiting, anorexia, paresthesias, maculopapular erythema
THIOGUANINE	Purine derivative antimetabolite antineoplastic agent; converted to 6-thioguanylic acid (TGMP) which interferes with synthesis of guanine nucleotides; inhibits *de novo* purine synthesis by inhibiting glutamine-5-phosphoribosyl-pyrophosphate amidotransferase	Acute Lymphatic Leukemia Acute Myelogenous Leukemia	Bone marrow depression Stomatitis
THIOTEPA (Thioplex)	Cell cycle non-specific alkylating agent	Breast Adenocarcinoma Ovarian CA Bladder CA	Nausea, vomiting, anorexia, dysuria, dizziness, headache, allergic reactions, hematopoietic toxicity
TOPOTECAN (Hycamtin)	Topoisomerase I inhibitor; causes DNA strand damage	Ovarian CA	Neutronpenia, leukopenia, thrombocytopenia, anemia, headache, fever, nausea, vomiting, diarrhea, dyspnea
VINBLASTINE (Velban, Velsar)	Vinca alkaloid derived from the periwinkle plant, *Vinca rosea* Arrests cell division in metaphase Inhibit assembly of microtubules Cells in S phase are most sensitive	Hodgkin's Disease Choriocarcinoma Breast Cancer Testicular Cancer Lymphoma	Myelosuppression (leukopenia, anemia, granulocytopenia), Neurotoxicity is rare

163

ANTINEOPLASTICS:

AGENT	MECHANISM OF ACTION	USES	TOXICITY
VINORELBINE (Navelbine)	Semisynthetic vinca alkaloid; interferes with microtubule assembly and mitosis at metaphase	Non-Small Cell Lung CA	Nausea, vomiting, anorexia, asthenia, peripheral neuropathy, AST elevation
VINCRISTINE (Oncovin, Vincasar)	Vinca alkaloid derived from the periwinkle plant (*Vinca rosea*) Arrest cell division in metaphase Inhibit assembly of microtubules Cells in S phase are most sensitive	Acute Lymphatic Leukemia Non-Hodgkin's Lymphoma Hodgkin's Disease Multiple myeloma Neuroblastoma Ewing's Sarcoma Wilms' Tumor	Dose limiting neurotoxicity or peripheral neuropathy which may manifest as muscular weakness or sensory impairment, constipation and paralytic ileus can occur

164

ANTIOSTEOPOROTICS:

AGENT	ORGAN SYSTEM EFFECTS	PHARMACOKINETICS	ADVERSE REACTIONS	THERAPEUTIC USE
ALENDRONATE (Fosamax)	Specific inhibitor of osteoclast-mediated bone resorption; synthetic analog of pyrophosphate, **binds hydroxyapatite in bone**	Given po, must take ½ hour prior to first food with water only; not metabolized; urine excretion	Mild, transient, asymptomatic decreases serum calcium and phosphate; MUST correct calcium prior to starting agent; hypocalcemia is **esophagitis;** contraindication; **Pregnancy category C**	**Osteoporosis** Paget's Disease of Bone
CALCITONIN (Calcimar, Miacalcin)	Decreases bone resorption; halts Paget's disease of bone	SubQ, IM, and nasal spray preparations	Rash, nausea, vomiting, diarrhea, facial flushing, malaise	**Paget's Disease of Bone** Bone Mineral Loss 2° to Hyperparathyroidism, Immobilization, and Malignancy
ETIDRONATE (Didronel)	Bisphosphonate with primary action on bone; inhibits bone resorption by inhibiting hydroxyapatite crystal dissolution	Not metabolized	GI complaints, bone pain, impaired renal function; **Pregnancy category B (po), C (parenteral)**	Paget's Disease of Bone Hypercalcemia of Malignancy
PAMIDRONATE (Aredia)	See Etidronate	Urine excretion	Mild temperature elevation, local soft tissue symptoms, fluid overload, pain, hypertension, abdominal pain, anorexia, constipatin, nausea, vomiting, UTI, bone pain, headache; **Pregnancy category C**	Paget's Disease of Bone Hypercalcemia of Malignancy
TILUDRONATE (Skelid)	Bisphosphonate with activity on bone; inhibits osteoclast activity	Taken with water, but not within 2 hours of food; peak plasma levels within 2 hours; excreted in urine	Nausea, diarrhea, dyspepsia; **Pregnancy category C**	Paget's Disease of Bone

165

ANTIPARKINSONIANS:

DRUG	ORGAN SYSTEM EFFECTS	PHARMACOKINETICS	ADVERSE REACTIONS	THERAPEUTIC USE
AMANTADINE (Symmetrel)	Synthetic stable amine; Prophylactic for influenza A2 virus; **increases DA release from neurons AND blocks DA** reuptake	Rapid and complete absorption with oral dose; peak plasma level within 2-4 hrs after dose; 90% urine excretion	Confusion, ataxia, sleep disorders, tremors, hallucination; anorexia, nausea, vomiting, orthostatic hypotension; occassionally see livedo reticularis, edema, slurred speech; anticholinergic effects	Parkinson's disease Influenza A epidemics
BENZTROPINE (Cogentin)	**Muscarinic antagonist; more for tremor** rather than rigidity or bradykinesia; counters excitatory effects of ACH neurons in CNS	No significant difference in onset of action after IV or IM dose, so IM is preferred, also given po	Dry mouth, blurred vision, drowsiness, euphoria, disorientation, urinary retention, postural hypotension, constipation, agitation; safety in pregnancy not established	Parkinson's Disease in conjunction with L-dopa Extrapyramidal Disorders
BIPERIDEN (Akineton)	Weak peripheral anticholinergic; has nicotinic receptor activity; centrally acting anticholinergic agents restore the distorted balance between excitatory (cholinergic) and inhibitory (dopaminergic) signals in the corpus striatum seen in Parkinsonism	Peak plasma levels within 1-1.5 hours; 29% oral bioavailability	Dry mouth, blurred vision, drowsiness, euphoria, disorientation, urinary retention, postural hypotension, constipation, agitation; **Pregnancy category C**	Parkinsonism Extrapyramidal Disorders
BROMOCRIPTINE (Parlodel)	**Direct dopaminergic agonist;** causes fewer abnormal involuntary movements than levodopa, but more mental aberrations possibly because of similarity to lysergic acid diethylamide (LSD)	30% oral absorption; high first pass effect leaves 6% to reach CNS; biliary excretion	Nausea, nasal congestion, orthostatic hypotension, constipation, headache, fatigue, hallucination; **Pregnancy category B**	Parkinson's disease Hyperprolactenemia Induced Amenorrhea and Galactorrhea
CARBIDOPA-LEVODOPA (Sinemet)	**Carbidopa inhibits dopa decarboxylase;** permits 75% reduction in L-dopa oral dose; faster improvement than with L-dopa; NO vitamin B6 antagonism	Dose requirement of L-dopa is reduced when combined with decarboxylase inhibitor carbidopa	Less peripheral side effects; CNS adverse effects are not reduced	Parkinson's disease
DIPHENHYDRAMINE (Benadryl)	Aminoalkylether that is competitive, reversible **H1 blocker;** antimuscarinic; local anesthetic (like Quinidine); aminoalkylether	ORAL; 30 min to onset; 4-6 hour duration; metabolized by DMMS (some tolerance to sedative effects)	Systemic use may cause sedation; agitation, nervousness, delirium, tremor, incoordination, hallucinations, convulsions; anorexia, nausea, vomiting, diarrhea or constipation, epigastric pain	Antimuscarinic Acute Type I allergy Sedative Motion sickness

166

ANTIPARKINSONIANS:

DRUG	ORGAN SYSTEM EFFECTS	PHARMACOKINETICS	ADVERSE REACTIONS	THERAPEUTIC USE
LEVODOPA (Larodopa)	The levo isomer of dopa, the precursor of dopamine; crosses blood brain barrier, while dopamine does not	Peak plasma levels within 2 hours	Safety in pregnancy not established; choreiform and/or dystonic movements, palpitations, orthostatic hypotension, mental changes, depression, anorexia, nausea, vomiting, dry mouth, dysphagia, headache, dizziness, numbness, bruxism	Parkinson's disease
PERGOLIDE (Permax)	Direct acting dopaminergic agonist at D_1 and D_2 receptors; as effective as bromocriptine, but with longer duration of action	50% absorption after oral dose; 90% plasma protein bound; renal excretion	Similar to Bromocriptine; **Pregnancy category B**	Parkinson's disease
PRAMIPEXOLE (Mirapex)	Non-ergot dopamine agonist with highest affinity for D_3 receptor subtypes, also has affinity for D_2 and D_4 receptors	May take with food	Nausea, dizziness, somnolence, insomnia, constipation, asthenia, dry mouth, dystonia, dyspepsia; **Pregnancy category C**	Idiopathic Parkinson's disease
PROCYCLIDINE (Kemadrin)	Synthetic antispasmodic compound of low toxicity; useful in symptomatic treatment of Parkinsonism and extrapyramidal dysfunction; atropine like effects; antispasmodic action on smooth muscle	po tablets	Dry mouth, mydriasis, blurred vision, lightheadedness, nausea, vomiting, epigastric pain, constipation; safety in pregnancy not established	Parkinsonism
SELEGILINE (Eldepryl)	**Selectively inhibits MAO-B;** given prior to MPTP is protective; **may delay need for L-dopa;** increases effects of endogenous and exogenous dopa(mine)	Rapid absorption after oral dose; some metabolism to (meth)amphetamine	Nausea, abdominal pain, dizziness, lightheadedness, confusion, hallucination; **POS drug screen for amphetamines;** Pregnancy category C	Slows progression of Parkinson's Disease
TRIHEXYPHENIDYL (Artane)	**Muscarinic antagonist;** more for tremor rather than rigidity or bradykinesia; counters excitatory effects of ACH neurons in CNS	Oral dose	Dry mouth, blurred vision, dizziness, nausea, nervousness are seen in 30-50% of patients	Parkinsonism Used with Levodopa Used with other Parasympathetic Inhibitors

ABBREVIATIONS:

ACH - acetylcholine
CV - cardiovascular
MAO-B - monoamine oxidase found in CNS
MPTP - designer synthetic heroine that induces Parkinsonian syndrome
BMAA - toxin found in seeds that caused Guam syndrome (Parkinsonian syndrome)

167

ANTIPROTOZOALS:

AGENT	ORGAN SYSTEM EFFECTS	PHARMACOKINETICS	ADVERSE REACTIONS	THERAPEUTIC USE
ATOVAQUONE (Mepron)	Antiprotozoal agent; analog of ubiquinone; has antipneumocystis activity with unknown mechanism; site of action in *Plasmodium* species is the cytochrome bc1 complex (Complex III); higher failure rate due to lack of response in Pneumocystis infection than Trimethoprim-Sulfamethoxazole (TMP-SMX, Bactrim)	Highly lipophilic; plasma levels have double peak kinetics; 1st peak plasma level occurs 1-8 hours after dosing, and 2nd peak occurs 24-96 hours after dosing	Rash, nausea, diarrhea, headache, vomiting, fever, insomnia, asthenia, pruritus, oral monilia, abdominal pain, constipation, dizziness; **Pregnancy category C**	*Pneumocystis carinii* pneumonia
EFLORNITHINE (Ornidyl)	Antiprotozoal agent of choice for *T. brucei gambiense* infections; Eflornithine is a fluorinated derivative of ornithine; **irreversible inhibitor of ornithine decarboxylase;** interferes with production of polyamines involved in DNA packaging, cell division and cellular differentiation	After IV dosage, 80% is eliminated unchanged in the urine; no significant plasma protein binding	Anemia (55%), leukopenia (37%) thrombocytopenia (14%); diarrhea, seizure, hearing impairment, vomiting, alopecia, abdominal pain, anorexia, headache, eosinophilia	*T. brucei gambiense* infection (African Sleeping Sickness)
PENTAMIDINE (NebuPent)	Antiprotozoal agent with activity against *Pneumocystis carinii*; mechanism of action is not fully known; may interfere with DNA, RNA, phospholipid and protein synthesis	Inhalation solution and IV	Fatigue, bad metallic taste, shortness of breath, decreased appetite, dizziness, rash, nausea, pharyngitis, chest pain or congestion; **Pregnancy category C**	*Pneumocystis carinii* pneumonia prophylaxis

168

ANTIPRURITICS:

AGENT	ORGAN SYSTEM EFFECTS	ADVERSE REACTIONS	THERAPEUTIC USE
CYPROHEPTADINE (Periactin)	Antihistaminic and antiserotonergic agent; has anticholinergic and sedative effects	Sedation, dizziness, confusion, restlessness, excitation, tremor, insomnia, blurred vision, diplopia, vertigo, tinnitus, hemolytic anemia, leukopenia, dry mouth, constipation, epigastric distress, nausea, vomiting, diarrhea, urinary frequency, urinary retention, early menses; **Pregnancy category B**	Perennial/Seasonal Allergic Rhinitis Vasomotor Rhinitis Allergic Conjunctivitis Urticaria/Angioedema Cold Urticaria Dermatographism
HYDROXYZINE (Atarax)	Bronchodilator, antihistaminic, antiemetic, and skeletal muscle relaxant effects have been demonstrated; potentiates sedative effects of CNS depressants such as narcotics, barbiturates and other analgesics	Dry mouth, drowsiness, tremor; **Contraindicated in early pregnancy**	Pruritus Symptoms of Psychoneurosis Sedative
TRIMEPRAZINE (Temaril)	A phenothiazine with antipruritic, antihistaminic, anticholinergic and sedative activity; phenothiazines are known to potentiate the CNS depressant and analgesic effects of narcotics; oral contraceptives, progesterone, and reserpine may potentiate effects of phenothiazine compounds	Drowsiness, **extrapyramidal reactions**, postural hypotension, anorexia, nausea, vomiting, GI distress, urinary frequency, dysurai; **Should not be used in women of childbearing potential**	Pruritic Symptoms of Urticaria Allergic Pruritus

ANTIPSORIASIS AGENTS:

AGENT	ORGAN SYSTEM EFFECTS	PHARMACOKINETICS	ADVERSE REACTIONS	THERAPEUTIC USE
ANTHRALIN (Anthra-Derm, Drithocreme)	Exact mechanism is not known; suggested to have antimitotic effect via inhibition of DNA synthesis	Minimal systemic absorption	Transient skin irritation; **Pregnancy category C**	Psoriasis *(topical use)*
CALCIPOTRIENE (Dovonex)	Topical synthetic vitamin D3 derivative shown to decrease psoriasis plaques	Some systemic absorption; may enter fetal circulation	Erythema, dry skin, peeling, rash, skin atrophy; **Pregnancy category C**	Plaque Psoriasis *(topical use)*
ETRETINATE (Tegison)	Decreases scale, erythema and thickness of lesions in psoriasis; unknown mechanism of action	High first pass effect; 99% plasma protein bound	Dry nose, chapped lips, alopecia, palm or sole skin peeling, hyperostosis, thirst, sore mouth, dry skin, itch, rash, fatigue, eye irritation, nosebleed, bruising, sunburn; **Pregnancy category X**	Severe Recalcitrant Psoriasis *(systemic use)*
METHOTREXATE	Folic acid analog; used as cancer chemotherapeutic at higher doses; lower dose is effective immunosuppressant; approved for treatment of severe Rheumatoid Arthritis; used in autoimmune diseases such as Polymyositis and Dermatomyositis; used to prevent both acute and chronic graft versus host disease in bone marrow transplant patients	Well absorbed from GI tract; peak plasma concentration after 1 hour; highest tissue levels found in kidney and liver; 50% plasma protein binding; penetrates blood brain barrier poorly; major route of excretion is renal	Most common side effects are ulcerative stomatitis, nausea, abdominal distress, liver toxicity; **Pregnancy category X**	Psoriasis *(systemic use)* Other Uses: Rheumatoid Arthritis Gestational Trophoblastic Disease

170

ANTIPSYCHOTICS:

DRUG	ORGAN SYSTEM EFFECTS	PHARMACOKINETICS	ADVERSE REACTIONS	THERAPEUTIC USE
CHLORPROMAZINE (Thorazine) aliphatic phenothiazine	Prototype antipsychotic agent that competitively blocks DA receptors in limbic cortex (primarily D2); disrupts temperature regulation; increases prolactin and increases lactation; blocks CTZ (antiemetic); reversibly blocks ovulation; anticholinergic; non-selective α1 and α2 blocker; histamine blocker	> 40 metabolites; h y d r o x y l a t i o n ; sulfoxylation; conjugation; p.o. and IM doses; 6-8 hour duration	HIGH sedation; HIGH α blocking (orthostatic hypotension); loss of temperature regulation; **galactorrhea;** increases MSH; inhibits ovulation; extra pyramidal reaction (EPR); neuroleptic malignant syndrome (NMS); tardive dyskinesia	Antipsychotic
CLOZAPINE (Clozaril)	An atypical antipsychotic agent; is a tricyclic dibenzodiazepine; binds to dopamine receptors, both D1 and D2; more active at limbic than striatal dopamine receptors which may explain less extrapyramidal side effects	95% plasma protein bound; 50% urine, 30% fecal excretion	Agranulocytosis, seizures, orthostatic hypotension, neuroleptic malignant syndrome, tardive dyskinesia, **Pregnancy category B**	Schizophrenia
FLUPHENAZINE (Prolixin)	Same as Chlorpromazine; LOW sedation; piperazine phenothiazine	p.o. 6-8 hour duration and IM in oil base (depot drugs) 2-3 week duration; **HIGH potency**	Same; **HIGH EPR**	Antipsychotic
HALOPERIDOL (Haldol)	Antipsychotic of choice; LOW sedation; butyrophenone	Rapid onset; high potency equal to fluphenazine	**SLOW onset, but severe EPR**	Antipsychotic
LOXAPINE (Daxolin)	Low sedation, low anticholinergic, low α blocker activities; dibenzoxazepine	High potency	High EPR	Antipsychotic
MESORIDAZINE (Serentil)	Phenothiazine tranquilizer that is effective in schizophrenia, organic brain disorders, alcoholism and psychoneuroses; acts indirectly on reticular formation to decrease neuronal activity	Oral dose tid	Drowsiness, hypotension, tremor, rigidity, dizziness, weakness, restlessness, dystonia, slurring, akathisia, dry mouth, nausea, vomiting, photophobia, impotence, rash; prolongs QT interval on EKG, extrapyramidal symptoms, tardive dyskinesia; safety in pregnancy not established	Schizophrenia Alcoholism Psychoneurosis
MOLINDONE (Moban)	Low sedation, low anticholinergic, low α blocker activities; dihydroindolone	High potency	**HIGH EPR with quick onset**	Antipsychotic

171

ANTIPSYCHOTICS:

DRUG	ORGAN SYSTEM EFFECTS	PHARMACOKINETICS	ADVERSE REACTIONS	THERAPEUTIC USE
PERPHENAZINE (Trilafon)	Piperazinyl phenothiazine with activity at all levels of CNS, especially the hypothalamus; mechanism is not known	Oral dose tid	Tardive dyskinesia, neuroleptic malignant syndrome, seizure; dry mouth, nausea, vomiting, galactorrhea, lactation, agranulocytosis, false positive pregnancy test	Psychotic Disorders
PIMOZIDE (Orap)	Orally active antipsychotic agent of piperidine series; blocks dopaminergic receptors in CNS; effective for controlling motor and phonic tics of Tourette's Disorder	Gradual increase in dose	Prolongs QT interval on EKG; extrapyramidal reactions, restlessness, dystonia, akathisia, hyperreflexia, oculogyric crisis; tardive dyskinesia neuroleptic malignant syndrome; **Pregnancy category C**	Tourette's Disorder
PROCHLORPERAZINE (Compazine)	Piperazine phenothiazine that is similar to Chlorpromazine; most potent antiemetic phenothiazine	**Suppository dose; 6-8 hour duration; HIGH potency** (but use low dose); also given po	Used at doses too low to cause EPR; (**high EPR at antipsychotic dose**)	Antiemetic
PROMAZINE (Sparine) aliphatic phenothiazine	Same as Chlorpromazine; HIGH anticholinergic effects; LEAST potent antipsychotic	6-8 hours; **LEAST potent antipsychotic**	Same; **LOW EPR**	Antipsychotic (least potent)
THIORIDAZINE (Mellaril) piperidine phenothiazine	Same as Chlorpromazine; HIGHEST anti-cholinergic effects; HIGH α blocking activity	6-8 hours	LOWEST EPR; eye lens pigmentation	Antipsychotic
THIOTHIXENE (Navane)	Thioxanthene derivative that is a psychotropic agent; effective in psychotic disorders; antiemetic effects	tid dosage	Drowsiness, tardive dyskinesia, neuroleptic malignant syndrome, safety in pregnancy not established	Psychotic Disorders
TRIFLUOPERAZINE (Stelazine)	Piperazine phenothiazine; similar to Prochlorperazine	6-8 hours; **HIGH potency**	**HIGH EPR**	Antipsychotic

ABBREVIATIONS:

MSH - melanocyte stimulating hormone
EPR - extrapyramidal reactions (dystonia, akathisia, parkinson-like syndrome)
CTZ - chemoreceptor trigger zone
NMS - neuroleptic malignant syndrome (hypotension, convulsions, ↓ muscle contractions)
Rx: phenytoin (antiepileptic), withdraw the antipsychotic agent

172

ANTIPSYCHOTICS, COMPARISON OF:

AGENT	CHEMISTRY	SED	ANTI-CHOL	α-BLOCKER	USE	POTENCY	EPR
CHLORPROMAZINE (Thorazine)	Aliphatic	HIGH	Moderate	HIGH	Antipsychotic 2nd most prescribed	Moderate	Moderate
FLUPHENAZINE (Prolixin)	Piperazine (depot)	LOW	Low	Low	Antipsychotic	HIGH	HIGH
HALOPERIDOL (Haldol)	Butyrophenone	LOW	Low	Low	Antipsychotic Most often prescribed	High (equal to Fluphenazine)	HIGH
LOXAPINE (Daxolin)	Dibnzoxazepine	Low	Low	Low	Antipsychotic	High	HIGH
MOLINDONE (Moban)	Dihydroindolone	Low	Low	Low	Antipsychotic	High	HIGH
PROCHLORPERAZINE (Compazine)	Piperazine	Mod	Low	Low	Antiemetic suppository (dose is low so no EPR)	HIGH	HIGH
PROMAZINE (Sparine)	aliphatic	Mod	HIGH	Mod	Antipsychotic	Moderate (least potent antipsychotic)	LOW
PROMETHAZINE (Phenergan)	Phenothiazene				Antihistaminic (antipsychotic at high dose, but not used for this indication)	High	NONE at antihistaminic dosage
THIORIDAZINE (Mellaril)	Piperidine	High	HIGHEST	HIGH	Antipsychotic	Moderate	LOW
TRIFLUOPERAZINE (Stelazine)	Piperazine	Low	Low	Low	Antipsychotic	HIGH	HIGH

173

ANTIPYRETICS:

DRUG	ORGAN SYSTEM EFFECTS	ADVERSE REACTIONS	THERAPEUTIC USE
ACETAMINOPHEN (Tylenol)	**Aspirin free;** 60% is conjugated through glucuronide; small amount metabolized to intermediate that requires -SH groups to be detoxified (role in hepatic toxicity in overdose); **NOT antiinflammatory**	Safe drug; has been traced to hepatic failure due to overdose, ties up IC glutathione SH groups of hepatic cells → **hepatocellular necrosis** (treat with **N-acetyl-cysteine**)	Analgesic Antipyretic
ASPIRIN	Original NSAID, first synthesized by Piria in 1838; Analgesic; antipyretic; antiinflammatory; mechanism of action is **cyclooxygenase inhibition**; **acetylation of platelets and decreases platelet aggregation;** NO known CV effects; GI ulceration due to decreased PG synthesis and salicylic acid is irritating (superficial erosions); **increases bleeding time,** NO effect on prothrombin time; **uricosuric;** potent platelet inhibitor	GI irritation (15%); frank ulcer (1%); Reye's syndrome in children following febrile, viral infection; **increases bleeding time;** small child poisoning (acidosis)	Antipyretic Analgesic Antiinflammatory
IBUPROFEN (Advil, Motrin)	Antipyretic; analgesic; antiinflammatory at higher dose; proprionic acid derivative	Nausea, vomiting, diarrhea, constipation, heartburn, and epigastric pain; less GI bleeding than seen with aspirin	Antipyretic Analgesic Antiinflammatory

174

ANTIRHEUMATICS:

AGENT	ORGAN SYSTEM EFFECTS	PHARMACOKINETICS	ADVERSE REACTIONS	THERAPEUTIC USE
AURANOFIN (Ridaura)	Gold compounds accumulate in macrophages	Oral dosage	Dermatitis, erythema urticaria, gastrointestinal disturbance; exfoliative dermatitis; nephrotoxic; **Pregnancy category C**	Severe Rheumatoid Arthritis
AUROTHIOGLUCOSE (Solganal)	See Auranofin	IM only	See Auranofin	Severe Rheumatoid Arthritis
GOLD SODIUM THIOMALATE (Myochrysine)	See Auranofin	IM only	See Auranofin	Severe Rheumatoid arthritis

Note: NSAIDs are the standard, first line antirheumatic agents.
        Gold salts are only used in severe cases of rheumatoid arthritis.

175

ANTISEBORRHEICS:

AGENT	ORGAN SYSTEM EFFECTS	PHARMACOKINETICS	ADVERSE REACTIONS	THERAPEUTIC USE
SELENIUM SULFIDE (Selsun)	Antiseborrheic, antifungal preparation; has cytostatic effect on cells of epidermis and follicular epithelium; reduces corneocyte production	Topical application	Skin irritation, hair discolorization, oily or dry hair/scalp; **Pregnancy category C**	Tinea Versicolor Seborrheic Dermatitis Dandruff

176

ANTISPASMODICS:

AGENT	ORGAN SYSTEM EFFECTS	PHARMACOKINETICS	ADVERSE REACTIONS	THERAPEUTIC USE
CLIDINIUM (Quarzan)	Anticholinergic agent with activity similar to that of Atropine against acetylcholine induced intestinal spasms; **decreases intestinal motility**	tid dosage	Dry mouth, blurred vision, urinary hestitancy and constipation; safety in pregnancy not established	Irritable Bowel Syndrome Irritable Colon Spastic Colon Mucous Colitis
HYOSCYAMINE (Levsin)	**Anticholinergic**, antispasmodic component of the belladonna alkaloids; inhibits acetylcholine activity on postganglionic cholinergic nerves and on smooth muscles that respond to acetylcholine but lack cholinergic innervation	Complete absorption given sublingually and orally	Dry mouth, urinary hesitancy and retention, blurred vision, tachycardia, mydriasis, cycloplegia, loss of taste, headache, drowsiness, insomnia, impotence, suppression of lactation; **Pregnancy category C**	Adjunct agent in Peptic Ulcer Gastric Secretion Control Visceral Spasm Hypermotility in Spastic Colitis Spastic Bladder Pylorospasm

<u>Note:</u>   There are several anticholinergic antispasmodics. The above represents commonly used agents.

177

ANTITHYROID DRUGS:

AGENT	ORGAN SYSTEM EFFECTS	PHARMACOKINETICS/ DYNAMICS	ADVERSE REACTIONS	THERAPEUTIC USE
METHIMAZOLE (Tapezole)	Antithyroid agent; **inhibits thyroid peroxidase**; inhibits synthesis of thyroid hormones; does not affect existing thryoxine or triodothyronine	Same as Propylthiouracil	Agranulocytosis, aplastic anemia, drug fever, lupus like syndrome, hepatitis, rash, urticaria, nausea, vomiting, arthralgia, alopecia, headache, drowsiness, vertigo; **Pregnancy category D**	Hyperthyroidism
PROPYLTHIOURACIL (PTU)	Antithyroid agent; **inhibits thyroid peroxidase** (blocks iodide → OI⁻ and coupling reaction); **blocks T4 → T3 conversion** outside of thyroid	ORAL dose; inactivated by liver; concentrated in thyroid; duration of activity increases during course of treatment	Skin rash, itching, fever, muscle pain; **agranulocytosis** (rare)	Hyperthyroidism; preferred in pregnancy and in thyroid storm
RADIOACTIVE IODINE .	Antithyroid agent; I¹³¹ emits ß particles that destroy thyroid tissue AND gamma rays used for monitoring; I¹²⁵ emits gamma rays for monitoring		Poor control of thyroid tissue destruction; **teratogen**	Thyroid Ablation (non surgical)

ANTITRICHOMONALS:

AGENT	ORGAN SYSTEM EFFECTS	PHARMACOKINETICS	ADVERSE REACTIONS	THERAPEUTIC USE
METRONIDAZOLE (Flagyl)	Synthetic antimicrobial agent introduced in 1960 for treatment of vaginal trichomoniasis; potent bactericidal action specific for obligate anaerobes; excellent activity against strict anaerobes, but is inactive against aerobic organisms	Oral and parenteral; 85% absorbed by oral dose; 10% plasma protein binding; lipid soluble; penetrates well into CSF in normal meninges and in meningitis; liver metabolized	Unpleasant metallic taste, anorexia, nausea, vomiting, neurotoxicity with sensory neuropathy, ataxia, encephalopathy and seizure is rare; **disulfiram reaction** with alcohol use; carcinogenic in mice and rat studies; **Pregnancy category B**	Anaerobic infections *B. Fragilis* Intraabdominal infections Pelvic infections Bacterial vaginosis *C. difficile* colitis Amebiasis Giardiasis Vaginal trichomoniasis

179

ANTITUSSIVES:

AGENT	ORGAN SYSTEM EFFECTS	PHARMACOKINETICS	ADVERSE REACTIONS	THERAPEUTIC USE
CODEINE SULFATE	Opioid agonist phenanthrene derivative similar to Morphine; alkaloids of the phenanthrene group have analgesic activity; Codeine is formed by addition of a methyl group to the oxygen atom at position 3 of Morphine; Codeine has lower affinity for opioid receptors than Morphine; about 30% potency of Morphine (given po); antitussive effect at the cough center in the vomiting center of medulla; causes histamine release	Higher lipid solubility and GI absorption than Morphine; readily crosses placenta; antitussive dose is less than analgesic dose	Nausea, vomiting, dizziness, pruritus, constipation, CNS depression; potential for tolerance, dependence and abuse; **Pregnancy category C**	Antitussive Analgesic
DEXTROMETHORPHAN	Methorphan is methylated derivative of Levorphanol called Levomethorphan which produces opioid like effects and is analgesic; the dextro isomer, Dextromethorphan is **not analgesic**, but has antitussive activity	Rapidly absorbed from GI tract; effects seen within 15-30 minutes; duration of action 4-6 hours; metabolized by liver	Central excitement and mental confusion; very high doses may cause respiratory depression; **Pregnancy category C**	Antitussive

Note: These drugs have potential for abuse, especially codeine. Dextromethorphan is thought to be non-addicting but is nevertheless abused.

180

ANTIULCER AGENTS:

AGENT	ORGAN SYSTEM EFFECTS	KINETICS	ADVERSE REACTIONS	THERAPEUTIC USE
ANTIBIOTICS	Used to treat *H. Pylori* infection Clarithromycin Erythromycin Tetracycline Commonly used in combination with H2-receptor blocker and bismuth	See each antibiotic for kinetics	See individual antibiotic descriptions	Peptic Ulcer Disease associated with *H. Pylori* infection
MISOPROSTOL (Cytotec)	Cytoprotective agent: prostaglandin E1 analog; major effect is cytoprotection of gastrointestinal mucosa; inhibits gastric acid secretion at higher dose; does not relieve symptoms of ulcer; not shown to prevent duodenal ulcers	Rapid and complete GI absorption; 80% urine excretion	Abdominal cramps, nausea, vomiting, flatulence, dyspepsia, diarrhea, increased uterine contractions; **Pregnancy category X**	Prevention of NSAID Induced Gastric Ulcers
SUCRALFATE (Carafate)	Cytoprotective agent; does not neutralize gastric acid or inhibit gastric acid secretion; major effect is cytoprotection of gastrointestinal mucosa; interacts with hydrochloric acid to form a viscous, negatively charged substance which reacts with positively charged proteins at the base of ulcers; binds preferentially to inflammed or abnormal mucosa; the viscous protective barrier prevents mucosal injury by gastric acid, pepsin, and bile	Insoluble in aqueous solution; poorly absorbed; 95% excreted unchanged	Constipation, diarrhea, nausea, vomiting, indigestion, flatulence; bezoar formation is reported in tube fed patients or patients with GI motility disorders; **Pregnancy category B** Alters absorption of the following drugs: Digoxin Warfarin Phenytoin Amitriptyline Cimetidine Ciprofloxacin Ranitidine Norfloxacin Tetracycline Ofloxacin	Duodenal Ulcer Reflux Esophagitis NSAID Induced Gastropathy
LANSOPRAZOLE (Prevacid)	Gastric acid pump inhibitor; suppresses gastric acid secretion through specific inhibition of the H+/K+ ATPase enzyme system of the gastric parietal cell	Rapid po absorption; peak plasma levels within 1.7 hours; metabolized by liver; 33% excreted in urine, 66% in feces	Headache, diarrhea, abdominal pain, nausea; **Pregnancy category B**	Duodenal Ulcer Erosive Esophagitis Pathologic Hypersecretory Conditions including Zollinger-Ellison Syndrome
OMEPRAZOLE (Prilosec)	Gastric acid pump inhibitor; see Lansoprazole	Rapid po absorption; peak plasma levels within 0.5-3.5 hours; 95% plasma protein bound; 77% excreted in urine	Headache, diarrhea, dizziness, rash, constipation, cough, back or abdominal pain; **Pregnancy category C**	Active Duodenal Ulcer Gastroesophageal Reflux Disease (GERD) Pathologic Hypersecretory Conditions including Zollinger-Ellison Syndrome

181

ANTIULCER AGENTS:

AGENT	ORGAN SYSTEM EFFECTS	KINETICS	ADVERSE REACTIONS	THERAPEUTIC USE
CIMETIDINE (Tagamet)	H₂ receptor reversible and competitive antagonist; no agonist activity; has no significant H₁ receptor activity; little effect on histamine release, synthesis or biotransformation; **inhibits gastric acid secretion**; markedly reduces both daytime and nocturnal basal gastric secretory volume; no effect on gastric motility or gastric emptying time; Cimetidine inhibits the P450 enzyme system	20% plasma protein bound; crosses the placenta; urine excretion; oral and IV doses	Headache, malaise, dizziness, constipation, diarrhea, skin rash, altered hepatic function; **gynecomastia**, reduced libido, and impotence (Cimetidine only); Cimetidine and Ranitidine may elevate serum prolactin; **Pregnancy category B**	Peptic Acid Disorders Duodenal Ulcer Disease Pathological Hypersecretion Zollinger-Ellison Syndrome Gastroesophageal Reflux Disease (GERD)
FAMOTIDINE (Pepcid)	H₂ receptor blocker; see Cimetidine	40-45% plasma protein bound; urine excretion; oral and IV doses	See Cimetidine; no anti-adrenergic effects; **Pregnancy category B**	Same as Cimetidine
NIZATIDINE (Axid)	H₂ receptor blocker; see Cimetidine	90-95% plasma protein bound; urine excretion; oral dose only	See Cimetidine; no anti-adrenergic effects; **Pregnancy category C**	Same as Cimetidine
RANITIDINE (Zantac)	H₂ receptor blocker; see Cimetidine	50-60% plasma protein bound; urine excretion; oral and IV doses	See Cimetidine; no anti-adrenergic effects; **Pregnancy category B**	Same as Cimetidine

182

ANTIVERTIGO AGENTS:

AGENT	ORGAN SYSTEM EFFECTS	PHARMACOKINETICS	ADVERSE REACTIONS	THERAPEUTIC USE
DIMENHYDRINATE (Dramamine)	Aminoalkylether that is competitive, reversible **H1 blocker**; no significant H2 effects; no effect on synthesis, release or metabolism of histamine	Good GI absorption; effects begin within 30 minutes, peak 1-2 hrs after dose	Sedation, dry mouth	Motion Sickness Sedation Acute Type I Hypersensitivity Antimuscarinic
DIPHENIDOL (Vontrol)	Specific antivertigo effect on the vestibular apparatus to control vertigo	Dosage every 4 hours	Hallucination, disorientation, confusion; use limited to patients that can be observed readily	Vertigo Nausea and vomiting Meniere's Syndrome
MECLIZINE (Antivert)	Piperazine that is competitive, reversible H1 blocker; same as Diphenhydramine	Given po	Drowsiness, dry mouth; **Pregnancy category B**	Motion Sickness Vertigo

183

ANTIVIRALS, SYSTEMIC AND TOPICAL:

DRUG	MECHANISM OF ACTION	KINETICS	ADVERSE EFFECTS	USE
ACYCLOVIR (Zorvirax)	Nucleoside analog of guanosine; **Acyclo-GTP** blocks **viral DNA polymerase**; gets incorporated into DNA and blocks elongation; "chain terminator"	**Prodrug**; acyclovir → acyclo-GTP (active); **topical, po, IV**; GI absorption is 15-30%; low plasma protein binding; renal excretion	**Topical**: transient burning and stinging, pruritus, rash; **Oral**: nausea, vomiting, headache, diarrhea, dizziness, anorexia, fatigue, edema, rash, leg pain, adenopathy, sore throat; **Pregnancy category C**	**Topical**: Herpes Simplex Virus **Oral**: Genital Herpes, Varicella and Shingles **IV**: Mucocutaneous and Severe Genital Herpes
AMANTADINE (Symmetrel)	Blocks adsorption of influenza A virus to cell membranes; Amantadine is weak base (influenza A needs acidic environment); blocks assembly of viral components (exact mechanism not known)	Rapid and complete oral absorption, peak plasma level within 2-4 hrs; urine excretion unchanged	Confusion, ataxia, sleep disorders, tremors, hallucinations; anorexia, nausea, vomiting, orthostatic hypotension; occassionally see livedo reticularis, edema, slurred speech; anticholinergic effects	Influenza A Prophylaxis Also used in Parkinson's Disease
FAMCICLOVIR (Famvir)	Metabolized to antiviral, penciclovir which inhibits Herpes Simplex virus 1 and 2	**Prodrug**; 95% urine excretion	Headache, nausea, fatigue, diarrhea; **Pregnancy category B**	Acute Herpes Zoster (Shingles)
FOSCARNET (Foscavir)	Analog of phosphonoacetic acid with potent antiviral activity against HSV types 1 and 2, CMV, VZ, HIV and influenza A virus; **inhibits DNA polymerase and reverse transcriptases of retroviruses**	IV dosing; urine excretion	Fever, nausea, diarrhea, anemia, nephrotoxicity, vomiting, headache are most common; granulocytopenia, genital ulceration and seizure are less frequent; **Pregnancy category C**	CMV Retinitis in AIDS Acyclovir resistant herpes simplex virus infection in immunocompromised patients

184

ANTIVIRALS, SYSTEMIC AND TOPICAL:

DRUG	MECHANISM OF ACTION	KINETICS	ADVERSE	USES
GANCICLOVIR (Cytovene)	Nucleoside analog of guanine structurally similar to Acyclovir; same mechanism of action as Acyclovir yet significantly more active against CMV	IV dose; 1-2% plasma protein binding; 90% kidney excretin unchanged	Usually more serious than Acyclovir; dose limiting toxcities are granulocytopenia and thrombocytopenia; anemia, fever, confusion, abnormal liver function, phlebitis, rash; **teratogenic, carcinogenic; Pregnancy category C**	CMV retinitis and other life threatening CMV infections of immunocompromised hosts
IDOXURIDINE (Herplex) OFF THE MARKET	Halogenated derivative of deoxyuridine; primary action is inhibition of DNA viral replication by inhibition of DNA polymerase	Limited to topical application	Severe adverse reactions if taken systemically; Topically: inflammatory edema of eyelid, photophobia, lacrimal duct occlusion, contact dermatitis	Herpres Simplex Virus Keratitis
RIBAVIRIN (Virazole)	Synthetic nucleoside analog effective *in vitro* against several DNA and RNA viruses, including respiratory syncytial virus (RSV), herpes simplex virus, and influenza A and B viruses	Administered via aerosol	Rash, headache, fatigue; **Pregnancy category X**	Respiratory Syncytial Virus (RSV) in infants and young children
RIMANTADINE (Flumadine)	Recently approved analog of Amantadine that is also active against influenza A		Lower incidence of CNS side effects; **Pregnancy category C**	Influenza A
TRIFLURIDINE (Viroptic)	Trifluorothymidine is a halogenated thymidine derivative used as an ophthalmic solution for Herpes Simplex Virus keratoconjunctivitis; inhibits DNA polymerase	Ophthalmic solution (topical use only)	Local burning or stinging; NO systemic effects are reported from topical use	HSV Keratoconjuntivitis

185

ANTIVIRALS, SYSTEMIC AND TOPICAL:

DRUG	MECHANISM OF ACTION	KINETICS	ADVERSE	USES
VALACYCLOVIR (Valtrex)	Effective in early treatment of Herpes Zoster in immunocompetent adults	Rapid GI absorption; low plasma protein bindng; rapidly converted to acyclovir via first pass intestinal or hepatic effect	Nausea, headache, vomiting, diarrhea, constipation, asthenia, dizziness, abdominal pain, anorexia; **Pregnancy category B**	Herpes Zoster (Shingles)
VIDARABINE (Vira-A)	Adenine arabinoside or Vidarabine is a stereoisomer of adenosine whose metabolite, vidarabine triphosphate, Inhibits viral DNA polymerase	**Prodrug;** triphosphate form is active metabolite; given IV or topical dosage; low solubility prohibits subcutaneous or IM use	Systemic: anorexia, nausea, vomiting, diarrhea; occasional tremor, dizziness, hallucination, confusion, psychosis, ataxia; Topical: burning and stinging	**Herpes simplex keratitis** (ophthalmology): systemic indications have largely been replaced by Acyclovir

186

ANTIVIRALS USED FOR HIV AND AIDS:

AGENT	MECHANISM OF ACTION	KINETICS	ADVERSE REACTIONS	USES
CIDOFOVIR (Vistide)	Suppresses cytomegalovirus (CMV) replication through inhibition of viral DNA synthesis	IV dosage; must be used with probenecid to achieve proper blood levels	Renal impairment, must prehydrate with saline and monitor serum creatinine with each dose	CMV Retinitis in AIDS
DIDANOSINE, ddI (Videx)	Nucleoside analog of deoxyadenosine; Dideoxyinosine or DDI is the second antiretroviral drug approved for treatment of AIDS; **HIV reverse transcriptase inhibitor**	Rapidly degraded by gastric acid; excretion is mostly renal but also involves biliary and GI tracts	Peripheral neuropathy: numbness, tingling, burning and pain in distal extremities; headache, confusion, rash insomnia, GI disturbances, hyperuricemia; leukopenia or thrombocytopenia may occur; **Pregnancy category B**	Indicated for treatment of advanced HIV infection in patients who cannot tolerate Zidovudine (AZT) or who are experiencing deterioration during Zidovudine therapy
FOSCARNET (Foscavir)	Analog of phosphonoacetic acid with potent antiviral activity against HSV types 1 and 2, CMV, VZ, HIV and influenza A virus; **inhibits DNA polymerase and reverse transcriptases of retroviruses**	IV dosing; urine excretion	Fever, nausea, diarrhea, anemia, nephrotoxicity, vomiting, headache are most common; granulocytopenia, genital ulceration and seizure are less frequent; **Pregnancy category C**	CMV Retinitis in AIDS and in Ganciclovir resistant CMV infection
INDINAVIR (Crixivan)	HIV protease inhibitor; HIV protease is an enzyme that cleaves viral protein precursors into funcitonal proteins found in infectious HIV	Rapid absorption; peak plasma levels within 1 hour; 60% plasma protein bound	Abdominal pain, asthenia, fatigue, nausea, diarrhea, vomiting, headache, insomnia, n e p h r o l i t h i a s i s , hyperbilirubinemia; **Pregnancy category C**	Treatment of HIV infection in adults
LAMIVUDINE, 3TC (Epivir)	Synthetic nucleoside analog with activity against HIV; **inhibits HIV reverse transcriptase**	Low plasma protein binding (36%); majority excretion in urine unchanged	Headache, malaise, fatigue, fever, chills, rash, nausea, diarrhea, anorexia, abdominal pian, dyspepsia, insomnia, pancreatitis, neutropenia; **Pregnancy category C**	Used in combination with Zidovudine and protease inhibitors in HIV infection

187

ANTIVIRALS USED FOR HIV AND AIDS:

AGENT	MECHANISM OF ACTION	KINETICS	ADVERSE REACTIONS	USES
NEVIRAPINE (Viramune)	Non-nucleoside **reverse transcriptase inhibitor**; blocks RNA-dependent and DNA-dependent DNA polymerase activity; does not disrupt eukaryotic DNA polymerase	Good po absorption; peak plasma levels within 4 hours; highly lipophilic; induces hepatic cytochrome P450 enzymes	Rash, fever, nausea, headache, abnormal liver function tests, diarrhea, abdominal pain, ulcerative stomatitis, peripheral neuropathy, paresthesia, myalgia, hepatitis; **Pregnancy category C**	Used with nucleoside analogs in HIV infection in adults (not used for monotherapy
RITONAVIR (Norvir)	**HIV protease inhibitor**; blocks processing of *gag-pol* protein precursor which causes production of non-infectious HIV particles	Peak plasma levels within 2-4 hours; 98% plasma protein bound	Asthenia, nausea, diarrhea, vomiting, anorexia, abdominal pain, taste perversion, circumoral and peripheral paresthesias; **Pregnancy category B**	Used with nucleoside analogs or as monotherapy for HIV infection
SAQUINAVIR (Invirase)	**HIV protease inhibitor**; which blocks cleavage of viral protein precursors that normally form functional proteins for HIV infected cells	80% excreted in feces; 98% plasma protein bound	Diarrhea, abdominal discomfort, nausea, buccal mucosa ulceration, paresthesia, peripheral neuropathy, asthenia, rash, lab abnormalities in creatine phosphokinase, glucose (low), AST, ALT and neutrophils (low); **Pregnancy category B**	Used in combination with other anti-HIV drugs in advanced HIV infection
STAVUDINE, d4T (Zerit)	Synthetic **thymidine nucleoside analog** active against HIV; inhibits replication of HIV in human cells *in vitro*; also inhibits cellular DNA polymerases	Rapid po absorption	Headache, fever, diarrhea, rash, nausea, vomiting, peripheral neuropathy, myalgia, insomnia, anorexia, allergic reaction, pancreatitis; **Pregnancy category C**	HIV Infected Adults with Prior Prolonged Zidovudine Therapy
ZALCITABINE, ddC (Hivid)	Dideoxycytidine or DDC is a pyrimidine nucleoside analog of deoxycytidine; active in triphosphate form and inhibits **HIV reverse transcriptase**	Good oral bioavailability; significantly reduced when given with food; renal excretion	Peripheral neuropathy, pancreatitis, GI disturbances, rash, headache, dizziness, myalgia; **Pregnancy category C**	Advanced HIV disease in patients with Zidovudine intolerance or failure; used in combination regimens

188

ANTIVIRALS USED FOR HIV AND AIDS:

AGENT	MECHANISM OF ACTION	KINETICS	ADVERSE REACTIONS	USES
ZIDOVUDINE, AZT (Retrovir)	Formerly azidothymidine or AZT; **Blocks RNA dependent DNA polymerase (viral reverse transcriptase)**; prolongs survival in AIDS, reduces frequency and severity of oportunistic infections; indicated when CD4 counts fall below 500/mm^3	**Prodrug**; AZT → triphosphate-AZT	Bone marrow suppression, anemia and neutropenia are dose limiting; nausea, anorexia, vomiting, headache, insomnia, confusion, agitation, seizure; myalgia, myositis; **Pregnancy category C**	Prophylaxis in HIV Infection First Line Agent in AIDS

189

APPETITE STIMULANTS:

AGENT	ORGAN SYSTEM EFFECTS	PHARMACOKINETICS	ADVERSE REACTIONS	INDICATIONS AND USAGE
DRONABINOL (Marinol)	Dronabinol is **delta-9-tetrahydrocannabinol** (delta-9-THC), a naturally occuring extract from *Cannabis sativa* (marijuana); also synthetic form available; orally active; central sympathomimetic activity in CNS; reversible effects on appetite, mood, cognition, memory and perception; tachyphylaxis and tolerance do not appear develop to appetite stimulant effects	Oral; 90-95% absorption after single oral dose; significant hepatic first pass effect; only 10-20% of oral dose reaches systemic circulation; 97% plasma protein bound; bile and urinary excretion	Tachycardia; conjunctival injection; orthostatic hypotension; syncope; potential for abuse; **Pregnancy category C**	Anorexia and weight loss in AIDS Nausea and vomiting of chemotherapy

190

BENZODIAZEPINE ANTAGONIST:

AGENT	ORGAN SYSTEM EFFECTS	PHARMACOKINETICS	ADVERSE REACTIONS	INDICATION AND USAGE
FLUMAZENIL (Romazicon)	**Benzodiazepine receptor antagonist;** works in CNS; competitive inhibitor at benzodiazepine site on GABA/benzodiazepine receptor complex (chloride ionophore)	Liver metabolized; clearance depends on hepatic blood flow	Dizziness, injection site pain, increased sweating, headache, blurred vision; risk of seizures; **Pregnancy category C;** effects on newborn unknown, thus not recommended during labor and delivery	Reversal of benzodiazpine sedation

191

BETA-LACTAM ANTIBACTERIALS: THE CEPHALOSPORINS, CARBAPENAMS, AND MONOBACTAMS

ASPECT	FIRST GENERATION	SECOND GENERATION	THIRD GENERATION	OTHERS
AGENTS	Cefazolin Cephalexin Cephalothin Cephradine Cefadroxil Cephapirin	Cefaclor Cefamandole Cefuroxime Cefoxitin Cefonicid Cefmetazole Cefotetan Cefprozil	Ceftriaxone Cefixime Ceftazidime Cefoperazone Cefpodoxime Cefotaxime Ceftizoxime	Carbapenams: Imipenem Monobactams: Aztreonam
SPECTRUM	Gram POS common gram NEG *S. aureus*	*B. fragilis* *Haemophilus influenzae* *N. gonorrhea* Proteus	Serratia Proteus Pseudomonas *Borrelia burgdorferi* (Lyme d.) resistant *N. gonorrhea* *H. influenzae*	**Carbapenams** (Imipenem) (broad spectrum, simple organisms through Pseudomonas) **Monobactams** (Aztreonam) (Gram NEG, especially *B. fragilis*) (Covers Pseudomonas)
PENICILLINASE	MOST sensitive	Less sensitive	NOT sensitive	Imipenem NOT sensitive
KINETICS	Cephalexin: po (NO phlebitis) Urine excretion Others are IM, IV	Cefaclor: po Others are IM, IV Urine excretion	IM, IV, some po available Ceftriaxone (10-12 hour duration) (bile excretion) (enterohepatic circulation))	Imipenem: IM, IV (metabolized by dipeptidase) (**use cilastatin**) Aztreonam: IM, IV
ADVERSE EFFECTS	Hypersensitivity reaction Nephritis **Phlebitis** (IM and IV doses)	Cefamandole (hypoprothrombinemia) (disulfiram reaction) Hypersensitivity	Hypersensitivity reactions Superinfections Diarrhea	Imipenem (Hypersensitivity reaction is low) (seizures reported) (Cross sensitivity with ß-lactams) Aztreonam (hypersensitivity reaction) (good if cephalosporin HS)
USES	Strep throat Middle ear infection Urinary Tract Infection **Staphylococcal infection**	Cefoxitin (Wide spectrum agent) Community acquired pneumonia Mixed aerobic-anaerobic infection	Lyme disease Gonorrhea Pseudomonas infections Meningitis	Imipenem covers Pseudomonas Aztreonam spectrum similar to aminoglycosides

192

BETA-LACTAM ANTIBACTERIALS: THE PENICILLINS

ASPECT	NATURAL PENICILLINS	PENICILLINASE RESISTANT	AMINOPENICILLINS	EXTENDED SPECTRUM
AGENTS	Penicillin G Penicillin V	Cloxacillin Methicillin Nafcillin Dicloxacillin Oxacillin	Amoxicillin Ampicillin	Carbenicillin Mezlocillin Piperacillin Ticarcillin Azlocillin
SPECTRUM	Streptococci Pneumococci Neisseria Treponema E. coli	Beta-lactamase producing Staphylococci	Gram NEG *E. coli* *Klebsiella* *Haemophilus influenzae* Less Gram POS	Gram NEG Pseudomonas Proteus Enterobacter NO gram POS activity
PENICILLINASE	Sensitive	Resistant	Sensitive	Sensitive
KINETICS	Penicillin G: IM, IV, po (acid unstable) Penicillin V: po (acid stable) kidney excretion	Dicloxacillin and Cloxacillin: po (acid stable; 95% ppb) Oxacillin and Nafcillin: IM, IV, po (bile and urine excretion) **(enterohepatic circulation)** (4-6 hour duration)	Ampicillin: po (bile and urine excretion) **(enterohepatic circulation)** Amoxicillin: po, IM, IV (better GI bioavailability)	IM, IV, NOT po urine excretion Ticarcillin (20% metabolized in liver) Mezlocillin (portion has bile secretion) **(enterohepatic circulation)** (slightly longer acting)
ADVERSE EFFECTS	Hypersensitivity reaction Convulsions (high dose) (Procaine Penicillin G) Hypernatremia (salt form of penicillin) (problem in CHF patients)	Hypersensitivity reaction Methicillin (hemorrhagic cystitis) (nephrotoxic) Nafcillin (bone marrow depression) (thrombocytopenia) (hepatotoxic)	Hypersensitivity reaction Ampicillin (diarrhea) **(HS independent rash)** Amoxicillin (less diarrhea) (seldom rash)	Hypersensitivity reaction Carbenicillin **(po OR parenteral)** (decreases platelet adhesiveness) (hypokalemia)
USES	Strep throat Pneumonia Middle ear infection Meningitis (Procaine Penicillin G) Gonorrhea **(Procaine Penicillin G)** Syphilis **(Benzathine Penicillin G)**	Staphylococcal skin abscesses Lung infections Heart infections	Gram NEG infections Urinary Tract Infection middle ear infections Meningitis Respiratory Infections	Severe gram NEG infections in hospital patients Carbenicillin for Urinary Tract Infection caused by Pseudomonas

BONE STABILIZERS:

AGENT	ORGAN SYSTEM EFFECTS	PHARMACOKINETICS	ADVERSE REACTIONS	THERAPEUTIC USE
ALENDRONATE (Fosamax)	Aminobisphosphonate that acts as specific **inhibitor of osteoclast mediated bone resorption**; bisphosphonate are synthetic analogs of pyrophosphate that bind to hydroxyapatite in bone; lowers vertebral fracture risk by 48%; 63% reduction in number of new vertebral fractures; 35% less overall height loss Note: patients in clinical trials all were supplemented with 500 mg calcium per day	MUST be taken at least one-half hours prior to the first food, beverage, or medication of the day with plain water; excreted in urine	**Esophagitis**; contraindicated in hypocalcemia; NOT recommended in patients with renal insufficiency; **Pregnancy category C**	**Osteoporosis** in postmenopausal women **Paget's disease of bone**
ETIDRONATE (Didronel)	Biphosphonate with action primarily on bone; inhibits normal and abnormal bone resorption by **slowing osteoclast activity**; inhibits bone formation	Oral and IV doses; significant reduction in serum calcium seen within 3 days; excreted unchanged in urine	Diarrhea and nausea, otherwise well tolerated; **Pregnancy category C**	**Paget's disease of bone** Parenteral form used to treat Hypercalcemia of Malignancy
PAMIDRONATE (Aredia)	Biphosphonate chemically related to Etidronate available for intravenous use to treat hypercalcemia associated with malignancy; slows osteoclast activity; see Etidronate	IV, excreted unchanged in urine	Transient mild elevation in body temperature, about 1°C (18% of patients); abdominal pain, anorexia, constipation, nausea, vomiting; **Pregnancy category C**	Paget's Disease of bone Hypercalcemia associated with malignancy

BRONCHODILATORS:

DRUG	MECHANISM OF ACTION	KINETICS	ADVERSE	USE
ALBUTEROL (Proventil)	Selective β2 adrenergic agent that stimulates adenyl cyclase which catalyzes reaction to form cAMP which mediates the cellular response; β2 receptors predominant in respiratory smooth muscle while cardiac muscle beta receptors are mostly β1	See improvement in pulmonary function within 5 minutes; maximal effects at 1 hour; duration is 3-4 hours; po tablets and syrup, inhalation solution available	Tremors (20%), dizziness (7%), nervousness, headache, insomnia, nausea, dyspepsia, tachycardia, hypertension, bronchospasm, cough; **Pregnancy category C**	Bronchospasm in Reversible Obstructive Airway Disease
AMINOPHYLLINE	Methylxanthine derivative See Theophylline	Oral, intravenous or suppository dosage	See Theophylline	Same as Theophylline
BITOLTEROL (Tornalate)	Selective β2 adrenergic agonist that produces bronchodilation	Inhalation dosage; onset within 3-4 minutes; duration 5-8 hours	Tremor, palpitation, tachycardia, shakiness, nervousness, dizziness, vertigo, headache, nausea, vomiting, cough, throat dryness or irritation; **Pregnancy category C**	Prophylaxis and treatment of Bronchial Asthma and Reversible Bronchospasm
DYPHYLLINE (Lufyllin)	Xanthine derivative bronchdilator; similar to Theophylline; has peripheral vasodilatory and smooth muscle relaxant activity	Excreted unchanged in urine	Nausea, vomiting, epigastric pain, diarrhea, headache, irritability, restlessness, insomnia, palpitation, tachycardia, tachypnea; **Pregnancy category C**	Bronchial Asthma Reversible Bronchospasm of Chronic Bronchitis and Emphysema
EPINEPHRINE	Direct acting catecholamine; **α and β adrenergic agonist;** β2 activity on respiratory smooth muscles causes bronchodilation	Respiratory action is rapid and short in duration as aerosol; duration of action is 1-3 hours	Palpitation, tachycardia, hypertension, anxiety, headache, tremor, arrhythmia	Bronchial Asthma Allergic Reaction (Histamine Release)
IPRATROPIUM (Atrovent)	Anticholinergic; bronchodilates with NO inhibition of mucociliary escalator; aka Isopropyl Atropine	Inhalational aerosol; duration of action is 3-4 hours	Dry mouth with improper aerosol administration, nervousness, dizziness, vomiting; **Pregnancy category B**	Bronchodilator Emphysema Chronic Bronchitis
ISOETHARINE (Bronkometer)	Sympathomimetic amine selective for β2 adrenergic receptors; relieves bronchospasm	Inhalational pocket nebulizer; duration of action is 1-3 hours	Tachycardia, palpitation, nausea, headache, blood pressure changes, anxiety, restlessness, insomnia, tremor; safety in pregnancy not established	Bronchial Asthma Reversible Bronchospasm of Chronic Bronchitis and Emphysema

195

BRONCHODILATORS:

AGENT	ORGAN SYSTEM EFFECTS	PHARMACOKINETICS	ADVERSE REACTIONS	THERAPEUTIC USE
ISOPROTERENOL (Isuprel)	Synthetic catecholamine with high selectivity for β adrenergic receptors; bronchodilation is prominent action of this agent via β2 receptors on pulmonary smooth muscle	Aerosol dosage; tablets for po; duration of action is 1-3 hours	Nervousness, headache, dizziness, tachycardia, palpitation, skin flushing, tremor; **Pregnancy category C**	Bronchospasm in Asthma Reversible Bronchospasm of Chronic Bronchitis and Emphysema
METAPROTERENOL (Metaprel)	Beta adrenergic agonist bronchodilator with rapid onset of action	Onset within 5-30 minutes; duration is 2-6 hours	Cough, headache, nervousness, tachycardia, tremor; **Pregnancy category C**	Bronchdilator in Asthma, Bronchitis, and Emphysema
OXTRIPHYLINE (Choledyl)	Methylxanthine derivative that relaxes smooth muscle of bronchi and pulmonary blood vessels; see Theophylline	Biotransformed by liver and excreted by kidneys	See Theophylline	Relief or prevention of bronchial asthma and reversible bronchospasm associated with chronic bronchitis and emphysema
PIRBUTEROL (Maxair)	Selective β2 adrenergic agonist that produces bronchodilation	Inhalational agent; onset of action within 5 minutes; duration of action is 5 hours	Shakiness, nervousness, tremor, palpitations, tachycardia, headache, nausea, vomiting, cough	Prevention and reversal of bronchospasm in patients with reversible bronchospasm including asthma
SALMETEROL (Serevent)	**Long acting β2 adrenergic agonist;** maximal effect within 3 hours; duration of action is 12 hours	Acts locally in lung, thus plasma levels do not predict effect	Tachycardia, palpitation, dental pain; rash, dysmenorrhea; **Pregnancy category C**	Chronic use for Asthma and Brochospasm; not for acute attacks of bronchospasm
TERBUTALINE (Brethine, Brethaire)	Most selective β2 adrenergic receptor agonist with bronchodilation as main effect; also widely used in preterm labor as uterine tocolytic agent (not FDA approved for this use)	Aerosol onset within 5 minutes, maximal effect by 1-2 hours, duration is 3-4 hours; subQ onset 5 minutes, maximal effect within 30-60 minutes, duration of action 1.5-4 hours	Tremor, nervousness, dizziness, headache, drowsiness, palpitation, tachycardia, dyspnea, chest discomfort, nausea, vomiting, flushing; **Pregnancy category B**	Bronchospasm in Reversible Obstructive Airway Disease Uterine Tocolysis (unlabeled use)

196

BRONCHODILATORS:

AGENT	ORGAN SYSTEM EFFECTS	PHARMACOKINETICS	ADVERSE REACTIONS	THERAPEUTIC USE
THEOPHYLLINE	Exact mechanism of Theophylline as a bronchodilator is not clear, but the methylxanthines are known inhibitors of cyclic AMP phosphodiesterase which causes an increase in cytosolic cAMP and subsequent relaxation of airway smooth muscle; this effect is NOT potent and the necessary *in vivo* concentrations may not be obtainable at therapeutic doses, thus other mechanisms may exist; also it is an **adenosine A_1 and A_2 receptor antagonist;** methylxanthine compound	Rapid and complete GI absorption; Theophylline and other xanthines cross the placenta; 50% plasma protein binding; blood level of 10-20μg/mL	Nausea/vomiting, anxiety, tremor, seizure, increased RR; increased HR, CO and increased O_2 use; vasodilation (except meningeal blood vessels, which constrict); increased gastric acid and pepsin secretion; renal loss of Na, K, Cl, and H2O; **Pregnancy category C** Drug interactions: Cimetidine Erythromycin Ciprofloxacin Troleandomycin Propranolol OCP's may levels	Chronic Obstructive Airway Disease Bronchial Asthma

Selectivity heirarchy of β2 adrenergic agonists:
   Terbutaline (most selective)
   Albuterol
   Metaproterenol
   Isoetharine (least selective)

Note: chronic therapy with beta-2 agonists is associated with bronchial hyperactivity

197

CALCIUM CHANNEL BLOCKERS:

AGENT	ORGAN SYSTEM EFFECTS	PHARMACOKINETICS	ADVERSE REACTIONS	THERAPEUTIC USE
AMLODIPINE (Norvasc, Lotrel)	Calcium channel blocker; dihydropyridine derivative; reduces peripheral vascular resistance	Peak effect at 2-3 hours; 90-95% plasma protein bound	Cough, edema, fatigue, GI upset, angioedema, orthostatic hypotension, hyperkalemia, palpitations, flushing; **Pregnancy category C/D** (in 2nd and 3rd trimesters)	Hypertension Vasospastic Angina Chronic Stable Angina
BEPRIDIL (Vascor)	Calcium channel blocker with well characterized anti-anginal properties but poorly characterized type I antiarrhythmic and antihypertensive properties; inhibits both slow calcium and fast sodium inward flux in myocardial and vascular smooth muscle; pyrrolidineethanamine derivative	Peak plasma levels within 2-3 hours; 99% plasma protein bound; 70% urine, 30% fecal excretion	Nausea, dyspepsia, diarrhea, dizziness, asthenia, nervousness; **Pregnancy category C**	Chronic Stable Angina
DILTIAZEM (Cardizem)	Calcium channel blocker; benzothiazepine drivative	Onset of action within 30-60 minutes; peak effect at 2-3 hours; 70-80% plasma protein bound	Edema, headache, dizziness, asthenia, 1st degree AV heart block, bradycardia, flushing, nausea, rash, CHF, liver enzyme elevation; **Pregnancy category C**	Hypertension Vasospastic Angina Chronic Stable Angina Unlabeled use as Antiarrhythmic agent
FELODIPINE (Plendil)	Calcium channel blocker; dihydropyridine derivative; reduces peripheral vascular resistance	Complete GI absorption; high 1st pass effect; onset of action within 2-5 hours; peak effect within 2.5-5 hours; 99% plasma protein bound	Peripheral edema, headache, flushing, dizziness, upper respiratory infection, asthenia, cough, paresthesia, dyspepsia, chest pain, nausea, muscle cramps; **Pregnancy category C**	Hypertension
ISRADIPINE (Dynacirc)	Calcium channel blocker; dihydropyridine derivative; reduces peripheral vascular resistance	Peak effect within 1.5 hours; 95% plasma protein bound	Dizziness, edema, palpitation, fatigue, flushing, dyspnea, GI upset, tachycardia, rash, polyuria, weakness, headache; **Pregnancy category C**	Hypertension

198

CALCIUM CHANNEL BLOCKERS:

AGENT	ORGAN SYSTEM EFFECTS	PHARMACOKINETICS	ADVERSE REACTIONS	THERAPEUTIC USE
NICARDIPINE (Cardene)	Calcium channel blocker; dihydropyridine derivative; inhibits transmembrane influx of calcium ion into cardiac muscle and vascular smooth muscle; reduces peripheral vascular resistance	Complete GI absorption; peak plasma levels within 30 minutes to 2 hours; >95% plasma protein bound	Pedal edema, dizziness, headache, asthenia, flushing, increased angina, palpitations, nausea, dyspepsia, dry mouth, somnolence, rash, tachycardia, myalgia; **Pregnancy category C**	Stable Angina Hypertension
NIFEDIPINE (Procardia)	Calcium channel blocker; dihydropyridine derivative; reduces peripheral vascular resistance	Onset of action within 20 minutes; peak effect within 30 minutes; 95-99% plasma protein bound	Edema, headache, fatigue, dizziness, constipation, nausea, palpitations, muscle cramps; **Pregnancy category C**	Hypertension Vasospastic Angina Chronic Stage Angina
NIMODIPINE (Nimotop)	Calcium channel blocker; inhibits calcium ion flux into cardiac and smooth muscle which inhibits contraction	Rapid oral absorption; peak plasma levels within 1 hour; >95% plasma protein bound	Decreased blood pressure; liver enzymes abnormalities; **Pregnancy category C**	Subarachnoid Hemorrhage Due to Ruptured Congenital Aneurysms (decreases ischemic)
VERAPAMIL (Calan)	Calcium channel blocker; diphenylalkylamine derivative; oldest of currently available calcium channel blockers	Onset of action within 30 minutes; peak effect within 1-2 hours; 80-90% plasma protein bound	Hypotension, impairs AV conduction, edema, bradycardia, CHF, constipation, dizziness, headache, fatigue, nausea, dyspnea, liver enzymes elevation, rash, flushing, ileus; **Pregnancy category C**	Hypertension Vasospastic Angina Chronic Stable Angina Atrial Flutter and Fibrillation Paroxysmal Atrial Tachycardia

199

CARDIAC GLYCOSIDES:

DRUG	ORGAN SYSTEM EFFECTS	PHARMACOKINETICS	ADVERSE REACTIONS	THERAPEUTIC USE
DIGITALIS *Digitalis purpura*	**Positive inotropic agent; blocks Na-K ATPase;** traps Na inside cell in phase 4; decreases Ca leaving cells; effects seen in failing hearts only (little effect on normal hearts); 4 ring structure; increases contraction, but also increases diastole; LESS oxygen use in failing heart; **decreases HR at SAN; increases RP at AVN;** decreases RP, increases ventricular irritability; increases PR segment; increases and depresses ST segment (more rapid decline of phase 2) Key to Digitalis: decreased HR at SAN; slow large contractions are superior to rapid, small contractions	Crude preparation no longer used; NOT an alkaloid	Nausea, vomiting, anorexia; blurred or **yellow vision** (yellow halo), headache, weakness, dizziness, apathy, psychosis; **heart block at AVN;** PVC's; hypokalemia, hypercalcemia, metabolic acidosis	<u>Historical use in:</u> Congestive Heart Failure Supraventricular Arrhythmia Atrial Fibrillation Atrial Flutter Limited use today, see Digoxin and Digotoxin
DIGITOXIN (Crystodigin) *Digitalis lanata and purpura*	See Digitalis; liver disease is concern; if alcoholic then MUST lower dose	> 90% oral bioavailability, t½ = 7-9 days; metabolized by liver DMMS; over 90% plasma protein bound; **excreted in feces;** rapidly passes into fetus; po dosage *Therapeutic drug level:* 9-25 ng/ml *Toxic blood level:* > 35 ng/ml	Anorexia, nausea, vomiting, abdominal discomfort, diarrhea, cardiac toxicity, CNS, ophthalmic toxicities; see Digitalis; **Pregnancy category C**	Congestive Heart Failure Atrial Flutter Paroxysmal atrial tachycardia (PAT) Cardiogenic Shock
DIGOXIN (Lanoxin) *Digitalis lanata*	See Digitalis	60-1CO% oral bioavailability, t½ = 33-51 hours; NOT biotransformed; less than 25% plasma protein bound; **excreted in urine;** rapidly passes into fetus; po or IV dosage *Therapeutic drug level:* 0.5-2 ng/ml *Toxic blood level:* > 2.5 ng/ml	Same as Digitoxin; **Pregnancy category C**	Congestive Heart Failure Atrial Flutter Paroxysmal atrial tachycardia (PAT) Cardiogenic Shock

200

CERVICAL RIPENING AGENTS:

AGENT	ORGAN SYSTEM EFFECTS	PHARMACOKINETICS	ADVERSE REACTIONS	THERAPEUTIC USE
DINOPROSTONE CERVICAL INSERT (Cervidil)	Prostaglandin which potentiates effects of Oxytocin; Ripens the cervix	PG E_2 impregnated tape that is placed in posterior fornix of vagina; MUST be removed before Oxytocin is started; can begin Oxytocin within 30 minutes of removal	Fever, nausea, vomiting, diarrhea and abdominal pain noted in less than 1% of patients; uterine hyperstimulation; **Pregnancy category C**	Cervical Ripening Induction of labor
DINOPROSTONE VAGINAL GEL (Prepidil Gel)	Prostaglandin derivative that ripens the unfavorable cervix in pregnant women at or near term	PG E_2 gel that is applied to the cervical os (opening); MUST wait 6-12 hours before starting oxytocin; must store under continuous refrigeration	Uterine hyperstimulation; safety has not been determined in patients with ruptured membranes; **Pregnancy category C**	Cervical Ripening Induction of labor
DINOPROSTONE VAGINAL SUPPOSITORY (Prostin E2)	Prostaglandin (PGE_2) which stimulates uterine smooth muscle contraction; cervical softener that facilitates dilation of the cervix (mechanism of action associated with increased collagenolysis)	PG E_2 vaginal suppository; half-life of action on uterus is about 30-60 minutes; MUST wait 3-5 hours prior to starting Oxytocin to avoid uterine hyperstimulation; must be stored at or below -20°C and brought to room temperature prior to insertion	Nausea, diarrhea, transient fever, headache and decreased diastolic blood pressure; **Pregnancy category C**	Induction of labor for fetal demise, missed abortion, benign hydatidiform mole, anencephalic fetus or elective abortion

CHELATING AGENTS:

AGENT	ORGAN SYSTEM EFFECTS	PHARMACOKINETICS	ADVERSE REACTIONS	THERAPEUTIC USE
DEFEROXAMINE (Desferal mesylate)	Powerful iron chelating agent derived from *Streptomyces pilosus*; will bind iron from transferrin, ferritin, and hemosiderin, but NOT from hemoglobin or the cytochromes; excess iron → hemosiderosis → hemochromatosis → fibrotic liver and pancreas damage; **give deferoxamine to chelate and prevent toxic levels of iron**	Poorly absorbed from GI tract; usually given via parenteral route; elimination half-life after IV use is about 1 hour; excreted by kidney *Contraindicated* in severe renal dysfunction or anuria	Allergic reactions commonly occur including pruritus, urticaria, skin rash, and less commonly anaphylaxis; dysuria, abdominal pain, diarrhea, cataract formation; **pregnancy category C**	Major use is removal of excess iron stores in patients with refractory anemia who require lifelong blood transfusion Treatment of Acute Iron Poisoning
DIMERCAPROL	Forms stable complex with arsenic, gold and mercury	Given IM; biotransformed in liver; excreted in urine	Nausea, vomiting, anxiety, restlessness, hypertension; high dose may cause convulsions	Lead toxicity High level mercury exposure Arsenic toxicity Gold toxicity
EDITATE CALCIUM DISODIUM	Salt of EDTA; binds to lead in a stable, soluble complex	Available po, parenteral; excreted in urine	Pain at injection site; renal toxicity; fevers	Diagnosis and treatment of: Lead toxicity Cadmium toxicity (but not demonstrated to work)
PENICILLAMINE (Cuprimine)	Disease modifying antirheumatic drug used to chelate heavy metal; binds copper, iron, mercury, and lead	Oral dose on empty stomach; excreted unchanged in urine	Contraindicated in pregnancy except for the treatment of Wilson's disease (copper toxicity); safety in breast feeding mothers not known; **teratogen**	Wilson's Disease Adjunct agent for: Lead toxicity Low level mercury exposure Arsenic toxicity Gold toxicity

CHOLINOMIMETICS:

DRUG	R	ORGAN SYSTEM EFFECTS	PHARMACOKINETICS	ADVERSE REACTIONS	THERAPEUTIC USE
ACETYLCHOLINE (Miochol)	M N_N N_M	Cardiovascular: decreases BP, HR (S-A node), TPR, atrial contractility, and effective refractory period (ERP) in atria; slows conduction through A-V node, minimal effect on ventricles, vasodilation (blood vessels have limited PNS innervation but do have M receptors); near sight accommodation (ciliary m.), bronchoconstriction, GI contraction, bladder contraction with increases urinary frequency, uterine contraction; Glands: increases salivation, lacrimation, bronchiole secretions, and sweating; NMJ: skeletal muscle contraction (physiological)	Short acting; given IV; metabolized by non-specific or plasma cholinesterase and acetylcholinesterase; highly polar ammonium ion; does NOT cross blood brain barrier well	Hypotension, bradycardia, flushing, sweating, dyspnea	Miotic agent (pupil constriction) in cataract surgery; short duration of action allows for rapid post operative recovery
AMBENONIUM		Increases acetylcholine at synapses	po	Similar to Neostigmine	Myasthenia gravis
BETHANECHOL (Urecholine)	M > N_N	Structural features of methacholine and carbachol; more selective action at muscarinic receptors of GI tract and bladder than other choline esters; carbachol with ß CH3 addition	Oral or subcutaneous dosage; resists hydrolysis; 30 minutes to onset, 2 hr duration of action	GI distress, abdominal cramping, sweating, flushing, hypotension, bronchoconstriction; Contraindications: peptic ulcer, bronchial asthma, bradycardia, hyperthyroid, CAD, parkinsonism	Post operative nonobstructive urinary retention; neurogenic atony of bladder
CARBACHOL	M, N	A.k.a. Carbamylcholine; same as acetylcholine; potent choline ester with muscarinic and nicotinic receptor activity, also stimulates autonomic ganglia and skeletal muscle; carbamate substituted for acetate on acetylcholine	Relative resistance to both esterases	Vasodilatation, reduced heart rate, increased tone and contraction of smooth muscle and stimulation of salivary, lacrimal, and sweat glands	Induction of **prolonged miosis**; limited uses
DEMECARIUM (Humorsol)		Indirect cholinesterase inhibitor; potentiates effect of acetylcholine on parasympathetic end organs	Ophthalmic solution used topical in eye; long duration of action	Iris cysts, burning, lacrimation, lid muscle twitching, conjunctival and ciliary redness, **Pregnancy category X**	Open-Angle Glaucoma

CHOLINOMIMETICS:

DRUG	R	ORGAN SYSTEM EFFECTS	PHARMACOKINETICS	ADVERSE REACTIONS	THERAPEUTIC USE
DONEPEZIL (Aricept)		Thought to enhance cholinergic function; increases concentration of acetylcholine through reversible inhibition of acetylcholinesterase	Good po absorption; peak plasma levels within 3-4 hours; food and time of dose (AM or PM) have no effect on absorption; metabolized by cytochrome P450	Headache, whole body pain, fatigue, nausea, diarrhea, vomiting, anorexia, muscle cramps, insomnia, dizziness, depression, abnormal dreams, ecchymosis, weight loss; **Pregnancy category C**	Alzheimer's disease
ECHOTHIOPHATE (Phospholine)		Organophosphate that is an **irreversible cholinesterase inhibitor**	Long acting; water soluble	Possible cataracts; irritation	Glaucoma
EDROPHONIUM (Tensilon)	N_M	Reversible cholinesterase inhibitor; direct N_M effects at low dose; differentiate myasthenic crisis (muscle weakness) and cholinergic crisis (paralysis)	Ultra short acting agent	Mild cholinomimetic effects due to short duration of action	Myasthenia Gravis (diagnostic agent) Anticurrare agent
MALATHION		Organophosphate that is an irreversible cholinesterase inhibitor; used as **insecticide**	High lipid sol; rapidly detoxified to **maloxon** inactive in humans; **Pralidoxime** is antidote	No adverse effects in humans	Insecticide
METHACHOLINE (Provocholine)	$M > N_N$	Acts primarily on muscarinic receptors in smooth muscle, glands, and heart, with little activity on nicotinic receptors of autonomic ganglia and skeletal muscle; acetylcholine with methyl substitution at the ß carbon	Metabolized ONLY by acetylcholinesterase; reaction is slower than that of ACH	Mild side effects including salivation	Used to diagnose bronchial hyperactivity in patients without clinically apparent asthma
MUSCARINE alkaloid	M	Toxin in various wild mushrooms, quaternary compound; historical agent without clinical use, muscarine was one of first cholinomimetic drugs to be systematically studied; NO nicotinic activity	More potent than ACH	Mushroom poisoning is fairly common medical emergency treated with atropine	Laboratory tool to investigate muscarinic receptors
NEOSTIGMINE (Prostigmine)		**Reversible cholinesterase inhibitor; synthetic; direct stimulation of M and N-II receptors; has a quaternary nitrogen**	Poor oral absorption; crosses BBB poorly	Salivation, perspiration, abdominal distress, nausea, vomiting; overdose may cause *cholinergic crisis*	Myasthenia gravis Anticurrare Post-op abdominal distension and urinary retention

CHOLINOMIMETICS:

DRUG	R	ORGAN SYSTEM EFFECTS	PHARMACOKINETICS	ADVERSE REACTIONS	THERAPEUTIC USE
PARATHION		Organophosphate that is an irreversible cholinesterase inhibitor used as **insecticide**	High lipid sol; slow metabolism to **paroxon** toxic in humans; **Pralidoxime** is antidote with Atropine along with respiratory support	Respiratory depression; death	Insecticide
PHYSOSTIGMINE (Antilirium)		Alkaloid that is a **reversible cholinesterase inhibitor;** increases acetylcholine; curare antidote effects; will reverse toxic dose effects of antimuscarinic agents such as Atropine, antihistaminics, and antipsychotics	Tertiary amine; crosses BBB; inactivated by plasma cholinesterase; topical and parenteral dosing; duration of action is 0.5-2 hours	Exacerbates peptic ulcer and bronchial asthma; ↓ HR; may cause bradyarrhythmias	Glaucoma; curare antidote; used in toxic overdose of anti-muscarinic agents
PILOCARPINE (Carpine)	M	Local application to eye causes miosis by contracting the circular muscle of the iris; contraction of ciliary muscle which relieves intraocular pressure; alkaloid, 3° amine	Crosses membranes readily; no effect on N receptors; onset in 15-30 minutes; 4-8 hr duration of action	Local burning or irritation; systemic effects from topical application are not common	Miotic Open Angle Glaucoma Chronic Glaucoma
PYRIDOSTIGMINE (Mestinon)		**Reversible cholinesterase inhibitor** with pharmacology same as neostigmine; direct stimulation of M and N_M receptors	Crosses BBB better than Neostigmine; poor oral absorption	Nausea, vomiting, diarrhea, miosis, ↑ bronchial secretion, muscle cramps, fasciculation, and weakness	Drug of choice for treatment of **Myasthenia gravis**; use in anesthesia to reverse skeletal m. blockade produced by curare-like agents
SARIN and **SOMAN**		Organophosphates that are irreversible cholinesterase inhibitor used in **gas warfare**	High lipid solubility; **undergoes aging**	Paralysis of respiratory muscles and death	**War gas** (no antidote or treatment)

205

CHOLINOMIMETICS:

DRUG	R	ORGAN SYSTEM EFFECTS	PHARMACOKINETICS	ADVERSE REACTIONS	THERAPEUTIC USE
TACRINE (Cognex)		Centrally acting reversible cholinesterase inhibitor; commonly referred to as THA; also acts as a partial agonist at muscarinic receptors in the CNS	Peak plasma levels within 1-2 hours; 55% plasma protein bound; extensive metabolism through cytochrome P450; undergoes first pass effect; smokers develop 1/3 plasma levels of non-smokers	Elevated liver enzymes, nausea, vomiting, diarrhea, dyspepsia, myalgia, anorexia, ataxia, headache, fatigue, chest pain, weight loss, agitation, depression, anxiety, flatulence, constipation, confusion, rash, facial flushing, cough; **Pregnancy category C**	Alzheimer's disease

ABBREVIATIONS:

R - receptor
ACH - acetylcholine
CAD - coronary artery disease
NMJ - neuromuscular junction

Cholinergic crisis - overdose of cholinesterase inhibitor may cause accumulation of acetylcholine at the end plate causing paralysis of transmission which results in weakness.
Must distinguish between cholinergic crisis and myasthenic crisis (both are causes of weakness)

CNS STIMULANTS

AGENT	ORGAN SYSTEM EFFECTS	PHARMACOKINETICS	ADVERSE REACTIONS	THERAPEUTIC USE
AMPHETAMINE (Adderall)	The Amphetamines are non-catecholamine agents with CNS stimulant and peripheral sympathomimetic activity; after oral administration patients feel more confident, alert, talkative, and have increased activity level; increases endurance and decreases fatigue; anorexic effect; IV dosage gives initial "rush"; produces euphoria and excitement	Lipophilic weak base; well absorbed orally; readily cross blood brain barrier; effects last several hours; metabolized in liver; urine excretion	Potential for tolerance, dependence and abuse; hyperthermia, profuse sweating, respiratory difficulty, tremor, cardiovascular effects including tachycardia, palpitation, arrhythmia, and hypertension; restlessness, dizziness, insomnia, dyskinesia, dysphoria, headache; **Pregnancy category C**	Attention Deficit Disorder Exogenous Obesity Narcolepsy
CAFFEINE	Methylxanthine derivative that is readily available and found in various beverages such as coffee, tea, and soda; CNS stimulant that decreases fatigue, elevates mood, increases work capacity, and prevents sleep; has effects on CNS, cardiovascular system and gastrointestinal system; promotes gastric acid and pepsin secretion in stomach	Undergoes purine oxidation via xanthine oxidase	Insomnia, tremor, nervousness, tachycardia, arrhythmia, increases gastric acid and pepsin secretion; convulsion at very high dose	CNS stimulant (OTC) Used in Combination with Other Agents for Pain, Headache and Migraine Respiratory Distress in Infants
DEXTROAMPHETAMINE (Dexedrine) **METHAMPHETAMINE** (Desoxyn)	See Amphetamine	See Amphetamine	Same as Amphetamine; **Pregnancy category C**	Narcolepsy Attention Deficit Disorder Exogenous Obesity
METHYLPHENIDATE (Ritalin)	Mild CNS stimulant; thought to stimulate the brain stem arousal system and cortex	Slow but complete GI absorption; tablet and sustained release tablet preparations	Potential for dependence and abuse; safety in pregnancy not established; nervousness, insomnia are most common side effects; rash, fever, arthralgia, anorexia, nausea, dizziness, palpitations, headache, dyskinesia, drowsiness, tachycardia, arrhythmia; **Pregnancy category C**	Attention Deficit Disorder Narcolepsy
PEMOLINE (Cylert)	Central nervous system stimulant; structure unrelated to Amphetamines and Methylphenidate; similar stimulants effects as Amphetamines, however, has minimal sympathomimetic effects	Rapidly absorbed from GI tract; 50% plasma protein bound; peak plasma levels within 2-4 hours; liver metabolism; urine excretion	Liver enzyme elevation, hepatitis and jaundice (reported); dizziness, irritability, headache, drowsiness, anorexia and weight loss, nausea, potential for dependence and abuse; **Pregnancy category B**	Attention Deficit Disorder

207

COAGULANTS:

AGENT	ORGAN SYSTEM EFFECTS	PHARMACOKINETICS	ADVERSE REACTIONS	THERAPEUTIC USE
AMINOCARPOIC ACID (Amicar)	**Fibrinolysis inhibitor:** inhibits plasminogen activators and has antiplasmin activity; useful for hemostasis when fibrinolysis contributes to bleeding	Available po and injectable; renal excretion is primary route of elimination	Nause, cramps, diarrhea, hypotension, dizziness, tinnitus, malaise, conjunctival suffusion, nasal stuffiness, headache, skin rash; **Pregnancy category C**	Hemostasis
OXIDIZED CELLULOSE (Interceed, Surgicel)	Sterile absorbable knitted fabric; **accelerates clotting** through unknown mechanism; after being saturated with blood, the fabric swells to form a gelatinous brown/black mass aiding the formation of clot	Topical barrier	Encapsulation of foreign body; may have stenotic effect when used around vessels, may block small hollow viscus such as ureter	Surgical Adjunct Agent for Hemostatis

Hemostatic Agents:

Aprotinin (Trasylol)
   given prior to cardiopulmonary bypass during coronary artery bypass graft surgery
   decreases perioperative blood loss

Tranexamic Acid (Cyklokapron)
   given prior to dental surgery

208

CONTRACEPTIVES, NON-ORAL:

AGENT	ORGAN SYSTEM EFFECTS	ADVERSE REACTIONS/DISADVANTAGES	THERAPEUTIC USE
LEVONORGESTREL (Norplant)	Synthetic progestin with no significant estrogenic activity; virtually 100% bioavailability: **prevents pregnancy by inhibiting ovulation and thickening cervical mucus;** implant contraceptive; small tubules containing Levonorgestrel are placed under skin with trocar and plunger - up to 5 year duration	Unpredictable menstrual bleeding; requires surgical placement and removal; visible under skin; headache; acne; weight change (more women gain than lose); breast pain; hirsutism; mood change; depression; **Pregnancy category X**	Long term pregnancy prevention (up to 5 years)
MEDROXYPROGESTERONE ACETATE, MPA (Provera, Depo-Provera)	Synthetic progestin; progesterone ↑ pituitary ↑ decreases FSH and LH ↑ decreases estrogen ↑ amenorrhea **Depot** form **inhibits ovulation providing** very **effective** contraceptive (0.3 failure rate with proper use); clinicians usually wait for menses and obtain a negative pregnancy test prior to administration; IM shot given every 3 months **Oral** form transforms proliferative into secretory endometrium and is indicated for secondary amenorrhea, abnormal uterine bleeding in absence of firbroids or uterine cancer	Menstrual irregularities (bleeding, amenorrhea or both), weight changes, headache, nervousness, abdominal pain or discomfort, dizziness, asthenia (weakness or fatigue) Contraindications: known or suspected pregnancy, undiagnosed vaginal bleeding, known or suspected breast cancer, active thrombophlebitis or history of thromboembolic disorder, liver dysfunction	Prevention of pregnancy
PARAGARD T380A (Copper T380A)	**Copper containing intrauterine device (IUD);** effective up to 10 years; T-shaped device; radiopaque polyethylene frame with 380 mm² of exposed copper surface area and a white polyethylene monofilament at the base; provides reversible long term contraception Recommended Patient Profile for IUD use: · parous woman (more than one full term birth) · low risk of sexually transmitted disease (STD) · stable, monogamous relationship · no history of pelvic inflammatory disease (PID)	Adverse effects of IUD: increased uterine bleeding, dysmenorrhea; increased vaginal discharge; actinomyces infection seen on PAP smears of up to 30% of IUD users (significance is not known) Disadvantages: abnormal uterine anatomy may prevent insertion; contraindicated in copper allergy or Wilson's disease If pregnancy occurs, must rule out ectopic pregnancy	Intrauterine Contraception
PROGESTERONE (Progestasert)	T-shaped intrauterine contraceptive device that releases a daily dose of progesterone; prevents pregnancy by creating spermicidal uterine cavity; uterus known to have sterile inflammatory reaction to this foreign body; associated with decreased menstrual flow and relief of dysmenorrhea; see ParaGard T380A for recommended patient profile for IUD use; provides reversible, long term, intrauterine contraception	See ParaGard T380A	Intrauterine Contraception

CONTRACEPTIVES, ORAL

MONOPHASIC (FIXED DOSE) PILLS	COMMON MONOPHASIC PILLS	MULTIPHASIC (VARIABLE DOSE)	COMMON MULTIPHASIC PILLS
Low dose pills that contain constant daily doses of estrogen and progestin throughout the menstrual cycle	**DESOGEN** Desogestrel 0.15 mg Ethinyl estradiol 30 μg **LO-ESTRIN 1.5/30** Norethindrone 1.5 mg Ethinyl estradiol 30 μg **LO-ESTRIN 1/20** Norethindrone 1.0 mg Ethinyl estradiol 20 μg **LO-OVRAL** Norgestrel 0.3 mg Ethinyl estradiol 30 μg **ORTHO-CEPT** Desogestrel 0.15 mg Ethinyl estradiol 30 μg **ORTHO-CYCLEN** Norgestimate 0.25 mg Ethinyl estradiol 35 μg **ORTHO-NOVUM 1/35** Norethindrone 1.0 mg Ethinyl estradiol 35 μg **OVRAL** Norgestrel 0.5 mg Ethinyl estradiol 50 μg *MINIPILLS:* (Progesterone only) **MICRONOR, NOR-Q.D.** Norethindrone 0.35 mg **OVRETTE** Norgestrel 0.075 mg	Low dose pills that contain constant or varied daily doses of estrogen while daily progestin dose is varied throughout the menstrual cycle Multiphasic pills are available as triphasic or biphasic preparations *Triphasic pills* have three varied progestin doses while estrogen dose is constant *Biphasic pills* have two varied progestin doses while estrogen dose is constant	*TRIPHASIC:* **ORTHO-NOVUM 7/7/7** Norethindrone 0.5 mg (7 days) Norethindrone 0.75 mg (7 days) Norethindrone 1.0 mg (7 days) Ethinyl estradiol 35 μg (21 days) **ORTHO-NOVUM 10/11** Norethindrone 0.5 mg (10 days) Norethindrone 1.0 mg (11 days) Ethinyl estradiol 35 μg (21 days) **ORTHO-TRI-CYCLEN** Norgestimate 0.180 mg (7 days) Norgestimate 0.215 mg (7 days) Norgestimate 0.250 mg (7 days) Ethinyl estradiol 35 μg (21 days) **TRIPHASIL** Levonorgestrel 0.05 mg (6 days) Ethinyl estradiol 30 μg Levonorgestrel 0.075 mg (5 days) Ethinyl estradiol 40 μg Levonorgestrel 0.125 mg (10 days) Ethinyl estradiol 30 μg *BIPHASIC:* **NELOVA 10/11** Ethinyl estradiol 35 μg Norethindrone 0.5 mg (10 days) Norethindrone 1.0 mg (11 days)

210

CONTRACEPTIVES, ORAL

ADVERSE REACTIONS TO OCP's	NON-CONTRACEPTIVE BENEFITS	HORMONE COMPONENT	ABSOLUTE CONTRAINDICATIONS

Nausea
Vomiting
Breast tenderness
Water retention
Amenorrhea
Gallstones
Cholestatic jaundice
Hepatocellular CA (rare)
Increased blood glucose
Increased triglycerides
Increased LDL
Decreased HDL
Deep vein thrombosis
Pulmonary embolism
Myocardial Infarction
Stroke
Growth of estrogen dependent tumors
Pregnancy category X
	Increased menstrual regularity
	Less anemia secondary to menses
	Less dysmenorrhea
	Less functional ovarian cysts
	   (50% reduction in incidence)
	Decreased rate of ectopic pregnancy
	Decreased fibroadenoma and fibrocystic
	   disease of breast
	Decreased uterine fibroids
	   (30% reduction in incidence)
	Decreased incidence of acute pelvic
	inflammatory disease (PID)
	Decreased endometrial carcinoma
	   (50% reduction in incidence)
	Decreased ovarian carcinoma
	   (40% reduction in incidence)
	Less rheumatoid arthritis
	Increased bone density
		Estrogen component:
		   Ethinyl estradiol
		   Mestranol
		
		Progestin component:
		   Desogestrel
		   Ethynodiol
		   Levonorgestrol
		   Norgestrel
		   Norgestimate
		   Norethindrone
			Thrombophlebitis
			Thromboembolic disorders
			Past personal history of deep venous thrombosis
			   (DVT) or thromboembolic disorder
			Cerebral vascular or coronary artery disease
			Known or suspected breast cancer
			Known or suspected carcinoma of the
			   endometrium or other estrogen-
			   dependent tissues
			Undiagnosed or unexplained vaginal bleeding
			Cholestatic jaundice or pregnancy or jaundice
			   with prior OCP use
			Hepatic adenoma or carcinoma
			Known or suspected pregnancy

Minor Effects of Estrogen:
   chloasma, nausea, weight gain, headache (migraine), breakthrough bleeding, amenorrhea, edema

Minor Effects of Progesterone:
   breast fullness, depression, delayed onset of menses, acne, hirsutism, increased appetite, weight gain, increased libido

Effects Common to Estrogen and Progesterone:
   vasomotor symptoms, irritibility, breakthrough bleeding, vaginal spotting

211

CORTICOSTEROIDS, SYSTEMIC :

DRUG	EFFECTS	KINETICS	ADVERSE	USE
ACTH	Increases cAMP leads to increased enzymes; cholesterol conversion to pregnenolone which is converted to hydrocortisone	IM, IV, subQ; t½ = 15 mins (IV)	Fluid retention, hypokalemic alkalosis, glucose intolerance, hypersensitivity reaction	Diagnostic for adrenocortical insufficiency
BECLOMETHASONE (Beclovent, Beconase)	Antiinflammatory inhaled corticosteroid	Inhalational; minimal water solubility	Known teratogen in rodent studies	Asthma Nonasthmatic Bronchitis
DEXAMETHASONE (Decadron) **BETAMETHASONE**	*Long acting* antiinflammatory agent; used in management of premature fetuses to promote lung maturity prior to preterm delivery	Undergoes reduction reaction in microsomal system then conjugation	See Hydrocortisone	Promotes Fetal Lung Maturity Arthritis Bronchial Asthma
FLUDROCORTISONE (Florinef)	High mineralocorticoid activity; short acting	Same as Dexamethasone	Fluid retention; hypersensitivity reaction	Adjunct in Adrenal Insufficiency
HYDROCORTISONE	*Short acting* antiinflammatory; increases serum neutrophils (from bone marrow), decreases migration of cells out of blood; decreases monocytes, eosinophils, basophils (increases migration into lymphoid tissue); decreases phospholipase A2 activity, decreases prostaglandins and leukotrienes through macrocortin (lipocortin); causes muscle wasting, increases gluconeogenesis, decreases peripheral glucose use; causes osteoporosis; increases lipogenesis in face, neck and supraclavicular area; increases lipolysis, decreases fat in extremities	Oral, injection, topically (eye, skin); metabolism by liver microsome system, reduced then conjugated with sulfate or glucuronic acid; binds to corticotropin binding globulin (CBG)	Iatrogenic Cushing's syndrome; acne; thinning of skin; decreases skeletal m. mass; hyperglycemia; edema; osteoporosis; psychosis; peptic ulcer; cataracts; increases susceptibility to infection	Acute or chronic adrenocortical insufficiency; congenital adrenal hyperplasia; status asthmaticus; severe allergic reactions; transplant rejection; lupus; leukemia; RA; skin and eye diseases
METHYLPREDNISOLONE (Medrol)	*Intermediate acting* antiinflammatory	Biological half life is 8-12 hours	See Hydrocortisone	Same as Hydrocortisone
PREDNISOLONE (Delta-Cortef)	*Intermediate acting* antiinflammatory; LOW mineralocorticoid activity	Oral and parenteral	See Hydrocortisone	Same as Prednisone
PREDNISONE (Deltasone)	*Intermediate acting* antiinflammatory; LOW mineralocorticoid activity	Oral and parenteral	See Hydrocortisone	2° adrenocortical insufficiency or congenital adrenal hyperplasia

DECONGESTANTS, NASAL, OCULAR, AND SYSTEMIC:

AGENT	ORGAN SYSTEM EFFECTS	ROUTE OF DOSE	ADVERSE REACTIONS	THERAPEUTIC USE
EPHEDRINE	Nasal decongestant; intended for use in allergy, and symptoms of cold and flu; CNS stimulant; often abused by athletes to increase alertness and enhance performance; present in *Ma Huang*	Topical Systemic	Arrhythmia, increased blood pressure; insomnia, nervousness, restlessness, dizziness, headache, lightheadedness, sweating, urinary difficulty, tremor, muscle weakness; prolonged use may causes symptoms resembling paranoid schizophrenia	Allergy Symptoms of Cold and Flu
NAPHAZOLINE (Privine)	Vasoconstriction of nasal blood vessels	Topical	If systemic absorption, see Ephedrine for side effects	Nasal Decongestant for Allergic Rhinitis and Common Cold
OXYMETAZOLINE (Afrin, Visine L.R.)	Topical nasal and ocular decongestant	Topical	If systemic absorption see side effects similar to Ephedrine	Nasal Decongestant Ocular Decongestant
PHENYLEPHRINE (Neo-Synephrine)	Nasal decongestant; similar to Ephedrine	Topical	See Ephedrine	Allergy Symptoms of Cold and Flu
PROMETHAZINE (Phenergan)	Phenothiazine derivative that differs slightly from antipsychotic phenothiazines and thus lacks significant dopaminergic action; has **H1 receptor blocking activity; sedative and antiemetic effects**	Well absorbed from GI tract; effects within 20 minutes; duration of action 4-6 hours; liver metabolized; po and IV dosage	Sedation, blurred vision, dry mouth, dizziness, extrapyramidal symptoms, change in blood pressure, rash, photosensitivity; **Pregnancy category C**	Seasonal Allergic Rhinitis Vasomotor Rhinitis Allergic Conjunctivitis Dermographism Anaphylactic Reactions Sedation Narcotic Adjunct Motion Sickness Antiemetic
PSEUDOEPHEDRINE (Sudafed)	Systemic decongestant; CNS stimulant similar to Ephedrine	Systemic	See Ephedrine	Allergy Symptoms of Cold and Flu
TETRAHYDROZOLINE (Tyzine, Visine)	Topical nasal and ocular decongestant	Topical	If systemic absorption see side effects similar to Ephedrine	Nasal Decongestant Ocular Decongestant
XYLOMETAZOLINE (Otrivin)	Nasal decongestant	Topical		Nasal Decongestant

Editor's Note: This table lists commonly used decongestants. There are several other agents not listed here.

DIURETICS:

DRUG	ORGAN SYSTEM EFFECTS	SITE of ACTION	ADVERSE REACTIONS	THERAPEUTIC USE
CHLOROTHIAZIDE (Diuril)	**Thiazide diuretic;** increases loss of sodium, chloride, potassium, **water,** and magnesium, while decreasing loss of calcium (parathyroid mechanism); enhances calcium reabsorption; moderate diuretic; 6 hour duration; decreases blood volume and decreases TPR (unknown mechanism); interfere with insulin secretion; LOW ceiling effect (safe); good oral absorption; NO biotransformation; kidney excretion (glomerular filtration, PT secretion) and in bile	Early segment of distal tubule	Nausea, vomiting, **hypokalemia** (CHF, increases risk of arrhythmia); **hyperglycemia**(interfere with insulin secretion); **hyperuricemia; hyperlipidemia;** increases activity of tubocurarine; thrombocytopenia (decreases megakaryocytes); photosensitivity; **Pregnancy category C**	Adjunct for Edema Hypertension Diabetes Insipidus Kidney stones (decreases formation)
HYDROCHLOROTHIAZIDE (Hydrodiuril)	Thiazide diuretic; see Chlorothiazide	Early segment of distal tubule	See Chlorothiazide; **Pregnancy category B**	See Chlorothiazide
CHLORTHALIDONE (Hygroton)	**Thiazide-related diuretic** with mechanism of action similar to thiazide diuretics; however, does NOT inhibit carbonic anhydrase; onset of action within 2 hours, duration of action 24-72 hours; high plasma protein binding; undergoes **enterohepatic circulation;** renal excretion through glomerular filtration and proximal tubule secretion	Early distal convoluted tubule	Similar to Chlorothiazide, except no hyperlipidemia	Diuresis Hypertension
INDAPAMIDE (Lozol)	**Thiazide-related diuretic;** see Chlorthalindone and Metolazone	Early segment of renal distal tubule	Same as Chlorthalindone; **Pregnancy category B**	Same as Chlorthalindone
METOLAZONE (Zaroxolyn)	**Thiazide-related diuretic;** similar to the thiazides EXCEPT does NOT cause hyperlipidemia; longer action (12-24 hours); undergoes **enterohepatic circulation**	Early segment of renal distal tubule	Same as thiazides EXCEPT **does NOT cause hyperlipidemia**	Diuresis Hypertension
BUMETANIDE (Bumex)	**Loop diuretic;** see Furosemide for mechanism of action and kinetics, some biotransformation	Loop of Henle	See Furosemide for adverse effects; **Pregnancy category C**	Edema (see Furosemide)
ETHACRYNIC ACID (Edecrin)	**Loop diuretic;** see Furosemide for mechanism of action and kinetics, some biotransformation	Loop of Henle	Same adverse effects as Furosemide, EXCEPT is **teratogenic**	Edema (see Furosemide)

214

DIURETICS:

DRUG	ORGAN SYSTEM EFFECTS	SITE OF ACTION	ADVERSE REACTIONS	THERAPEUTIC USE
FUROSEMIDE (Lasix)	**Prototype loop diuretic**; oral onset within 30 minutes with 6 hour duration, IM and IV onset within 5 minutes with 2 hour duration), low biotransformation; excreted mostly unchanged by kidney via glomerular filtration and proximal tubule secretion; loop diuretics are MOST potent class of diuretics; HIGH ceiling effect; decreases response to NE driven hypertension; helps control blood pressure with antihypertensive drugs	Loop of Henle	Hypokalemia, hyperuricemia, hyperglycemia, ototoxicity (tinnitus, deafness); does not cause hyperlipidemia Drug interactions:: increases salicylate toxicity; NSAIDs decrease diuretic and antihypertensive response; **Pregnancy category C**	Edema associated with: Congestive Heart Failure Cirrhosis of the Liver Nephrotic Syndrome Chronic Heart Failure Renal Failure Hypertension Acute Hypercalcemia Acute Pulmonary Edema
TORSEMIDE (Demadex)	**Loop diuretic**; pyridine-sulfonylurea derivative; see Furosemide for mechanism of action and kinetics, biotransformed	Loop of Henle	See Furosemide for adverse effects; **Pregnancy category B**	Edema (see Furosemide) Hypertension
AMILORIDE (Midamor)	**Potassium sparing diuretic**; increases sodium, decreases potassium, and increases chloride excretion; adequate gastro-intestinal absorption; onset of action within 2 hours; excreted unchanged by kidney CONTRAINDICATED IN HYPERKALEMIA	Late renal distal tubule and collecting duct	Headache, weakness, fatigability, muscle cramps, dizziness, hyperkalemia; nausea, vomiting, anorexia, diarrhea; less common are orthostatic hypotension, dry mouth, paresthesia, confusion and insomnia; **Pregnancy category B**	Adjunct for Edema Hypertension Mainly used to treat diuretic induced hypokalemia
SPIRONOLACTONE (Aldactone)	**Potassium sparing diuretic**; increases Na, decreases K, and increases Cl excretion; NOT used in presence of hyperkalemia; **competitive inhibitor of aldosterone** in collecting duct region (binds cytoplasmic receptor); active metabolite is camrenone CONTRAINDICATED IN HYPERKALEMIA	Renal collecting duct and late distal tubule	Lethargy, drowsiness, ataxia, headache, mental confusion; diarrhea, GI disturbances; hypermenstruation in females); gynecomastia in males Contraindicated in hyperkalemia; should NOT be given with potassium supplements; caution when given with ACE inhibitors which also cause hyperkalemia Not recommended in pregnancy or nursing mothers	Edema Hypertension Hirsutism in Women (agent of choice) Treatment of Hypokalemia

215

DIURETICS:

DRUG	ORGAN SYSTEM EFFECTS	SITE OF ACTION	ADVERSE REACTIONS	THERAPEUTIC USE
TRIAMTERENE (Dyrenium)	**Potassium sparing diuretic**; pyrazine derivative that inhibits sodium reabsorption and prevents potassium excretion in the collecting duct; onset of action within 2-4 hours; liver and renal excretion via proximal tubular secretion CONTRAINDICATED IN HYPERKALEMIA	Renal collecting duct and late distal tubule	Hyperkalemia, ECG changes, decreases glomerular filtration rate (GFR); use with cyclooxygenase inhibitors has been reported to cause renal failure; **Pregnancy category C**	Adjunct for Edema Hypertension
ACETAZOLAMIDE (Diamox)	**Carbonic anhydrase inhibitor** that acts in renal tubule; produces an alkaline urine with increased excretion of sodium, potassium, bicarbonate, and phosphate; peak plasma level within 2 hours; structure is aromatic sulfonamide	Renal proximal tubule; alters HCO_3 reabs	Flushing, headache, drowsiness, dizziness, fatigue, irritability, excitability; polydypsia, polyria, paresthesia, ataxia, hyperpnea, anorexia, vomiting and GI distress have all been reported; may cause fever and blood dyscarsia as any other of the sulfonamides; **Pregnancy category C**	Edema (promote diuresis) Glaucoma Absence seizures Premenstrual tension Altitude or Mountain Sickness
MANNITOL (Osmitrol)	**Osmotic diuretic**; given in solution to maintain urine flow; prevents anuria; decreases intraocular pressure; decreases elevated CSF pressure	Not reabsorbed by kidney, remains in lumen with fluid	Contraindicated in CHF as given in solution (so is addition of fluid)	To Increase Urine Output Decreases Intracranial Pressure Decreases Intraocular Pressure

216

ESTROGENS:

DRUG	CLASS/MECHANISM OF ACTION	PHARMACOKINETICS	ADVERSE EFFECTS	USE
ESTRADIOL, ESTRONE (Depo-Estradiol)	**Prototype estrogens;** non-synthetic, have steroid nucleus; orally active estrogen preparations **ALL** estrogens, natural, synthetic, and nonsteroidal act on estrogen receptors in the nucleus; (synthetic estrogens LACK steroid nucleus) **POTENCY of estrogens:** estradiol > estrone > estriol **EFFECT OF ESTROGENS:** development and maintenance of 2° sex characteristics; increased muscle mass; increased HDL; antagonize PTH	Well absorbed via skin and mucous membranes, subcutaneously and intravenously; systemic effects may occur from transdermal absorption; oral absorption has HIGH liver 1st pass effect; Variety of tissues such as fat, muscle, liver, skin, endometrium and hypothalamus have aromatase enzyme to convert C-19 steroids to estrogen	Nausea, dizziness, vomiting, edema, headache, hypertension, jaundice, increases clotting factors, thrombophlebitis, stroke, myocardial infarction	Estrogen Replacement Therapy Atrophic Vaginitis
CHLOROTRIANISENE (Tace)	Nonsteroidal estrogen; see Estradiol	LONG duration; goes into fat; 1 month duration	Gynecomastia, impotence in men; fluid retention	Palliative treatment of advanced Prostatic carcinoma
CONJUGATED ESTROGENS (Premarin)	Natural estrogen; orally active estrogen preparation; see Estradiol Hormone Replacement Therapy (HRT) in: •Moderate to severe vasomotor symptoms associated with menopause •Atrophic vaginitis •Osteoporosis •Hypoestrogenism due to hypogonadism, castration or primar ovarian failure •Palliative therapy in metastatic breast cancer •Palliation therapy for advanced androgen-dependent prostatic carcinoma	Oral, parenteral, vaginal dosage	Breakthrough bleeding, vaginal spotting, change in menstrual flow, dysmenorrhea, PMS-like syndrome, vaginal candidiasis, change in cervical secretion; breast tenderness/enlargement; nausea, vomiting, abdominal cramps, bloating, cholestatic jaundice; chloasma or melasma, rash; alopecia, hirsutism; **contact lens intolerance;** headache, migraine, dizziness, depression, chorea; weight change; **Pregnancy category X** (teratogen)	Hormone Replacement Therapy (HRT) in Postmenopausal women Must be used with progestin such as Provera if patient has intact endometrium Hypogonadism Atrophic Vaginitis

217

ESTROGENS:

DRUG	CLASS/MECHANISM OF ACTION	PHARMACOKINETICS	ADVERSE EFFECTS	USE
DIENESTROL (DV)	Synthetic nonsteroidal estrogen used topically for localized therapy; see Estradiol	Intravaginal use	Vaginal candidiasis; cystitis-like syndrome; systemic adverse effects may occur, otherwise well tolerated	Atrophic Vaginitis Atrophic Vulva
DIETHYLSTILBESTROL, DES (Stilphostrol)	Synthetic nonsteroidal estrogen capable of producing all activity and response as natural estrogen; see Estradiol; not recommended as "morning after pill"; has limited therapeutic use	Administered orally	Nausea, vomiting; **females exposed in utero may have increased risk of developing a rare form of vaginal or cervical cancer later in life**	Palliation for Metastatic Breast Cancer in Men and Women Palliative Therapy for Advanced Prostatic Carcinoma
ESTROPIPATE (Ogen)	See Estradiol	po dosing	Estrogen increases risk of endometrial CA in postmenopausal women, increases risk of gallbladder disease; nausea, vomiting, bloating, headache, migraine, dizziness; **Pregnancy category X**	Vasomotor symptoms of menopause Vulval and Vaginal Atrophy Hypoestrogenism Female Hypogonadism Castration Ovarian Failure Prevention of Osteoporosis
ETHINYL ESTRADIOL	Synthetic estrogen; common estrogen compoenent in oral contraceptive preparations	Potent oral form	See Estradiol	Common Estrogen in Many Estrogen/Progestin Oral Contraceptives
MESTRANOL (Norinyl 1/50 21-day and 28-day regimens)	Synthetic estrogen; see Conjugated Estrogens for activity; used as estrogen component in some oral contraceptive preparations	**Prodrug**; demethylated in liver to ethinyl estradiol	See Conjugated Estrogens	Oral Contraceptive Component
QUINESTROL (Estrovis)	Synthetic estrogen; derivative of ethinyl estradiol; effective as conjugated estrogens in treating vasomotor flushes in menopausal women	**Prodrug**; de-esterified in liver to ethinyl estradiol; 1 week duration; goes into adipose	Nausea, breast tenderness, headache, dizziness, blurred vision, vaginal discharge and spotting are reported	Hormone Replacement Therapy (HRT)

218

EXPECTORANTS:

AGENT	ORGAN SYSTEM EFFECTS	ADVERSE REACTIONS	THERAPEUTIC USE
ACETYLCYSTEINE (Mucomyst)	Mucolytic agent; also decreases hepatotoxicity following Acetaminophen overdose by maintaining glutathione levels	Stomatitis, nausea, vomiting, fever, rhinorrhea, drowsiness, clamminess, chest tightness, rash, bronchoconstriction, bronchospasm; **Pregnancy category B**	Nebulizer Treatments Acetaminophen Overdose Antidote
AMMONIUM CHLORIDE	Expectorant found in combination cough and cold preparations		Expectorant
GUAIFENESIN (Robitussin)	Glyceryl guaiacolate is a mucoregulator, emetic expectorant	Nausea and drowsiness occur rarely; **Pregnancy category C**	Expectorant
IODINATED GLYCEROL	Elixir, solution and tablets		Expectorant

219

FLUOROQUINOLONES, THE:

AGENT	ORGAN SYSTEM EFFECTS	PHARMACOKINETICS	ADVERSE REACTIONS	THERAPEUTIC USE
CIPROFLOXACIN (Cipro)	Fluoroquinolones are potent bactericidal agents that inhibit **DNA gyrase** (topoisomerase II) concentration dependent bactericidal action; highly active against *N. gonorrhea*, *N. meningitidis* and *Moraxella catarrhalis*; excellent activity against Enterobacteriaceae including *E. Coli, Klebsiella, Enterobacter, Proteus, Morganella, Providencia, Citrobacter, Serratia, Salmonella, Shigella* and *Yersinia enterocolitica*; active against other gram negatives: *Eikenella corrodens, Pasteurella multocida, Aeromonas hydrophila, Campylobacter jejuni, Vibrio, Helicobacter pylori, Hemophilus influenza, Hemophilus ducreyi* and *Legionella*; quinolones have good activity against Methicillin-susceptible *S. aureus* and coagulase negative Staphylococci	Good GI absorption; peak plasma levels within 1-2 hours; chelates with metal cations thus avoid taking with antacids containing magnesium, aluminum and calcium and Sucralfate; 30% plasma protein bound; IV and po	CNS stimulation, dizziness, lightheadedness, GI upset, headache, restlessness, rash, eosinophilia, liver enzymes elevation, **photosensitivity**, Stevens-Johnson syndrome, tendinitis, tendon rupture; **Pregnancy category C**; fluoroquinolones have been shown to have adverse effects on fetal animal cartilage and thus should be avoided in pregnancy, nursing women and prepubertal children	Urinary Tract Infection Lower Respiratory Infection Cellulitis Bone and Joint Infection Also has use in *Mycobacteria tuberculosis* therapy
ENOXACIN (Penetrex)	Flouroquinolone; see Ciprofloxacin	40% plasma protein bound; taken 1-2 hours after meals	Nausea, vomiting, abdominal pain, diarrhea, dizziness, headache; **Pregnancy category C**	Uncomplicated Cystitis Complicated Cystitis Uncomplicated Gonorrhea
LEVOFLOXACIN (Levaquin)	Flouroquinolone; see Ciprofloxacin	See Ciprofloxacin; taken po at least 2 hours before or after antacids or Sucralfate, iron or multivitamins	See Ciprofloxacin; **Pregnancy category C**	Chronic Bronchitis (Acute Exacerbation) Community Acquired Pneumonia Acute Maxillary Sinusitis Uncomplicated UTI Acute Pyelonephritis
LOMEFLOXACIN (Maxaquin)	Flouroquinolone; see Ciprofloxacin	12% plasma protein bound; taken po without regard to meals	Photosensitivity, CNS stimulation, dizziness, GI upset, headache, tenditis, tendon rupture; **Pregnancy category C**	Lower Respiratory Infection Urinary Tract Infection

220

FLUOROQUINOLONES, THE:

AGENT	ORGAN SYSTEM EFFECTS	PHARMACOKINETICS	ADVERSE REACTIONS	THERAPEUTIC USE
NORFLOXACIN (Noroxin)	Fluoroquinolone; see Ciprofloxacin	15% plasma protein bound; taken po with water	Nausea, headache, dizziness, asthenia, rash, abdominal pain, dyspepsia, somnolence, insomnia, constipation, dry mouth, fever, tendinitis, photosensitivity; **Pregnancy category C**	Urinary Tract Infection Sexually Transmitted Disease Uncomplicated Gonorrhea
OFLOXACIN (Floxin)	Fluoroquinolone; see Ciprofloxacin	30% plasma protein bound	Nausea, insomnia, headache, dizziness, diarrhea, vomiting, rash, pruritus, dysgeusia (bad taste); tendinitis, tendon rupture, photosensitivity; **Pregnancy category C**	Lower Respiratory Infection Cellulitis Sexually Transmitted Disease Uncomplicated Gonorrhea Chlamydial infection Prostatitis

NOTE: The fluoroquinolones have been shown to have adverse effects on fetal animal cartilage and thus should be avoided in pregnancy, nursing women and prepubertal children.

221

GASTRIC ACID PUMP INHIBITORS:

AGENT	ORGAN SYSTEM EFFECTS	PHARMACOKINETICS	ADVERSE REACTIONS	THERAPEUTIC USE
LANSOPRAZOLE (Prevacid)	Antisecretory compound; not anticholinergic or antihistaminic; decreases gastric acid secretion via inhibition of **gastric proton pump** (H$^+$/K$^+$ ATPase); shown to have significant effect on basal gastric acid output and mean gastric pH	Peak plasma levels within 1.7 hours; rapid GI absorption; liver metabolized; urine excretion	Abdominal pain, diarrhea, nausea; **Pregnancy category B**	Active Duodenal Ulcer Erosive Esophagitis Pathological Hypersecretory Conditions
OMEPRAZOLE (Prilosec)	*Prototype* member of new class of **gastric antisecretory** agents, the substituted benzimidazoles; inhibits the gastric acid proton pump (H$^+$/K$^+$ ATPase inhibitor); decreases stomach acid; has NO anticholinergic or H2 blocking properties	Oral; onset of action within 1 hour of dose; maximal effect within 2 hours; duration of action is 72 hours	Headache; diarrhea; rash; nausea, constipation; **Pregnancy category C**	Active Duodenal Ulcer Gastroesophageal Reflux Disease (GERD) Severe Erosive Esophagitis Pathological Hypersecretory Conditions

222

GI STIMULANTS:

AGENT	ORGAN SYSTEM EFFECTS	PHARMACOKINETICS	ADVERSE REACTIONS	THERAPEUTIC USE
CISAPRIDE (Propulsid)	GI stimulant thought to act by increasing release of acetylcholine at the myenteric plexus; does not act on muscarinic or nicotinic receptor sites; increases lower esophageal sphincter tone and peristalsis; accelerates gastric emptying; reduces symptoms of heartburn associated with gastroesophageal reflux disease (GERD)	Rapid oral absorption; onset of action within 30-60 minutes	Abdominal pain; headache; nausea, diarrhea; **Pregnancy category C**; excreted in human breast milk	Nocturnal Heartburn associated with Gastroesophageal Reflux Disease (GERD)
METOCLOPRAMIDE (Reglan)	Stimulates upper gastrointestinal motility without stimulating gastric, biliary or pancreatic secretion; thought to sensitize tissues to acetylcholine as its actvity is inhibited by anticholinergic agents; increases gastric contraction, relaxes pyloric sphincter and duodenal bulb; increases peristalsis in duodenum and jejunum; accelerates gastric emptying and intestinal transit time; increases lower esophageal sphincter resting tone; little effect on colon or gall bladder motility	Rapid and complete GI absorption	Restlessness, drowsiness, fatigue and lassitude in 10%; acute dystonic reactions in 0.2%; **Pregnancy category B**; excreted in human breast milk	Gastroesophageal Reflux Diabetic Gastroparesis Antiemetic in Chemotherapy Post Operative Antiemetic Small Bowel Intubation Radiological Examination

223

GONADOTROPIN INHIBITORS and GnRH AGONISTS:

AGENT	ORGAN SYSTEM EFFECTS	PHARMACOKINETICS	ADVERSE REACTIONS	THERAPEUTIC USE
DANAZOL (Danocrine)	Antiestrogen synthetic derivative of 17α-ethinyl testosterone; **suppresses midcycle gonadotropin (FSH, LH) surge from pituitary**; hypoestrogenism is seen at higher doses; antiestrogen action causes regression of normal and ectopic endometrial tissue in endometriosis, and decreases growth of abnormal breast tissue in fibrocystic breast disease; only the Danazol-androgen receptor complex binds nuclear DNA; in endometriosis, Danazol makes normal and ectopic endometrial tissue inactive and atrophic	Oral absorption; undergoes hepatic transformation	Water and electrolyte retention; headache, dizziness, sleep disorders, behavioral changes; may cause hirsutism, acne, voice deepening, clitoral enlargement, changes in libido; **Pregnancy category X**	Endometriosis Fibrocystic Breast disease Hereditary Angioedema
GONADORELIN (Lutrepulse)	Synthetic gonadotropin releasing hormone (GnRH) used for **ovulation induction**; causes increased release of FSH and LH from the anterior pituitary gland	Pulsatile Intravenous Injection	Ovarian hyperstimulation; multiple pregnancy; **Pregnancy category B**	Primary Hypothalamic Amenorrhea
GOSERELIN (Zoladex)	Synthetic **decapeptide analog of lutenizing hormone releasing hormone (LHRH)** which inhibits pituitary gonadotropin (FSH, LH) secretion; initial effect is increased LH, FSH and testosterone; **chronic effects are decreased LH, FSH, and testosterone** to levels seen in castrated males; in women chronic effects are decreased FSH and LH with **reduction of estradiol to** levels seen in postmenopausal women	About 2-4 weeks to see decreased testosterone in males; about 3 weeks to see decreased estradiol in women; cylinder shaped implant (1.5 mm diameter) is delivered subcutaneously via supplied syringe	**Males:** hot flashes, sexual dysfunction, lethargy, rash, anorexia, insomnia, nausea, **Females:** hot flashes, amenorrhea, vaginitis, decreased libido, depression, acne, breast atrophy, injection site reactions; **Pregnancy category X**	Prostatic CA Palliation Endometriosis Advanced Breast Cancer
LEUPROLIDE (Lupron)	Synthetic nonapeptide analog of gonadotropin releasing hormone (GnRH); greater potency than naturally occurring hormone; see Goserelin effects	Depot form is long acting	See Goserelin **Pregnancy category X**	Endometriosis Uterine Leiomyomata (Fibroids)
NAFARELIN (Synarel)	Potent agonist analog of gonadotropin releasing hormone (GnRH) which stimulates FSH and LH production by pituitary with short term use	Nasal spray; rapid systemic absorption	Acne, transient breast enlargement, vaginal bleeding, emotional lability, transient increase in pubic hair, body odor; **Pregnancy category X**	Central Precocious Puberty in Both Sexes

HAIR GROWTH STIMULATOR:

AGENT	ORGAN SYSTEM EFFECTS	PHARMACOKINETICS	ADVERSE REACTIONS	INDICATION
MINOXIDIL (Rogaine)	A direct acting peripheral vasodilator that decreases systolic and diastolic blood pressure when taken by mouth; found to have hair growth stimulating effect po and topically	Applied topically to scalp	NOT recommended for children under 18 years, in pregnancy, or breast feeding women; dermatitis Systemic side effects: chest pain, tachycardia, faintness, dizziness, edema, weight gain	Hair growth stimulator Post menopausal indication in women with frontoparietal hair loss or thinning in women with family history of hair loss

225

HEAVY METALS, THE:

DRUG	EXPOSURE TO HEAVY METALS	SYMPTOMS OF TOXICITY	THERAPY
ARSENIC	Used as tonic stimulant; defoliant, found in insecticides; variable absorption; **pentavalent arsenics** uncouple oxidative phosphorylation; trivalent arsenics tie up sulfhydryl (SH) groups); **stored in tissues with cumulative effects of small dose chronic exposure**	Immediate large dose: CV collapse; encephalopathy; neuropathy (foot drop, paresthesia)	Acute overdose: Supportive Therapy **Dimercaprol** **Penicillamine**
CADMIUM	Inhalation exposure in industry; poor oral absorption; **binds avidly to tissues; t½ ≈ 10-30 years**	Kidney toxicity (failure); lung toxicity (pulmonary edema and fibrosis)	**Chelator Therapy is poorly effective** Editate Calcium Disodium
GOLD	Gold salts are used IM for rheumatoid arthritis; oral gold is available BUT causes diarrhea; mechanism of action is unknown; accumulates in reticuloendothelial system; idiosyncratic toxicity (NOT predictable)	**Idiosyncratic toxicity:** skin rash; itching; mouth lesions; shock-like signs; Stevens Johnson syndrome (erythema multiforme bullosum); bone marrow depression (agranulocytosis or pronounced leukopenia)	Treat idiosyncratic toxicity with **Dimercaprol** and **Penicillamine**
IRON	Unsupervised children may ingest ferrous sulfate tablets (a common and potentially fatal poisoning seen in pediatrics practice); iron is NEVER free form in blood; free iron is VERY toxic	Acute CV collapse	Supportive measures + **Deferoxamine** both orally AND IV doses together
LEAD	Unsupervised children may ingest lead paint chips found in old buildings; acidic food increases lead absorption; 10% adult bioavailability; 40% child bioavailability; 90% absorption of lead vapors; phase I distribution to soft tissues; in phase II lead acts like calcium and is deposited in hydroxyapatite of bone; t½ ≈ 1-2 months	High dose: encephalopathy with coma and convulsion (rare); chronic low level lead exposure: GI stimulation; lead colic (cramps); peripheral neuropathy (foot drop); CNS accumulation; interferes with porphyrin metabolism of hemoglobin; kidney toxicity	Supportive measures **Editate Calcium Disodium** **Dimercaprol** **Penicillamine**
MERCURY	Industrial exposure; elemental mercury poorly absorbed; vaporized mercury is well absorbed; organic mercury has 90% bioavailability (inorganic 10%); believed to have medicinal value in some cultures	Acute exposure: CV collapse, anemia, renal toxicity Chronic exposure: mercury deposit in brain resulting in psychosis, salivation, and gingivitis; methyl mercury shows selective peripheral nervous system toxicity	Supportive measures **Dimercaprol** for high level mercury exposure **Penicillamine** for low level mercury exposure

HEMATINICS:

DRUG	SYSTEM EFFECTS	CHARACTERISTICS	ADVERSE REACTIONS	THERAPEUTIC USE
FERROUS SULFATE (Feosol, Fer-In-Sol, Slow Fe)	Two forms of Ferrous sulfate: **hydrated salt** containing **20% elemental iron** by weight, **and desiccated form containing 80% anhydrous FeSO4**; ORAL dose; 200 mg iron/day (absorb 20%) to **restore red cell production, restore storage supply** (takes 3-6 months); ↑ 0.1 g/dL Hb/day; indicated when **MCV < 80 μ^3**	20% elemental iron; as ↑ storage, ↑ mucosal block; overdose can overload transferrin and ↑ free iron which is corrosive	GI irritation; gastroenteritis; hypotension; shock; acidosis; kidney and liver damage Rx for toxicity: HCO3- converts iron to ferric form NOT absorbed	Iron Deficiency Anemia Post Partum Replacement
IRON DEXTRAN INJECTION (Imferon)	Parental dose (IM, IV); contains 50 mg of elemental iron per mL; indicated in patients who cannot tolerate oral iron such as those with ulcerative colitis, regional enteritis, colostomy, or extensive bowel resection	High dose IM or IV	Skin staining at injection site, thrombophlebitis, arthralgia, fever, myalgia, hypotension, bradycardia, headaches, abdominal pain, nausea, vomiting, dizziness	Microcytic Anemia (In patients who cannot tolerate oral iron) Severe Iron Deficiency

Abbreviations: MCV - mean corpuscular volume   RDA - recommended daily allowance

CLASSIFICATION OF THE ANEMIAS:

Anemia Secondary to Blood Loss
    Acute blood loss leading to symptoms of hypovolemia and hypoxia
    Chronic occult blood loss resulting in iron-deficiency anemia

Anemia Secondary to Decreased Red Blood Cell Production
    Microcytic Anemias
        Iron-deficiency anemia
        Sideroblastic anemia
        Thalassemias
    Macrocytic Anemias
        Vitamin B12 deficiency
        Folate deficiency
    Normocytic Anemias
        Anemia of chronic disease
    Hemolytic Anemias

227

HEMORHEOLOGIC AGENT:

AGENT	SYSTEM EFFECTS	PHARMACOKINETICS	ADVERSE REACTIONS	THERAPEUTIC USE
PENTOXIFYLLINE (Trental)	Pentoxifylline and its metabolites improve flow properties of blood by decreasing viscosity; in chronic peripheral vascular disease (PVD) increases blood flow and enhances oxygen delivery; exact mechanism of action not known	Oral dosage; almost complete oral absorption; undergoes **first pass effect**; peak plasma levels of parent and metabolites within 1 hour; almost total urine excretion	Dyspepsia, nausea, vomiting, belching, flatus, bloating; agitation, headache; **Pregnancy category C**	Intermittent claudication associated with Peripheral Vascular Disease

HEPARIN ANTAGONIST:

AGENT	ORGAN SYSTEM EFFECTS	PHARMACOKINETICS	ADVERSE REACTIONS	THERAPEUTIC USE
PROTAMINE SULFATE	Simple protein of low molecular weight rich in arginine and **strongly basic**; occurs in salmon and other fish; given alone Protamine has anticoagulant effect; but given in presence of Heparin (strongly acidic), a stable salt forms stopping the anticoagulant effects of both	Rapid onset of action; neutralization of Heparin occurs within 5 minutes of IV dosage	Sudden hypotension and bradycardia; transitory flushing and feeling of warmth; dyspnea, nausea, vomiting; lassitude; overdosage may cause bleeding; **Pregnancy category C**	Heparin Overdosage

HISTAMINE H$_2$-BLOCKERS:

DRUG	MECHANISM OF ACTION	PHARMACOKINETICS	ADVERSE EFFECTS	THERAPEUTIC USE
CIMETIDINE (Tagamet)	1st H2 receptor antagonist, introduced in 1977; decreases gastric acid secretion; **reversible and competive inhibition of histamine activity on H2 receptors** in dose dependent fashion; pure antagonist, NO agonist properties; NO significant H1, β adrenergic or muscarinic receptors; NO effect on gastric motility or gastric emptying time	Does NOT cross BBB; t½ = 2-3 hours; long duration; LOW plasma protein binding (20%); undergoes extensive first pass biotransformation; long duration of action (bid dosing); excreted in urine	Safe agents; may cause headache, malaise, dizziness, constipation, diarrhea, skin rash, and altered liver function; CNS disturbances have been reported (somnolence, insomnia, confusion, hallucination); gynecomastia has been reported; **Pregnancy category B** 50% liver metabolism by cytochrome P$_{450}$ which inhibits this enzyme; will increase effects of agents also metabolized by P$_{450}$ (see below)	Peptic Ulcer Disease (PUD) Gastroesophageal Reflux Disease (GERD) Zollinger-Ellison syndrome (gastrin secreting pancreatic tumor) Stress Ulcer Prophylaxis in pre and post operative patients who are npo (nothing per mouth)
FAMOTIDINE (Pepcid)	See Cimetidine	20% plasma protein binding; half life 3-4 hours; minimal first pass effect; long duration of action (bid dosing) excreted in urine	See Cimetidine; does not inhibit cytochrome P$_{450}$; **Pregnancy category B**	Same as Cimetidine
NIZATIDINE (Axid)	See Cimetidine	35% plasma protein binding; half life 1-2 hours; minimal first pass effect; long duration of action (bid dosing); excreted in urine; NOT available by injection	See Cimetidine; does not inhibit cytochrome P$_{450}$; **Pregnancy category C**	Same as Cimetidine
RANITIDINE (Zantac)	See Cimetidine	15% plasma protein binding; half life 2-3 hours; minimal first pass effect; long duration of action (bid dosing); excreted in urine	See Cimetidine; does not inhibit cytochrome P$_{450}$; **Pregnancy category B**	Same as Cimetidine

Some agents metabolized by P$_{450}$:

Benzodiazepines
Warfarin (Coumadin)
Propranolol (Inderal)
Nifedipine (Procardia)
Digitoxin

HYPOCALCEMICS:

DRUG	MECHANISM OF ACTION	KINETICS	ADVERSE EFFECTS	THERAPEUTIC USE
CALCITONIN (Calcimar)	Secreted by parafollicular or C cells of the thyroid gland in response to hypercalcemia; salmon and human Calcitonin have been isolated for human use; Calcitonin has **hypocalcemic and hypophosphatemic** effects; major site of action is bone where it **inhibits osteoclast function**; also inhibits PTH-stimulated bone resorption; at pharmacologic doses it has a **direct calciuric effect**	Subcutaneous, IM; onset within **24-48** hours, duration of action is short due to tachyphylaxis that may develop within several days	Nausea and vomiting are most common (50% of patients), facial flushing; abdominal cramps, diarrhea, itching, urinary frequency, urticaria may occur less frequently; **Pregnancy category C**	Paget's disease of bone Bone Mineral Loss in Hyperparathyroidism, Immobilization, and Malignancy
GALLIUM NITRATE	Hypocalcemic effect produced by preventing resorption of calcium by bone; may decrease bone turnover; exact mechanism is not known, but no cytotoxic effect on bone cells	IV by continuous infusion	Nephrotoxic, not to be given with other nephrotoxic drugs such as aminoglycosides	Malignancy related hypercalcemia not responsive to hydration therapy

231

HYPOGLYCEMIC AGENTS:

AGENT	ORGAN SYSTEM EFFECTS	PHARMACOKINETICS	ADVERSE REACTIONS	THERAPEUTIC USE
ACETOHEXAMIDE (Dymelor)	Same as Tolbutamide; 1st generation oral hypoglycemic agent	ORAL; 1-2 hours to onset; 12-24 hour duration	Same as Tolbutamide	Type II NIDDM
CHLORPROPAMIDE (Diabinese)	Same as Tolbutamide; 1st generation oral hypoglycemic agent	ORAL; 1-3 hours to onset; 24-60 hour duration	Same as Tolbutamide; **Pregnancy category C**	Type II NIDDM
GLIMEPIRIDE (Amaryl)	Sulfonylurea; used as adjunct to diet control in Type II diabetes mellitus OR in cases of uncontrolled patients on insulin therapy	ORAL	Hypoglycemia, dizziness, asthenia, headache, nausea, allergic skin reaction, blood dyscrasia **Pregnancy category C**	Type II NIDDM
GLIPIZIDE (Glucotrol)	Same as Tolbutamide; 2nd generation oral hypoglycemia agent	ORAL; 1-1.5 hours to onset; 12-24 hour duration	Same as Tolbutamide; **Pregnancy category C**	Type II NIDDM
GLYBURIDE (Diabeta, Micronase)	Same as Tolbutamide; 2nd generation oral hypoglycemia agent	ORAL; 2-4 hours to onset; 16-24 hour duration	Same as Tolbutamide; **Pregnancy category C**	Type II NIDDM
METFORMIN (Glucophage)	Oral anthyperglycemic agent; NOT related to sulfonylureas; improves glucose tolerance in NIDDM; lowers post prandial and basal plasma glucose	50-60% oral absorption; excreted unchanged in urine	Diarrhea, nausea, vomiting, bloating, flatulence, anorexia; metallic taste, lactic acidosis (rare); **Pregnancy category B**	Type II NIDDM
TOLAZAMIDE (Tolinase)	Same as Tolbutamide; 1st generation oral hypoglycemia agent	ORAL; 4-6 hours to onset; 12-24 hour duration	Same as Tolbutamide; **Pregnancy category C**	Type II NIDDM
TOLBUTAMIDE (Orinase)	**1st generation oral hypoglycemic agent** introduced along with Acetohexamide and Chlorpropamide; **lowers blood glucose;** binds K channel and alters flux; open Ca channels; Ca influx, insulin efflux; **REQUIRES circulating insulin**	ORAL; 1-4 hours to onset; 6-12 hour duration	Hypoglycemia is most common; less commonly see nausea, vomiting, dyspepsia, rash, pruritus, exfoliative dermatitis, hemolytic anemia and bone marrow aplasia; **Pregnancy category C**	Type II NIDDM
TROGLITAZONE (Rezulin)	Antidiabetic agent that lowers plasma glucose levels by decreasing target cell insulin resistance; improves insulin sensitivity in muscle and adipose tissue; inhibits gluconeogenesis; REQUIRES presence of insulin for activity	ORAL	Asthenia, dizziness, gastrointestinal upset, reversible liver enzymes elevation; **Pregnancy category B**	Type II NIDDM not controlled with Insulin therapy

232

HYPOLIPIDEMICS:

DRUG	ORGAN SYSTEM EFFECTS	PHARMACOKINETICS	ADVERSE REACTIONS	THERAPEUTIC USE
LOVASTATIN (Mevacor)	*Prototype* **HMG CoA reductase inhibitor;** decreases synthesis of cholesterol → decreases liver cholesterol → increases liver uptake of plasma cholesterol; **decreases LDL, increases HDL, decreases TG;** up to 50% reduction of cholesterol	**Prodrug;** lactone group converted to active group; crosses BBB; oral dose; 80% excreted in feces; 10% in urine	Generally well tolerated; increased liver transaminase (liver toxic); myalgia and myopathy (0.5%); increases creatinine phosphokinase activity (renal toxic); **Pregnancy category X**	Hypolipidemic
ATORVASTATIN (Lipitor)	**HMG-CoA reductase inhibitor;** selective, competitive inhibitor that lowers plasma cholesterol and lipoprotein levels	Rapid po absorption; max plasma levels within 1-2 hours; bile excretion	Headache, abdominal pain, diarrhea, rash, arthralgia, paresthesia; **Pregnancy category X**	1° Hypercholesterolemia Mixed Dyslipidemia
PRAVASTATIN (Pravacor)	**HMG CoA reductase inhibitor;** same as Lovastatin	Has active group without conversion; will NOT cross BBB	Same as Lovastatin; **Pregnancy category X**	Hypolipidemic
SIMVASTATIN (Zocor)	**HMG CoA reductase inhibitor;** same as Lovastatin	**Prodrug**	Same as Lovastatin; **Pregnancy category X**	**Hypolipidemic**
CHOLESTYRAMINE	**Bile acid binding resin;** binds bile acids which are then excreted in feces; decreases LDL; may increase TG; loss of cholesterol causes increased hepatic production of cholesterol and up regulation of hepatic LDL receptors	Water insoluble, NOT absorbed; LARGE dose (12-24 g/day)	LOW toxicity but poorly tolerated; constipation, bloating, steatorrhea; interferes with absorption of fat soluble vitamins (K,A,D,E); tend to increase TG early in treatment; caution in pregnancy	1° Hypercholesterolemia
COLESTIPOL (Colestid)	**Bile acid binding resin,** same as Cholestyramine	See Cholestyramine	Constipation, bloating; interferes with absorption of fat soluble vitamins	Same as Cholestyramine
CLOFIBRATE (Atromid-S)	**Fibric acid derivative;** decreases LDL synthesis by liver, decreases TG; LESS effects on HDL (may increase LDL in some patients called **ß shift**)	Almost total oral absorption; hydrolyzed to clofibric acid which is active and highly plasma protein bound (95%); excreted in urine	Weight gain, skin rash, alopecia, weakness, impotence, breast tenderness, loss of libido; elevation of liver transaminases; long term use increases risk of gallstones and cholecystitis	Type IIb (high TG) and Type III (high IDL, chylomicrons) Hyperlipoproteinemia

233

HYPOLIPIDEMICS:

DRUG	ORGAN SYSTEM EFFECTS	PHARMACOKINETICS	ADVERSE REACTIONS	THERAPEUTIC USE
GEMFIBROZIL (Lopid)	Fibric acid derivative; see Clofibrate	Excellent GI absorption; peak plasma levels within 1-2 hours; excreted in urine	Similar to Clofibrate but less long term side effects; commonly see: GI upset, blurred vision, impotence, gallstones; **Pregnancy category C**	**Hypertriglyceridemia** in adults with plasma leverls greater than 1000 mg/dL
PROBUCOL (Lorelco)	Lowers plasma cholesterol with little to no effect on triglycerides; LDL fraction decreases, but proportionally greater decrease in HDL fraciton; mechanism may be associated with potent **antioxidant property;** use was largely replaced by Lovastatin	POOR oral bioavailability; highly lipophilic and distributes into adipose; 20% may remain in plasma after 6 months	Prolongation of QT interval on EKG; arrhythmogenic in animals; diarrhea and loose stools are common; nausea, vomiting, flatulence will decrease with continued use; less frequently see skin rash, thrombocytopenia, peripheral neuritis, and angioneurotic edema	**Type IIa and IIb hyperlipoproteinemia** in patients who failed to respond to diet and weight reduction
NICOTINIC ACID (Niacin)	Large doses of Niacin aka vitamin B3, in the form of **nicotinic acid lowers plasma cholesterol and triglycerides;** NOT due to vitamin activity as nicotinamide has not hypolipidemic effect; mechanism appears to be via reduction of VLDL production by liver, which results in decreased IDL and LDL, and raised HDL levels; synthesis of Lp(a) is reduced	2-6 g/day dosage; well absorbed from GI tract; excreted in stool	**Intense cutaneous vasodilation (flushing),** aspirin may reduce this, EtOH increases flushing; vomiting, diarrhea, dyspepsia, increased acidity are common; peptic ulceration is reported; most serious toxicity is elevated liver transaminases, and jaundice is reported	Lowers both cholesterol and triglycerides from 10-30%

IMMUNOSUPPRESSANTS:

DRUG	MECHANISM OF ACTION	KINETICS	ADVERSE EFFECTS	THERAPEUTIC USE
AZATHIOPRINE (Imuran)	**Blocks purine synthesis;** interferes with nucleic acid synthesis through enzyme inhibition and may be incorporated into DNA; inhibits delayed type hypersensitivity (Type IV); suppresses T > B-cells; best just prior and just after immune challenge; NO effect on established graft rejection; cytotoxic activity	**Prodrug;** converted to 6-mercaptopurine (anti-metabolite); well absorbed from GI tract; peak plasma level 1-2 hours after dose; metabolized to 6-thiouracil by xanthine oxidase; eliminated in urine	LESS adverse than 6-MP; nausea, vomiting, diarrhea, bone marrow suppression (1 week delay); 2° infection; ↑ risk of neoplasm; use with **Allopurinol** (xanthine oxidase inhibitor) will increase activity of azathioprine	Main immunosuppresive agent in all types of transplants, especially in **renal allografts** Other uses include: Rheumatoid Arthritis Wegener's Granulomatosis Systemic Lupus Ulcerative Colitis
CYCLOSPORINE (Sandimmune)	Binds cyclophilin in T cells; blocks production of IL-2 (interleukin) from T-helpers; **peptidyl-cis-trans-isomerase** is believed to be cyclophilin; works in G$_o$ and G$_1$ phase of cells	POOR oral bioavailability (30%); t½ = 6 hours; **endocytosis uptake into cells;** crosses BBB; biotransformed by P$_{450}$ in liver; excretion via bile	NO myeloid depression; HIGH nephrotoxicity, tremor, hirsutism, hypertension, gum hyperplasia	Kidney, Heart, Liver Transplant in conjunction with prednisone Rheumatoid Arthritis Glomerulonephritis Psoriasis Crohn's Disease
MYCOPHENOLATE (Cellcept)	Active metabolite, MPA is potent reversible inhibitor of inosine monophosphate dehydrogenase which inhibits *de novo* guanosine nucleotide synthesis	Rapid po absorption; undergoes complete metabolism to MPA which is active form; 97% plasma protein bound; excreted in urine	Diarrhea, leukopenia, sepsis, vomiting, pain, abdominal pain, fever, headache, asthenia, chest pain, back pain, hypertension, anemia, renal impairment; **Pregnancy category C**	Prophylaxis of Organ Rejection
TACROLIMUS (FK506) (Prograf)	**Macrolide immunosuppressant;** prolongs survival of host and transplanted graft; inhibits the activation of T-lymphocytes; exact mechanism not known	IV infusion or oral dosage	Tremor, headache, hypertension, nausea, renal dysfunction, insomnia, paresthesia, constipation, anorexia, vomiting, anemia, leukocytosis, thrombocytopenia, rash hyperglycemia, pruritus, abdominal pain; increased risk of malignancy; **Pregnancy category C**	Prophylaxis of Organ Rejection

235

INOTROPIC AGENTS:

DRUG	ORGAN SYSTEM EFFECTS	PHARMACOKINETICS/DYNAMICS	ADVERSE REACTIONS	USE
AMRINONE (Inocor)	Increases cardiac contractility without increasing oxygen use; does NOT decrease heart rate; phosphodiesterase III isoenzyme inhibitor (increases cAMP, which increases Ca uptake by myocardial cells); 2nd line inotropic agents for short term use; increases cardiac output, decreases peripheral vascular resistance, decreases pulmonary capillary wedge pressure in congestive heart failure	Oral and Intraveous dosage; 10-50% plasma protein binding; therapeutic plasma level: 2.4 μg/mL	Cardiac arrhythmias and hypotension are most common; high incidence of dose-related, reversible thrombocytopenia; headache, nausea, vomiting, abdominal distress; hypersensitivity after 2 weeks of therapy manifests as pericarditis, pleuritis and ascites; may elevate liver enzymes	Congestive Heart Failure (CHF)
MILRINONE (Primacor)	Same as Amrinone	Oral ONLY; 65-70% plasma protein binding; therapeutic plasma level: 0.2 μg/mL	39-66% mortality rate with chronic use	CHF
DIGITOXIN (Crystodigin)	See Digitalis and Cardiac Glycosides; liver disease is concern; if alcoholic then MUST lower dose; made from *Digitalis lanata and purpura*	>90% oral bioavailability, half-life is 7-9 days; metabolized by liver DMMS; **excreted in feces**; rapidly passes into fetus; po dosage	Anorexia, nausea, vomiting, abdominal discomfort, diarrhea, cardiac toxicity, CNS and ophthalmic toxicities, see Digitalis; **Pregnancy category C**	CHF
DIGOXIN (Lanoxin)	See Digitalis and Cardiac Glycosides; made from *Digitalis lanata*	60-100% oral bioavailability, half-life is 33-51 hours; NOT biotransformed; less than 25% plasma protein bound; **excreted in urine**; rapidly passes into fetus; po or IV dosage	Same as Digitoxin; **Pregnancy category C**	CHF

<u>Editor's Note:</u> All adrenergic beta agonists are inotropic agents but are useful only in acute situations. In congestive heart failure, vasodilators are useful to reduce preload and increase myocardial contractility indirectly. Commonly used vasodilators include nitroglycerin (preload), ACE inhibitors (afterload) and sodium nitroprusside (preload and afterload).

236

INSULINS, THE:

DRUG	MECHANISM OF ACTION	KINETICS	ADVERSE EFFECTS	USE
INSULIN INJECTION (REGULAR)	Insulin Injection a.k.a. Regular Insulin has rapid onset	IV onset within 5 minutes; **subcutaneous onset with 15 minutes**; duration of action is 4-6 hours	Hypoglycemia; local or systemic allergic reaction, may cause atrophy or hypertrophy of subcutaneous fat tissue	Type I IDDM Gestational Diabetes Mellitus Type A2 (GDMA2)
ISOPHANE INSULIN (NPH)	Use regular insulin + Isophane Insulin to get **rapid onset with long duration**	**1-1½ hours to onset; 24-48 hour duration**; insulin to protamine ratio is 1:1	LESS hypersensitivity than Protamine Zinc Insulin; hypoglycemia	Same as Regular Insulin Injection
LENTE	Combination of Semilente + Ultralente; RAPID onset with LONG duration	**2 hours to onset; 22-26 hour duration**		Type I IDDM
PROTAMINE ZINC INSULIN		4-8 hours to onset; 36 hour duration	**Hypersensitivity** to excess free protamine; hypoglycemia	Type I IDDM
SEMILENTE	SMALL crystals	**½-1 hours to onset; 12-16 hour duration**	Hypoglycemia	Type I IDDM
ULTRALENTE	LARGE crystals	4-8 hours to onset; **36 hour duration**	Hypoglycemia	Type I IDDM

LAXATIVES:

AGENT	ORGAN SYSTEM EFFECTS	PHARMACOKINETICS	ADVERSE REACTIONS	THERAPEUTIC USE
CASTOR OIL	Irritant (contact) laxative; action through ricinoleic acid; increases cAMP to promote Na, K, Cl and water secretion	1-3 hours to onset		Irritant Laxative
DOCUSATE SODIUM (Colace)	Emollient or stool softener	Some absorption	Liver toxic	Emollient Laxative
GLYCERIN	An alcohol which absorbs water and irritate the bowel; increases peristalsis when given rectally; onset to action within 2-6 hours	Rectal suppository or enema	Rectal discomfort	Osmotic Laxative
LACTULOSE (Chronulac)	Hyperosmotic laxative; acts by drawing water into intestinal lumen; once in colon, is broken down into low molecular weight acids which further increase osmotic load and stimulate colonic motility; intestinal contents become acidic which draws ammonia (NH3) into lumen which is then trapped as NH4; disaccharide containing galactose and fructose	Oral dosage; not absorbed; not metabolized until reaches colon	Should be avoided in those lactose intolerant; occasionally see abdominal cramps, diarrhea, bloating, flatulence, nausea and vomiting	Osmotic Laxative Hepatic Encephalopathy (via ammonia trapping action)
MAGENESIUM CITRATE MAGNESIUM HYDROXIDE	Saline laxatives	Insoluble	POOR taste	Saline Laxatives
MALT SOUP EXTRACT (Maltsupex)	Bulk laxative			Bulk Forming Laxative
MINERAL OIL	Loosens stools; decreases fat soluble vitamin absorption		VERY loose stools	Lubricant Laxative
PHENOLPHTHALEIN (Ex-Lax)	Irritant (contact) laxative; increases cAMP to promote Na, K, Cl and water secretion	6-8 hours to onset	Diarrhea	Irritant Laxative
PSYLLIUM (Perdiem Fiber)	Bulk forming laxative; absorbs water and increases stool bulk			Bulk Forming Laxative
SENNA CONCENTRATE (Senokot)	Irritant (contact) laxative	po		Irritant Laxative

238

LEPROSTATICS:

AGENT	ORGAN SYSTEM EFFECTS	PHARMACOKINETICS	ADVERSE REACTIONS	THERAPEUTIC USE
CLOFAZIMINE (Lamprene)	Antileprosy agent; has slow bacteriocidal effect on *Mycobacterium leprae*; binds to mycobacterial DNA; has antiinflammatory activity in Erythema Nodosum Leprosum reactions; unknown mechanism of action	Oral dosage with variable absorption; **highly lipophilic** and deposits in fatty tissue and in reticuloendothelial system cells; taken up by macrophages throughout body; should be taken with meals	**Pregnancy category C**; skin pigmentation (from pink to brownish-black), ichthyosis and dryness, rash and pruritus; abdominal pain, diarrhea, nausea, vomiting, GI intolerance (40-50%); corneal pigmentation, eye dryness, burning, itching, and irritation; discoloration of urine, feces, sweat, sputum; elevates serum glucose; elevates ESR	Lepromatous leprosy (including Dapsone resistant lepromatous leprosy)
DAPSONE (DDS)	A sulfone with structural resemblance to para-aminobenzoic acid (PABA). Like sulfa drugs, Dapsone inhibits folic acid synthesis; is both bacteriocidal and bacteriostatic against *Mycobacterium leprae*; mechanism of action against *Dermatitis herpetiformis* is not known	Rapid and complete GI absorption; peak serum concentration within 4-8 hours; given daily at least 8 days to achieve plateau blood level	**Pregnancy category C**; may exaggerate hemolysis and Heinz body formation in patients with glucose-6-phosphate dehydrogenase (G6PD) deficiency; peripheral neuropathy; nausea, vomiting, abdominal pain, pancreatitis; vertigo, blurred vision, tinnitus, insomnia; fever, headache	Dermatitis herpetiformis Leprosy

NOTE: The usual drug regimen for leprosy combines Dapsone, Rifampin (see Tuberculostatics) and Clofazamine.

239

NEUROMUSCULAR BLOCKERS:

AGENT	ORGAN SYSTEM EFFECTS	PHARMACOKINETICS	ADVERSE REACTIONS	THERAPEUTIC USE
ATRACURIUM (Tracrium)	Nondepolarizing skeletal muscle relaxant, action at N-II; causes hypotension, vasodilation, and alterations in heart rate	Short acting < 30 minutes; rapid metabolism by plasma cholinesterase, spontaneous degradation at blood pH	Apnea; allergic reaction, hypotension, bronchospasm	Bronchoscopy, laryngoscopy; adjuvant in general anesthesia; orthopedic procedures
DOXACURIUM (Nuromax)	*Long acting*, nondepolarizing skeletal muscle relaxant; competitive binding to N-II receptors on motor end plate antagonizing Ach; action is antagonized by reversible acetyl-cholinesterase inhibitors	IV; 2.5-3 times more potent that Pancuronium; 10-12 times more potent than Metocurine	Most common adverse reaction is effects lasting beyond time needed for surgery; **Pregnancy category C**	Adjunct to general anesthesia; Skeletal muscle relaxant for use in endotracheal intubation
METOCURINE (Metubine)	Nondepolarizing skeletal muscle relaxant; also blocks N-I receptors; causes histamine release	Prolongation of drug's effects beyond time necessary for procedures	Effects beyond time necessary for procedures; allergic reaction; histaminic effects; **Pregnancy category C**	Same as Doxacurium Adjunct in Electroshock Therapy
MIVACURIUM (Mivacron)	*Short acting* nondepolarizing skeletal muscle relaxant; binds competitively to N-II receptors on motor end plate of skeletal muscle	Hydrolyzed by plasma cholinesterase; half-life is 2-3 minutes	Flushing; apnea; hypotension, bronchospasm; **Pregnancy category C**	Anesthesia Adjunct Tracheal Intubation Skeletal Muscle Relaxation
PANCURONIUM (Pavulon)	Nondepolarizing skeletal muscle relaxant; action at N-II; Cardiovascular effects: blocks NE uptake, increases NE release; increases HR, increases cardiac output, increases blood pressure, N-I agonist	Biotransformed to 3-OH-pancuronium which is active; excreted by kidney	Apnea; cardiac effects; increased heart rate and blood pressure	Same as Tubocurarine
PIPERCURONIUM (Arduan)	Nondepolarizing skeletal muscle relaxant	Excreted by kidney	Apnea	Skeletal Muscle Relaxation Endotracheal Intubation
SUCCINYLCHOLINE (Anectine)	Depolarizing blocker (blocks depolarization); some increased histamine release at high dose; stimulates N-I receptors and cardiac muscarinic receptors	Very short acting (5-10 minutes); rapid metabolism by both cholinesterases, cleaved to succinylmonocholine (active) which is cleaved to succinic acid and choline (inactive); may act longer in some patients	Hyperkalemia, muscle pain, bradycardia, tachycardia, apnea	Bronchoscopy, laryngoscopy; adjuvant in general anesthesia; orthopedic procedures; used in **electroshock therapy** to prevent dangerous muscle contractions

240

NEUROMUSCULAR BLOCKERS:

AGENT	ORGAN SYSTEM EFFECTS	PHARMACOKINETICS	ADVERSE REACTIONS	THERAPEUTIC USE
TUBOCURARINE	Nondepolarizing skeletal muscle relaxant; action at N-II receptors;; N-I blocker and increases histamine release at high dose; decreases blood pressure; first affects eye muscles, then face muscles, then limbs, then trunk muscles, then intercostal muscles, and finally the diaphragm	Long acting (1-2 hours); will not cross BBB; excreted unchanged by kidney	Apnea; bradycardia, tachycardia, blood pressure changes, bronchospasm, hypersensitivity reactions are rare	Skeletal Muscle Relaxation Endotracheal Intubation
VECURONIUM (Norcuron)	Nondepolarizing skeletal muscle relaxant; action at N-II; NO cardiovascular effects; purest skeletal muscle relaxant; NO effect on histamine release; derivative of Pancuronium	Intermediate acting; some metabolism; main excretion route is renal	See Tubocurarine	Endotracheal Intubation

Note   nondepolarizing skeletal muscle relaxants are also known as *nondepolarizing curariform agents*

241

NICOTINIC RECEPTOR AGONISTS:

DRUG	ORGAN SYSTEM EFFECTS	PHARMACOKINETICS	ADVERSE REACTIONS	THERAPEUTIC USE
DECAMETHONIUM	N-II blocker; compound contains 10 carbons	No oral absorption		No therapeutic use — Pharmacologic Research Tool
HEXAMETHONIUM	**Ganglionic blocking agent** (antidepolarizing); **decreases BP**; synthetic compound containing 6 carbons	No oral absorption	High toxicity	No therapeutic use — Pharmacologic Research Tool
LOBELINE (Bantron)	**Ganglionic stimulant** (depolarizing agent); identical to nicotine; LESS potent; secondary ganglionic blocker at high dose	Same as Nicotine, except LOWER mg potency	Same as Nicotine	Same as Nicotine
MECAMYLAMINE (Inversine)	**Ganglionic blocking agent** (antidepolarizing); ONLY ganglionic blocker used for anti-hypertensive effects	Lipid soluble, effective orally, GI absorption is variable	CNS effects	Antihypertensive
NICOTINE (Habitrol, Nicoderm) transdermal patch **NICOTINE POLACRILEX** (Nicorette) gum preparation	**Ganglionic stimulant** (depolarizing agent) **Respiration:** small dose (2 mg or less), stimulation of carotid and aortic bodies to increase respiration (peripheral effect); increased dose, more crosses BBB, direct stimulation of medulla to increase respiration (central effect); high dose, blocker action at carotid and aortic bodies and in medulla decreases respiration; **Nausea and vomiting:** acts on **chemoreceptor trigger zone (CTZ)** on floor of 4th ventricle which has direct input to vomiting center; **CNS effects:** tremors (at N-II receptors) and convulsions, increases alertness and exerts positive effect on the limbic reward system; **Cardiovascular:** increases HR, increases TPR, and increases BP; **GI tract:** increases secretions, increases GI motility	Liquid alkaloid from tobacco, weak base, **high lipid solubility**; NO activity at M receptors; penetrates skin and mucous membranes; <u>cigar smoke</u> is lipid soluble with uptake occurs through buccal, stomach, intestinal mucosa; <u>cigarette smoke</u> is acidic thus nicotine is in water soluble form but is still absorbed rapidly in lungs (reaches brain in 8 seconds); biotransformed by liver and is eliminated by kidney, $t_{1/2}$ = 2 hours	Nausea, vomiting, may exacerbate peptic ulcer, diarrhea, **nicotine toxicity** causes ↓ HR, ↓ TPR, ↓ BP, respiratory failure (and paralysis of respiratory m.) and cardiac collapse; crosses placenta, appears in breast milk <u>Patch:</u> erythema, pruritus, or irritation at site of administration; <u>Gum:</u> hiccups, increased salivation, diarrhea	Transdermal Patch — Provides constant blood level Gum — Nicotine release with chewing **Smoking Cessation Aids** — HIGH placebo effect

242

NSAIDs:

DRUG	ORGAN SYSTEM EFFECTS	PHARMACOKINETICS	ADVERSE REACTIONS	THERAPEUTIC USE
ASPIRIN	Analgesic; antipyretic; antiinflammatory; mechanism of action is **cyclooxygenase inhibition; acetylation of platelets** and decreases platelet aggregation; NO known CV effects; GI ulceration due to decreases PG synthesis and salicylic acid is irritating (superficial erosions); **increases bleeding time,** NO effect on prothrombin time; **uricosuric;** potent platelet inhibitor	t½ ≈ 15 minutes; loss of acetyl group to form **salicylic acid** (t½ = 2-4 hours)	GI irritation (15%); frank ulcer (1%); Reye's syndrome in children following febrile, viral infection; increased bleeding time; small child poisoning (acidosis); salicylism; hypersensitivity reactions	Analgesic Antipyretic Antiinflammatory Myocardial Infarction and Cerebrovascular Infarction Prophylaxis
DICLOFENAC SODIUM (Voltaren) **DICLOFENAC POTASSIUM** (Cataflam)	Analgesic; antipyretic; antiinflammatory; increases platelet aggregation time, no effect on bleeding time, no clinically evident effect on PT/PTT; **prostaglandin synthetase inhibitor**	Po dosing; half-life is 2 hours	Nausea, dyspepsia, diarrhea, **peptic ulceration, GI bleeding;** liver enzyme elevations; hypersensitivity: fluid retention and edema; all NSAIDs have been associated with reduced renal blood flow and renal papillary necrosis in elderly; avoid use in hepatic porphyria, tinnitus in 3-9%; **Pregnancy category B**	Rheumatoid Arthritis Osteoarthritis Ankylosing Spondylitis Dysmenorrhea
DIFLUNISAL (Dolobid)	Non-steroidal drug with analgesic, antiinflammatory and antipyretic properties; peripherally acting non-narcotic analgesic; it is a salicylic acid derivative; weakly inhibits cyclooxygenase	Completely absorbed po; peak plasma level within 2-3 hours; excreted in urine; half-life is 8-12 hours	Nausea, vomiting, dyspepsia, GI pain, diarrhea, constipation, flatulence; somnolence, insomnia; dizziness; tinnitus; rash; headache, fatigue	Mild to Moderate Pain Osteoarthritis Rheumatoid Arthritis
ETODOLAC (Lodine)	Analgesic; antiinflammatory; antipyretic; inhibits prostaglandin synthesis	Half-life is 7-8 hours; peak plasma level within 1-2 hours po; 99% plasma protein bound	GI ulceration and bleeding Dyspepsia (10%); Precaution in impaired renal function, heart failure, and hepatic dysfunction; false-positive urine bilirubin and/or ketone; **pregnancy category C**	Osteoarthritis Pain Management

243

NSAIDs:

DRUG	ORGAN SYSTEM EFFECTS	PHARMACOKINETICS	ADVERSE REACTIONS	THERAPEUTIC USE
FLURBIPROFEN (Ansaid)	Nonsteroidal antiinflammatory agent with analgesic and antipyretic properties	Well absorbed po with peak plasma levels within 1.5 hours; urine excretion; >99% plasma protein binding	Dyspepsia, diarrhea, abdominal pain, nausea; headache; edema	Rheumatoid Arthritis Osteoarthritis
IBUPROFEN (Motrin)	Nonsteroidal antiinflammatory agent that has analgesic, antipyretic, and antiinflammatory actions	Good po absorption; urine excretion; half-life is 2 hours	Nausea, epigastric pain, heartburn; dizziness; rash; risk of gastric or duodenal ulcer with bleeding and/or perforation, GI hemorrhage and melena; caution in pregnancy	Rheumatoid Arthritis Osteoarthritis Mild to Moderate Pain Primary Dysmenorrhea
INDOMETHACIN (Indocin)	Nonsteroidal drug with antiinflammatory, antipyretic and analgesic activity that should NOT be considered or used as a simple analgesic; **potent inhibitor of prostaglandin synthesis**	Po and pr (per rectum) dosing; urine and fecal excretion; **enterohepatic circulation;** 99% plasma protein binding	Dizziness; nausea, dyspepsia; risk of GI ulceration and hemorrhage; not recommended in pregnancy or nursing mothers; use in pregnancy may cause oligohydramnios, premature closure of the ductus arteriosus, and neonatal pulmonary hypertension	Rheumatoid Arthritis Ankylosing Spondylitis Osteoarthritis Acute Shoulder Bursitis/Tendinitis Acute Gouty Arthritis Patent Ductus Arteriosus (IV) Uterine Tocolysis (unlabeled use)
KETOPROFEN (Orudis, Oruvail)	Nonsteroidal antiinflammatory drug with analgesic and antipyretic properties; Orudis capsules release drug in stomach; Oruvail capsules resist low pH of stomach and release drug at controlled rate in higher pH environment of duodenum; NOT recommended for acute pain because of controlled release design	Well absorbed po; peak plasma levels within 0.5-2 hours; steady state concentrations are reached with 24 hours after continuing dosing; 80% urine excretion	Dyspepsia, nausea, abdominal pain, diarrhea, constipation, flatulence; headache, insominia, nervousness; impaired renal function; **Pregnancy Category B**	Rheumatoid Arthritis Osteoarthritis
KETOROLAC (Toradol)	Nosteroidal antiinflammtory drug with analgesic and antipyretic properties; inhibits synthesis of prostaglandins and is considered a peripherally acting analgesic; indicated for short term pain management (up to 5 days); Dose adjustment is required in elderly and renal impairment	IM or po; time to peak plasma level IM is 50 minutes, and for po is 44 minutes; 99% plasma protein binding; 90% urine excretion	Nausea, dyspepsia, GI pain, diarrhea; edema; pruritus; drowsiness, dizziness; risk of GI ulceration, perforation and bleeding; nephrotoxicity especially in elderly; **Pregnancy category B**	**Short Term Pain Management** Effective adjunct agent for use with narcotic rescue doses for breakthrough pain Itching (topical use in allergy)

244

NSAIDs:

DRUG	ORGAN SYSTEM EFFECTS	PHARMACOKINETICS	ADVERSE REACTIONS	THERAPEUTIC USE
MECLOFENAMATE SODIUM (Meclomen)	Nonsteroidal antiinflammatory agent; potent antiinflammatory agent	Half-life is 2 hours; peak plasma level within 30-60 minutes	Diarrhea, gastrointestinal irritation, ulcers	Mild to Moderate Pain Rheumatoid Arthritis Osteoarthritis
NAPROXEN (Naprosyn)	Nonsteroidal antiinflammatory drug with analgesic, antiinflammatory, and antipyretic properties	Complete GI absorption; peak plasma levels with 2-4 hours; steady state concentrations achieved after 4-5 doses; >99% plasma protein bound; 95% urine excretion	Constipation, heartburn, abdominal pain, nausea; headache, dizziness, drowsiness; pruritus, skin eruptions, ecchymosis; tinnitus; edema, dyspnea; **Pregnancy category B**	Rheumatoid Arthritis Osteoarthritis Juvenile Arthritis Ankylosing Spondylitis Tendinitis Bursitis Acute Gout Mild to Moderate Pain Primary Dysmenorrhea
OXAPROZIN (Daypro)	Nonsteroidal antiinflammatory drug with analgesic and antipyretic properties; analgesia acheived after single dose; antiinflammatory effect requires more than single dose	Peak plasma levels po within 3-5 hours; 99.9% plasma protein bound; metabolized by liver; urine (65%) and fecal (35%) excretion; steady state acheived after several days	Constipation, diarrhea, dyspepsia, nausea; rash; risk of GI ulceration and hemorrhage; **Pregnancy category C**	Osteoarthritis Rheumatoid Arthritis
PHENYLBUTAZONE	Pyrazolon derivative; action similar to other NSAIDs, but use limited due to side effects; not recommended for use longer than 1 week; used in severe Ankylosing Spondylitis after less toxic NSAIDs have not been effective	po dosage; half-life is 60-100 minutes; biotransformed to oxyphenbutazone	Most serious adverse effect is agranulocytosis, both idiosyncratic, irreversible and dose related, reversible agranulocytosis is seen; serious GI ulceration and bleeding may occur; liver and kidney toxic; contraindicated in elderly and in pediatric patients less than 15 yrs old	Severe Ankylosing Spondylitis

245

NSAIDs:

DRUG	ORGAN SYSTEM EFFECTS	PHARMACOKINETICS	ADVERSE REACTIONS	THERAPEUTIC USE
PIROXICAM (Feldene)	Antiinflammatory, analgesic and antipyretic properties; edema, erythema, tissue proliferation, fever and pain can all be inhibited	Well absorbed po; peak plasma levels within 3-5 hours; steady state concentrations within 7-12 days; urine and fecal excretion (2:1)	Epigastris distress, nausea; decreases hemoglobin and hematocrit; **not recommended in pregnancy** or nursing mothers	Osteoarthritis Rheumatoid Arthritis
SULINDAC (Clinoril)	NSAID with analgesic, antipyretic and antiinflammatory properties	po dosage; half-life 7-18 hours; peak plasma level within 2 hours; active product is its sulfide form	GI toxicity like all other NSAIDs; skin rash, tinnitus, edema, renal toxicity	Osteoarthritis Rheumatoid Arthritis Ankylosing Spondylitis Acute Painful Shoulder Acute Gouty Arthritis
TOLMETIN (Tolectin)	Nonsteroidal antiinflammatory agent with analgesic and antipyretic activity; expected therapeutic response within a few days to one week after first dose	Rapid and complete po absorption; peak plasma levels within 30-60 minutes; biphasic elimination	Dyspepsia, GI distress, abdominal pain, diarrhea, flatulence, vomiting; headache, asthenia; increased blood pressure, edema; dizziness; weight gain or loss; **Pregnancy category C**	Rheumatoid Arthritis Juvenile Rheumatoid Arthritis

246

OPIOID ANTAGONISTS:

DRUG	ORGAN SYSTEM EFFECTS	PHARMACOKINETICS	ADVERSE REACTIONS	THERAPEUTIC USE
NALOXONE (Narcan)	Antagonist at μ, k, and δ receptors; NO agonist activity; **reduced opioid induced respiratory depression**; NO effect on non-opioid (alcohol, sedative-hypnotic, benzodiazepine) induced respiratory depression); Naloxone also reverses other opioid actions such analgesia, GI effects, biliary duct spasm, pupillary constriction and release of antidiuretic hormone	SHORT acting, with immediate onset; HIGH water solubility; injectable; t½ ≈ 1 hour; NOT orally effective, HIGH first pass effect in liver	Must continually dose long acting opioid overdose patient; **Pregnancy category B**	Opioid Induced Respiratory Depression Diagnosis of Opioid Dependence Post-partum Neonatal Respiratory Depression
NALTREXONE (Trexan)	Antagonist at μ, k, and δ receptors; NO agonist activity; used for opioid abusers after withdrawal from opioids has occurred; will block euphoria and thus decreases temptation to resume opioid abuse; if use during opioid addiction, will precipitate withdrawal reaction	LONG acting (24-72 hours); orally active; metabolized to ß-naltrexol; action may last for several days	Precipitates withdrawal in active opioid abusers; difficulty sleeping, anxiety, nervousness, abdominal pain, nausea, vomiting, low energy, joint and muscle pain, headache; **Pregnancy category C**	Post Opioid Withdrawal Prophylaxis in Narcotics Addiction Suppression of Ethanol Drinking in Alcoholism

247

OPIOID AGONIST-ANTAGONISTS:

DRUG	ORGAN SYSTEM EFFECTS	PHARMACOKINETICS/DYNAMICS	ADVERSE REACTIONS	THERAPEUTIC USE
BUPRENORPHINE (Buprenex)	**High affinity agonist at mu receptors;** antagonist at kappa receptors; also partial agonist at mu receptor NO ceiling effect; analgesia via activity at mu receptors	Given IM is 25-50x's potency of morphine; duration of action is 6 hours	Abuse potential; Naloxone may fail to antagonize respiratory depression caused by Buprenorphine because of its high affinity for mu receptor; **pregnancy category C**	Moderate to Severe Pain
BUTORPHANOL (Stadol)	Mixed agonist-antagonist; VERY potent analgesic; highly sedative; used as anesthetic adjunct; **ceiling effect on respiratory depression;** analgesia mediated through kappa receptor activity	IV or intramuscular dosage; given IM is 5x's potency of morphine; peak plasma level within ½ -1 hour; nasal spray available for use in migraine	Low potential for abuse; sedation, dizziness, GI upset, respiratory depression, diaphoresis, change in blood pressure, rash, palpitations, tinnitus; **Pregnancy category C**	Preoperative Agent Anesthesia Supplement Labor Analgesic Migraine Headache
DEZOCINE (Dalgan)	Synthetic opioid agonist-antagonist; greater affinity for mu than kappa receptors; antagonist activity at mu greater than Pentazocine; analgesia via kappa activity; **ceiling effect for respiratory depression occurs quickly**	Intramuscular and IV doses equal potency to morphine; urine excretion; should adjust dose in renal or hepatic disease	Nausea, vomiting; sedation; injection site reactions; low dependence liability; **Preganancy category C**	Postoperative Pain (Not a controlled substance)
NALBUPHINE (Nubain)	Mixed agonist-antagonist; **ceiling effect for respiratory depression;** analgesia mediated through activity on kappa receptors	Parenteral dosage only; intramuscular dose potency equal to morphine	Sedation; less cardiovascular effects; less post operative nausea and vomiting than Morphine	Obstetric Analgesic Labor Post Partum Post Operative
PENTAZOCINE (Talwin)	Mixed agonist-antagonist; analgesia mediated through activity on kappa receptors	Active orally and parenterally; given IM is 1/3 potency of morphine; well absorbed from GI tract, but has HIGH first pass effect	Common effects are: dizziness, sweating, nausea, and vomiting; tachycardia, hypertension, dysphoria, psychotomimetic effects are seen with large doses; **pregnancy category C**	Moderate to severe pain Labor analgesia

248

OVULATION STIMULANTS:

AGENT	MECHANISM OF ACTION	CONDITIONS FOR USE	ADVERSE REACTIONS
CLOMIPHENE (Clomid)	Oral non-steroidal with some estrogenic activity; **Ovulation induction agent** with exact mechanism not known; appears to involve pituitary to stimulate release of pituitary gonadotropins to mediate ovulation; increases incidence of multiple gestation	Ovulatory failure Fertile husband or partner Normal liver function Normal endogenous estrogen Normal pituitary and ovary function Absence of gynecologic neoplasm	Vasomotor flushing Ovarian enlargment Abdominal discomfort Breast tenderness Nausea, Vomiting Nervousness Insomnia Visual disturbances Increased midcycle pain (*mittelschmerz*) Increases incidence of multiple pregnancy

OXYTOCICS:

AGENT	ORGAN SYSTEM EFFECTS	PHARMACOKINETICS	ADVERSE REACTIONS	THERAPEUTIC USE
ERGONOVINE (Ergotrate)	Causes strong uterine contraction with long duration (hours); used in attempt to control post partum hemorrhage; acts as serotonin antagonist	po, IM, IV routes	Tetanic uterine contraction; may cause transient but severe hypertension; blurred vision, convulsion; contraindicated during pregnancy	Postpartum Hemorrhage Uterine Atony Uterine Subinvolution
METHYLERGONOVINE (Methergine)	Same as Ergonovine	po, IM, IV routes	Contraindicated during pregnancy	Postpartum Hemorrhage Uterine Atony Uterine Subinvolution
OXYTOCIN (Pitocin, Syntocinon)	Used during third stage of labor (after delivery of placenta) to maintain a firmly contracted uterus; also used in labor induction and augmentation of inadequate uterine contractions	IM, IV routes	<u>Maternal:</u> Postpartum hemorrhage, uterine rupture, arrhythmia, water intoxication, uterine hypertonicity (tetanic uterine contraction) <u>Fetal:</u> has been associated with bradycardia, low APGAR score, anoxia, death <u>Contraindications:</u> cephalopelvic disproportion, unfavorable fetal lie (position), fetal distress, uterine hypertonicity, placenta previa, vasa previa	Oxytocic agent used in 3rd stage of labor; Induction agent used in management of 1st or 2nd stages of labor

250

PENICILLIN ADJUNCT AGENTS:

AGENT	ORGAN SYSTEM EFFECTS	PHARMACOKINETICS	ADVERSE REACTIONS	PURPOSE
CILASTATIN	**Dipeptidase** inhibitor used in combination with Imipenem (in Primaxin); has no antimicrobial activity; inhibits biotransformation of imipenem	t ½ = 1 hour; peak plasma level within 1 hour	Nausea and vomiting	PRIMAXIN: Imipenem, Cilistatin
CLAVULANIC ACID	Naturally occurring **β-lactamase inhibitor** used in combination with Amoxicillin in (Augmentin)	t ½ = 1 hour; 30% plasma protein bound	Well tolerated	AUGMENTIN: Amoxicillin, Clavulanic Acid
PROBENECID	Decreases penicillin excretion; used in combination with Ampicillin; also uricosuric effect	Total GI absorption	Well tolerated	Used with Ampicillin to increase blood levels and duration of action Gout
SULBACTAM	Semisynthetic **β-lactamase** inhibitor used in combination with Ampicillin in (Unasyn)	t ½ = 1 hour; approximately 80% excreted unchanged in urine	Well tolerated	UNASYN: Ampicillin, Sulbactam Used for beta-lactamase producing organisms

251

PLATELET AGGREGATION INHIBITORS:

AGENT	ORGAN SYSTEM EFFECTS	PHARMACOKINETICS	ADVERSE REACTIONS	THERAPEUTIC USE
DIPYRIDAMOLE (Persantine)	Platelet inhibitor; platelet adhesion inhibitor; may increase thromboxane A_2 formation	Peak plasma levels within 75 minutes; highly plasma protein bound	Dizziness, abdominal distress, headache, rash; **Pregnancy category B**	Adjunct to Coumarin anticoagulants to prevent thromboembolic complications of cardiac **valve** replacement
TICLOPIDINE (Ticlid)	Platelet aggregation inhibitor; time and dose dependent inhibition of both platelet aggregation and release of platelet clot promoting factors; prolongs bleeding time; platelet inhibition is **irreversible for the life of the platelet**	Peak plasma levels within 2 hours; 98% plasma protein bound; extensive liver metabolism; 60% urine excretion and 25% in feces	Neutropenia, thrombocytopenia, cholesterol elevation, diarrhea, nausea, dyspepsia, rash; **Pregnancy category B**	Thrombotic Stroke Prophylaxis (in patients intolerant to aspirin) Unstable Angina Pectoris

252

POSTERIOR PITUITARY HORMONES:

AGENT	ORGAN SYSTEM EFFECTS	PHARMACOKINETICS	ADVERSE REACTIONS	THERAPEUTIC USE
DESMOPRESSIN (DDAVP)	Antidiuretic hormone; synthetic analog of 8-arginine vasopression; increases plasma levels of factor VIII activity in patients with hemophilia and von Willebrand's disease Type I	Activity is rapid and occurs within 30 minutes; peak effects within 90-120 minutes; 10 times more potent IV than intranasal dosage	Headache, nausea, abdominal cramps, vulvar pain; water intoxication and hyponatremia; **Pregnancy category B**	Hemophilia A von Willebrand's Disease Diabetes Insipidus
LYPRESSIN (Diapid)	Lysine-8-vasopressin is a naturally occurring polypeptide form of the posterior pituitary antidiuretic hormone	Nasal spray; short acting	Rhinorrhea, nasal congestion, irritation and pruritus of nasal passages, headache; **Pregnancy category C**	Diabetes Insipidus
OXYTOCIN (Pitocin, Syntocinon)	Used during third stage of labor (after delivery of placenta) to maintain a firmly contracted uterus; also used in labor induction and augmentation of inadequate uterine contractions	Intramuscular or intravenous dosage	<u>Maternal:</u> Postpartum hemorrhage, uterine rupture, arrhythmia, water intoxication, uterine hypertonicity (tetanic uterine contraction) <u>Fetal:</u> Bradycardia, low APGAR score, anoxia, death <u>Contraindications:</u> cephalopelvic disproportion, unfavorable fetal lie (position), fetal distress, uterine hypertonicity, placenta previa, vasa previa	Oxytocic agent used in 3rd stage of labor Induction agent used in 1st or 2nd stages of labor
VASOPRESSIN	Hormone produced in the **anterior hypothalamus** that acts to conserve body water by concentrating the urine; enhances osmotic flow of water from renal collecting tubule lumens to medullary interstitium; deficiency of Vasopressin results in **Diabetes Insipidus** which is a state of excessive thirst, increased fluid intake (polydypsia) and output of dilute urine (polyuria)	Administered IM, IV, intranasal, subcutaneouly; t ½ = 20 minutes	Caution in cardiovascular disease; hyponatremia, allergic reaction, abdominal cramping	Diabetes Insipidus

253

PROGESTINS:

AGENT	ORGAN SYSTEM EFFECTS	ADVERSE REACTIONS	THERAPEUTIC USE
PROGESTINS Desogestrel Levonorgestrel Norethindrone Norgestimate Norgestrel	The term progestin (or progesterogen) includes progesterone and other agents with the same physiologic effects; Progesterone is the active hormone secreted by the corpus luteum and placenta; Progestins induce secretory changes in the uterine glandular epithelium and decidual changes in the uterine stroma; normal menstruation occurs when the corpus luteum stops producing progesterone 14 days after ovulation; progestational agents given 6-7 days after ovulation will delay menses until 2-3 days after the hormone is stopped Progestins cause induction of a secretory endometrium and decrease myometrial contractility Progesterone induces an elevation of basal body temperature (clinically useful method to detect ovulation)	Headache, weight gain, depression, disruption of menstrual cycle, fluid retention, increased appetite, fatigue, hypertension, increased total cholesterol, increased LDL, decreased HDL	Menstrual Abnormalities Endometriosis Dysmenorrhea Components of combination oral contraceptives (see Oral Contraceptives) Levonorgestrel Implants are for long term contraception that last up to 5 years (see Non-Oral Contraceptives)
MEDROXYPROGESTERONE (Provera, Depo-Provera)	Synthetic progestin; acts on pituitary → decreased FSH, LH → decreased estrogen → amenorrhea **Depot form inhibits ovulation providing very effective** contraceptive (0.3 failure rate with proper use); 1st dose given just after menses or a negative pregnancy test; IM shot given every 3 months **Oral form transforms proliferative into secretory endometrium** and is indicated for secondary amenorrhea, abnormal uterine bleeding in absence of fibroids or uterine cancer	Menstrual irregularities (bleeding, amenorrhea or both), weight changes, headache, nervousness, abdominal pain or discomfort, dizziness, asthenia (weakness or fatigue) Contraindications: known or suspected pregnancy, undiagnosed vaginal bleeding, known or suspected breast cancer, active thrombophlebitis or history of thromboembolic disorder, liver dysfunction	Injectable Contraceptive (for 3 months) Abnormal Uterine Bleeding Adjunctive therapy and palliative treatment of advanced endometrial and renal carcinoma
NORETHINDRONE	19-nortestosterone derivative progestin commonly found as the progestational component of oral contraceptive pills (OCP's)	Irregular bleeding depression, hirsutism	Progestin component of many oral contraceptive preparations, also used alone in "minipill" preparations

PSYCHOTOMIMETIC DRUGS:

DRUG	ORGAN SYSTEM EFFECTS	PHARMACOKINETICS/DYNAMICS	ADVERSE REACTIONS	THERAPEUTIC USE
LYSERGIC ACID DIETHYLAMIDE (LSD)	Tryptophan derivative (serotonin precursor); 4 ring structure; **directly excitatory on S2 receptors in limbic system; blocks 5-HT reuptake;** 50 μg dose achieves hallucinations; **somatic, sensory, psychosis reactions;** treat overdose with Buspirone (antianxiety agent)	Oral dose; good absorption; HIGH 1st pass effect; high protein binding; HIGH lipid solubility; **LOWEST dose drug (μg)**; < 1% of 50 μg dose reaches brain; 10-12 hour duration; $t\frac{1}{2}$ = 2-3 hours; **DMMS hydroxylation;** eliminated in feces; duration of action is 12 hours	Flashbacks; questionable teratogen; sympathetic overtone; tolerance; little or no dependence	NONE
MARIJUANA (THC) *Cannabis sativa*	▴9-tetrahydrocannabinol (prodrug) and 11-OH-▴9-THC-COOH (metabolite) are inactive; mechanism NOT known; slow leeching out of adipose; mood changes; potent cardiac stimulation; potent bronchodilation; blocks chemoreceptor trigger zone (CTZ); increases adrenal cortex output; decreases intraocular pressure; decreases testosterone production in males, decreases sperm count; BP remains normal	Once in blood, 90% protein bound; $t\frac{1}{2}$ = 2-3 hours; **rapid onset (30-40 seconds) by smoking;** hashish, a resin of marijuana contains 10% THC; peak effects within 30-90 minutes; duration of action is 2-4 hours	Impairs attention and learning, anxiety, increased heart rate, **conjunctival vascular reaction ("red eyes"),** ataxia, nystagmus, fine tremor, dry mouth, paranoid reaction, decreased testosterone in males; <u>chronic use:</u> amotivational syndrome, tolerance and dependence	Controversial Antiemetic in Cancer Chemotherapy and AIDS Patients
PHENCYCLIDINE (PCP)	Shorter somatic effects than LSD; longer sensory and psychosis effects than LSD; treat overdose with antipsychotic agents	po, inhalation, intranasal, injection routes; high gastro-blood recirculation; DMMS hydroxylation; eliminated in urine	NO flashback; NO teratogenic effects; **irreversible brain damage;** sympathetic overtone; tolerance and dependence	Veterinarian IV anesthetic

255

SCABICIDES:

AGENT	ORGAN SYSTEM EFFECTS	PHARMACOKINETICS	ADVERSE REACTIONS	THERAPEUTIC USE
CROTAMITON (Eurax)	Scabicidal and antipruritic agent available as cream or lotion for topical use; mechanisms of action are not known	Applied topically	Allergic sensitivity or primary irritation reactions may occur; **Pregnancy category C**	Eradication of Scabies Treatment of Pruritic Skin
LINDANE (Kwell)	Ectoparasiticide and ovicide effects against *Sarcoptes scabiei* (scabies)	Applied topically; penetrates human skin; reported 10% skin absorption	**Pregnancy category B**; central nervous stimulation ranging from dizziness to convulsion (usually via accidental oral ingestion)	Topical Scabicide
PERMETHRIN (Elimite, Nix)	Topical scabicidal agent for treatment of infestation with *Sarcoptes scabiei* (scabies); active against a broad range of pests: lice, ticks, fleas, mites, and other arthropods; disrupts sodium channel current in nerve cell membranes	Applied topically; less that 2% skin absorption	**Pregnancy category B**; mild and transient burning and stinging following application; pruritus, erythema, numbness, tingling ans rash are reported	Scabies infestation

256

SEDATIVES and HYPNOTICS:

DRUG	MECHANISM OF ACTION/EFFECTS	CLASSIFICATION BY ACTION	ADVERSE REACTIONS	THERAPEUTIC USE
AMOBARBITAL (Amytal)	Same as Phenobarbital	Short acting (4-6 hours)	Same as Phenobarbital	Sedation and Hypnosis
BUTABARBITAL (Butisol)	Short to intermediate acting barbiturate	Short/intermediate acting	Same as Phenobarbital	Sedation and Hypnosis
CHLORAL HYDRATE	**Activated by ADH to trichloroethanol**; little REM suppression; little effect on respiration and blood pressure; action probably similar to ethanol	Intermediate acting (4-9 hours)	Tolerance and dependence; low TI; irritates GI (gastritis); metabolite will displace other drugs bound to albumin; rebound depression	**Mickey Finn;** elderly and children
DOXYLAMINE (Unisom)	Antihistamine of the ethanolamine class which has high incidence of sedation; onset of action within 30 minutes; for nighttime use only	Intermediate	Occasional anticholinergic effects seen; should not be taken by pregnant women or those breast feeding	Nighttime Sleep Aid
ESTAZOLAM (Prosom)	Slow onset benzodiazepine with intermediate duration of action	Intermediate; t½ = 18 hours	See Flurazepam	Insomnia
ETHCHLORVYNOL (Placidyl)	Fast onset; similar to short acting barbiturates	Short acting (4-6 hours)	**Addictive;** low therapeutic index; CNS depression; hypersensitivity reactions	Anticonvulsant Skeletal Muscle Relaxant
FLURAZEPAM (Dalmane)	**Facilitates inhibitory action of GABA;** increases stage 2 sleep; NO decrease in REM; decreases stage 3 and mostly 4 sleep; Flurazepam is pro-drug that MUST be metabolized to desalkyl and hydroxyethyl-flurazepam, active metabolites	Long acting; **prodrug**	Daytime **residual sedation** or motor impairment; **rebound insomnia;** anterograde amnesia; paradoxical anxiety, psychoses	Antianxiety; Anticonvulsant; sedative-hypnotics; Skeletal Muscle Relaxant; Night Terror; Bed Wetting
HYDROXYZINE (Vistaril)	Antihistamine; has bronchodilator activity, antihistaminic, antiemetic and analgesic effects; potentiates effects of meperidine and barbiturates	4-6 hours duration of action	Contraindicated in early pregnancy	Antianxiety Analgesic Adjuvant Antihistamine
MEPHOBARBITAL	Long acting barbiturate	Long acting; duration 16 hours	Same effects as barbiturates; **Pregnancy category D**	Sedative-Hypnotic Antiepileptic
MIDAZOLAM (Versed)	Rapid onset benzodiazepine with ultrashort duration of action	Ultrashort acting; duration 2 hours	See Flurazepam for side effects; main adverse effect is respiratory depression	Preoperative sedation Induction of Anesthesia

SEDATIVES and HYPNOTICS:

DRUG	MECHANISM OF ACTION/EFFECTS	CLASSIFICATION BY ACTION	ADVERSE REACTIONS	THERAPEUTIC USE
PARALDEHYDE (Paral)	Active without metabolism; broken down by Krebs cycle to $CO_2 + H_2O$; 48% exhaled in lung; unknown mechanism of action	Onset of action within 10-15 minutes	Malodorous, irritating to throat, acidosis, respiratory depression	Sedation and Hypnosis Alcohol Withdrawal
PENTOBARBITAL (Nembutal)	Same as Phenobarbital	Intermediate acting (lasts 4-6 hours)	Same as Phenobarbital	Insomnia Sedation
PHENOBARBITAL (Luminal)	Non-specific effect on CNS membranes; hyperpolarizes neurons in CNS through GABA interaction (GABA is *required* for low dose barbiturate activity at the chloride ionophores); high dose barbiturates are GABA-mimetic and directly activate chloride channels; increases stage 2 sleep; suppresses REM; anticonvulsant	Long acting (6-12 hours); $t_½ > 100$ hours	**Respiratory depression**; enzyme induction of DMMS; pharmacokinetic or metabolic tolerance; pharmacodynamic tolerance; LOW TI and LOW margin of safety; drug interactions with other CNS depressants; hypersensitivity; contraindicated in porphyria; physical withdrawal; status epilepticus; **Pregnancy category D**	Daytime Sedation Insomnia Anticonvulsant Antiepileptic
PROMETHAZINE (Phenergan)	Phenothiazine derivative with antihistaminic, sedative, antimotion-sickness, antiemetic and anticholinergic effects; blocks dopamine (D_2) receptors	Lasts 4-6 hours	Safe use in early pregnancy NOT established; drowsiness; tachycardia, bradycardia, dizziness; safe for use in obstetric analgesia; toxic reactions similar to the phenothiazines	Allergic reactions; Anaphylaxis as adjunct to epinephrine; Motion sickness; pre and post operative and obstetric sedation; antiemetic; adjunct to analgesics
QUAZEPAM (Doral)	Benzodiazepine derivative that is an active drug with active metabolites; **facilitates inhibitory action of GABA**; increases stage 2 sleep; NO decrease in REM; decreases stage 3 and mostly 4 sleep	Long acting $t½ = 39$ hours	Same as Flurazepam, including respiratory depression	Insomnia
SECOBARBITAL (Seconal)	Same as Phenobarbital	Short acting (1-2 hours)	Same as Phenobarbital	Sedation and Hypnosis
TEMAZEPAM (Restoril)	Benzodiazepine derivative that facilitates inhibitory action of GABA; increases stage 2 sleep; NO decrease in REM; increases stage 3 and mostly 4 sleep; LEAST adverse effects	Intermediate acting (lasts 4-6 hours)	Same as Flurazepam	Sedative-Hypnotic

258

SEDATIVES and HYPNOTICS:

DRUG	MECHANISM OF ACTION/EFFECTS	CLASSIFICATION BY ACTION	ADVERSE REACTIONS	THERAPEUTIC USE
TRIAZOLAM (Halcion)	Benzodiazepine derivative that facilitates inhibitory action of GABA; increases stage 2 sleep; NO decrease in REM; decreases stage 3 and mostly 4 sleep	Short acting t½ = 1-5 hours	Same as Flurazepam; Triazolam has been associated with violent, hostile, paranoid, and psychotic reactions at high doses	Hypnotic
ZOLPIDEM (Ambien)	Non-benzodiazepine hypnotic; unrelated to barbiturate or benzodiazepine structure; selectively binds to benzodiazepine receptor site, GABA$_A$, but is NOT muscle relaxant or anticonvulsant; good GI absorption	t½ = 2 hours	Headache, confusion, drowsiness, ataxia and vertigo, diarrhea; overdose symptoms include respiratory depression and cardiovascular collapse	Short term treatment of insomnia

ABBREVIATIONS:

    DMMS - drug microsomal metabolizing system
    TI - therapeutic index

Note: Barbiturates at high dose are GABA-mimetic and directly increase the *duration* of chloride channel openings via GABA$_A$ receptors. Barbiturates at low dose require GABA for activity. Benzodiazepines require GABA for activity and increase the *frequency* of chloride channel openings via GABA$_A$ receptors.

Benzodiazepines superior to barbiturates because:

- have higher therapeutic index
- no DMMS induction
- less addictive
- less tolerance
- do not decrease REM
- no REM rebound
- little or no respiratory depression

Other miscellaneous sedative-hypnotics:

- Ethinamate (Valmid)
- Glutethimide (Doriden)
- Methyprylon (Nodular)

259

SKELETAL MUSCLE RELAXANTS:

DRUG	ORGAN SYSTEM EFFECTS	PHARMACOKINETICS/DYNAMICS	ADVERSE REACTIONS	THERAPEUTIC USE
ATRACURIUM (Tracrium)	Nondepolarizing skeletal muscle relaxant; action at N-II; NO cardiovascular effects	Short acting < 30 minutes; rapid metabolism by **plasma cholinesterase, spontaneous degradation at blood pH**	Apnea, hypotension, bronchospasm	Bronchoscopy, laryngoscopy; adjuvant in general anesthesia; orthopedic procedures
BACLOFEN (Lioresal)	Centrally acting skeletal muscle relaxant; works at level of spinal cord, NO significant peripheral effects; spasmolytic best in patients with muscle spasms; inhibitory activity (like GABA) on $GABA_B$ R (not a chloride channel); NO effect on $GABA_A$ R (chloride channel); derivative of GABA	Oral activity as spasmolytic agent; 30% plasma protein binding; 70-85% excretion unchanged by kidney; duration of action 4-6 hours	Sedation; dizziness; weakness, fatigue; headache	Oral spasmolytic agent; relieves muscle spasticity due to muscular sclerosis, clonus, and muscular spasticity
CYCLOBENZAPRINE (Flexeril)	Centrally acting skeletal muscle relaxant; works at level of CNS (brainstem); unknown mechanism; similar to tricyclic anti-depressants	Absorbed well orally; significant first pass effect; 93% plasma protein binding; t ½ 1-3 days	Sedation; xerostomia; dizziness	Skeletal muscle relaxant
DANTROLENE (Dantrium)	Direct acting skeletal muscle relaxant, works directly on the muscle fiber, blocks calcium release from sarcoplasmic reticulum (appears to be mechanism in reversal of malignant hyperthermia as well); will not achieve complete muscle relaxation; spasmolytic;	Oral dose; outpatient use t ½ = 8 hours	Muscle weakness; sedation; hepatitis (rare)	Spasmolytic; given prior to or during anesthesia to stop or prevent **malignant hyperthermia (hyperpyrexia)**
DIAZEPAM (Valium) benzodiazepine	Centrally acting skeletal muscle relaxant; binds benzodiazepine receptor; enhances GABA inhibitory activity by increasing *frequency* of channel openings; decreases neurotransmission in spinal cord; does NOT effect spinal cord reflex arc	t ½ = 30-60 hours	Sedation, amnesia, fatigue, ataxia, skin rash	Skeletal Muscle Relaxant
GALLAMINE (Flaxedil)	Nondepolarizing skeletal muscle relaxant; <u>Cardiovascular effects</u>: muscarinic blocker, increases NE release, increases HR, increases CO, slightly increases BP; NO effect at N-I; NO histamine effect	Long acting (1-2 hours); excreted unchanged by kidney	Apnea; mild hypertension	Same as Tubocurarine

260

SKELETAL MUSCLE RELAXANTS:

DRUG	ORGAN SYSTEM EFFECTS	PHARMACOKINETICS/DYNAMICS	ADVERSE REACTIONS	THERAPEUTIC USE
METHOCARBAMOL (Robaxin)	Centrally acting skeletal muscle relaxant; no direct effect on contractility, the motor end plate or nerves of muscle	IV, po, IM; duration of action 6-8 hours	Dizziness, vertigo, dyspepsia, headache, fever	Musculoskeletal Conditions
PANCURONIUM (Pavulon)	Nondepolarizing skeletal muscle relaxant; action at N-II; Cardiovascular effects: blocks NE uptake, M blocker, increases NE release, increases HR, increases CO, increases BP, N-I agonist; biotransforms to 3-OH-pancuronium (active metabolite)	Biotransformed to 3-OH-pancuronium which is active; t ½ = 3 hours	Apnea, hypotension	Same as Tubocurarine
SUCCINYLCHOLINE (Anectine)	*Very short acting* depolarizing blocker (causes depolarization, then prevents depolarization); some increase in histamine release at high dose; NO other significant activity	Very short acting (5-10 minutes); rapid metabolism by both cholinesterases, cleaved to succinylmonocholine (active) which is cleaved to succinic acid and choline (inactive); may act longer in some patients	Apnea in the case of atypical PCE; cardiac arrhythmias, muscle pain, hyperkalemia	Bronchoscopy, laryngoscopy; adjuvant in general anesthesia; used in orthopedic procedures; **electroshock therapy** to prevent dangerous muscle contractions
TUBOCURARINE	Nondepolarizing skeletal muscle relaxant; action at N-II; N-I blocker and increases histamine release at high dose; decreases BP, bronchospasm; first affects eye muscles, then face muscles, then limbs, then trunk muscles, then intercostal muscles, and finally the diaphragm	Long acting (1-2 hours); will not cross BBB; excreted unchanged by kidney	Apnea, histamine release, hypotension	Skeletal Muscle Relaxant during surgery of moderate or long duration
VECURONIUM (Norcuron)	Nondepolarizing skeletal muscle relaxant; action at N-II; NO cardiovascular effects; purest skeletal muscle relaxant; NO effect on histamine release; derivative of Pancuronium	Intermediate acting; some metabolism	No release of histaimine	Endotracheal Intubation Surgery

NOTES: Reversal of skeletal muscle relaxation (paralysis) is possible with Neostigmine or Edrophonium (indirect acting cholinomimetics)
PCE - plasma cholinesterase
nondepolarizing skeletal muscle relaxants are also known as *nondepolarizing curariform agents*

261

SULFONAMIDE ANTIBACTERIALS:

ASPECT	SULFONAMIDES
Agents:	Sulfacetamide (eye drops) Sulfadiazine (topical for burns) Sulfamethizole Sulfamethoxazole - Trimethoprim (Bactrim) Sulfanilamide Sulfinpyrazone Sulfisoxazole Sulfone
Mechanism of Action:	**Dihydropteroate synthetase inhibitors** blocks folic acid synthesis HIGH selectivity
Spectrum:	Actinomyces Chlamydia Nocardia Pneumocystis carinii Toxoplasmosis E. coli (even though resistant)
Resistance Mechanism:	Alteration of dihydropteroate synthetase

Kinetics:	Some are acetylated (**crystaluria**)
	Some are partially secreted by renal proximal tubule
	Acetylated sulfisoxazole is soluble
	Patient should be well hydrated
	Concentrates in bladder (excellent for urinary tract infection)
	Sulfasalazine
	    POORLY absorbed, remains in bowel lumen
	    Used for local GI effects

Use:	Urinary tract infection (UTI)

Adverse Effects:	Serious toxicity in 5% of patients
	    Hemolytic anemia (especially with G6PD deficiency)
	    Aplastic anemia
	    Erythema multiform
	    Stevens Johnson syndrome (large bullous skin lesions)

THROMBOLYTICS:

DRUG	ORGAN SYSTEM EFFECTS	ADVERSE REACTIONS	THERAPEUTIC USE
ALTEPLASE, RECOMBINANT (Activase)	Synthetic tissue plasminogen activator produced via DNA recombinant technology; **serine protease inhibitor** that promotes conversion of plasminogen to plasmin in presence of fibrin (in thrombi)	See Urokinase; **Pregnancy category C**	Acute Myocardial Infarction Pulmonary Embolism Acute Ischemic Stroke
ANISTREPLASE (Eminase)	Derivative of Lys-Plasminogen-Streptokinase activator complex that is blocked by an anisoyl group; deacylation forms active drug form which promotes production of plasmin from plasminogen; t ½ = 70-90 minutes	See Urokinase; bleeding, arrhythmias secondary to reperfusion, hypotension, allergic reactions, **Pregnancy category C**	Acute Myocardial Infarction
STREPTOKINASE (Kabikinase)	**Activates plasminogen → plasmin**; plasmin lyses formed clots; causes LEAST amount of cerebral hemorrhage of all fibrinolytic agents; t ½ = 80 minutes	See Urokinase	Deep Venous Thrombosis Pulmonary Emboli Acute Myocardial Infarction
TISSUE PLASMINOGEN ACTIVATOR (tPA)	Made through recombinant DNA techniques; activates plasminogen to plasmin by splitting bond at arg(560) - valine(561)	Same as Urokinase; MOST expensive agent in class	Pulmonary Emboli Coronary Artery Thrombus
UROKINASE (Abbokinase)	Enzyme found in urine that is produced by kidneys; thrombolytic agent that acts on the fibrinolytic system; increases fibrinolytic activity	<u>Precautions:</u> recent (within 10 days) surgery or obstetrical delivery, organ biopsy, serious GI bleed; SBE, pregnancy, cerebrovascular disease, diabetic hemorrhagic retinopathy <u>Contraindications:</u> active internal bleed, history of stroke, recent CNS surgery, recent trauma, intracranial tumor, aneurysm, or AV malformation, bleeding disorder, uncontrolled arterial hypertension	Pulmonary Embolism Coronary Artery Thrombus IV Catheter Clearance

NOTES: SBE - Subacute Bacterial Endocarditis
Anisoylated Plasminogen Streptokinase Activated Complex (APSAC) is a recently introduced fibrinolytic agent

263

THYROID HORMONES:

DRUG	MECHANISM OF ACTION	KINETICS	ADVERSE	USE
LEVOTHYROXINE (L-T$_4$) (Levothroid) (Synthroid)	Replacement of thyroxine (L-T$_4$)	Oral; IV (for myxedema coma); 99% plasma protein binding; t½ = 7 days; levels do NOT fluctuate daily	Increased blood pressure, increased sweating, palpitations, weight loss, tachycardia; thyrotoxicosis	Agent of choice for chronic treatment of Hypothyroidism
LIOTHYRONINE (L-T$_3$) (Cytomel)	Replacement of triiodothyronine (L-T3)	Faster onset, shorter duration; 4x's more potent than L-T4; better oral absorption; 99% plasma protein binding; t½ = 1 day; IV for myxedema coma	Arrhythmias, headache, sweating, angina; thyrotoxicosis	Acute and short term use to establish necessary L-T4 dosage; **diagnosis of thyroid function**
LIOTRIX (L-T$_3$ and L-T$_4$) (Thyrolar)	Replacement of thyroxine and triiodothyronine	Oral dosage, T$_4$:T$_3$ ratio is 4:1 in this preparation	Same adverse effects as Liothyronine	Chronic hormone replacement for Hypothyroidism
THYROID (Armour Thyroid)	Desiccated thyroid hormone derived from beef or pork	Oral dosage	Same adverse effects as Liotrix, hypersensitivity to proteins in the preparation	Hypothyroidism

Iodism (iodine poisoning)
· metallic taste in mouth
· burning in mouth
· salivary gland swelling
· increased salivation
· GI irritation, bloody diarrhea
· headache, depression

264

TUBERCULOSTATICS:

AGENT	SYSTEM EFFECTS / HISTORY	PHARMACOKINETICS	ADVERSE REACTIONS	THERAPEUTIC USE
CAPREOMYCIN (Capastat)	Macrocyclic polypeptide antibiotic isolated from *Streptomyces capreolus*; Active only against Mycobacteria	Not absorbed orally; must be given IM; 60-80% of dose is excreted unchanged in urine	Nephrotoxic, vestibular effects and ototoxicity (vertigo, tinnitus, and deafness) are the most serious side effects; should NOT be given in combination with Streptomycin or other aminoglycosides; **Pregnancy category C**	2nd Line Agent
CYCLOSERINE (Seromycin)	Antibiotic isolated from *Streptomyces orchidaceus*; interferes with 1st stage of cell wall synthesis	Well absorbed orally; widely distributed to tissues and body fluids, including CSF; 65% excreted unchanged in urine; serum concentrations should be monitored during therapy	High serum concentration may precipitate focal or tonic-clonic seizures; psychic disturbances such as excitement, aggression, confusion, and depression are not infrequent; NOT to be taken with alcohol; **Pregnancy category C**	2nd Line Agent
ETHAMBUTOL (Myambutol)	Discovered 1961; bacteriostatic action against *Mycobacterium tuberculosis* via unknown mechanism; appears to inhibit RNA synthesis; all other bacteria are resistant	80% oral absorption; widely distributed throughout body and enters macrophages; penetration through normal meninges is poor; in meningitis, 25-50% of serum level is achieved in CSF; crosses the placenta in pregnancy; 20-30% plasma protein bound; 65% excreted unchanged in urine	Generally well tolerated; **retrobulbar neuritis** is the most important adverse effect, symptoms include decreased visual acuity, central scotoma, and **color blindness** (↓ red-green vision) may be unilateral or bilateral, completely reversible; other adverse effects: allergic reactions, drug fever, GI upset, hyperuricemia, arthralgia, and perihperal neuritis; use in pregnancy has no detectable effect on the fetus	1st Line Agent
ETHIONAMIDE (Trecator-SC)	Derivative of isonicotinic acid active against *Mycobacterium tuberculosis*; and *M. leprae*	80% GI tract absorption; wide body distribution including CSF; metabolized in liver and excreted in urine	Most poorly tolerated antituberculosis agent; nausea, vomiting, abdominal pain are universal and severe; diarrhea, bitter metallic taste (may cause profound anorexia), hepatotoxic (5%), neurotoxicity (may be relieved by giving pyridoxine); teratogenic effects in animal studies	2nd Line Agent

265

TUBERCULOSTATICS:

AGENT	SYSTEM EFFECTS / HISTORY	PHARMACOKINETICS	ADVERSE REACTIONS	THERAPEUTIC USE
ISONIAZID (INH)	Synthetic antituberculous agent introduced in 1953; bactericidal activity against *Mycobacterium tuberculosis*; inhibits the synthesis of mycolic acid, a component of mycobacterial cell wall	Available in oral and parenteral doses; wide body tissue and fluid distribution; achieve serum levels in CSF in meningitis; readily crosses placenta and fetus; 10% plasma protein bound; metabolized by liver, excreted in urine	**Peripheral neuropathy** seen as parasthesia may be prevented by co-administration of pyridoxine (vitamin B6); asymptomatic liver transaminase elevation in 10-20%; hepatitis is much less frequent but is more common in rapid acetylators, routine monitoring of liver enzymes during therapy is not necessary, patient should be followed clinically for symptoms of hepatitis; drug fever; agranulocytosis; **Pregnancy category C**	Drug of choice for chemoprophylaxis in persons at risk of developing tuberculosis; 1st Line Agent
KANAMYCIN (Kantrex)	Isolated in 1957 from *Streptomyces kanamyceticus*; the most commonly used aminoglycosde in the 1960's is seldom used today	Poorly absorbed po; given parenterally	Ototoxic; nephrotoxic; may cause neuromuscular blockage with respiratory paralysis at high serum levels	2nd Line Agent
PARA-AMINOSALICYLIC ACID (Sodium PAS)	Weak bacteriostatic activity against *Mycobacterium tuberculosis*	85% GI absorption; excreted 20% and 80% as metabolites in urine	High frequency of GI intolerance often causing poor patient compliance	2nd Line Agent
PYRAZINAMIDE	Derivative of nicotinamide synthesized in 1952; bactericidal in vitro; MOST active agent against intracellular tubercle bacilli; only used during first two months of therapy; mechanism of action not known	Complete GI absorption; wide body distribution, penetrates macrophages, attains good CSF levels in meningitis	Hepatotoxic, asymptomatic liver transaminase elevations are common, overt hepatits is infrequent; hyperuricemia 2° to interfering with tubular secretion of uric acid, which may cause gout	1st Line Agent

TUBERCULOSTATICS:

AGENT	SYSTEM EFFECTS / HISTORY	PHARMACOKINETICS	ADVERSE REACTIONS	THERAPEUTIC USE
RIFABUTIN (Mycobutin)	Inhibitis DNA-dependent RNA polymerase in *E. Coli* and *Bacillus subtilis*, but antimycobacterial mechanism of action is not clear; one year survival rates vs. placebo was not found to be statistically significant	Good GI absorption t ½ = 45 hours	Abdominal pain, dyspepsia, eructation, nausea, headache, vomiting, myalgia, rash, taste disturbance, discolored urine; **Pregnancy category B**	*Mycobacterium avium* Complex Prophylaxis in Advanced HIV Infection
RIFAMPIN (Rifadin)	DNA dependent RNA polymerase inhibitor (lacks affinity for human enzyme); bactericidal activity against *Mycobacterium tuberculosis* and a wide range of gram positive and negative bacteria; 2°resistance occurs via single step mutations in the RNA polymerase; 1° resistance in < 1% of cases in United States	Rapid and complete GI absorption; 80% plasma protein bound; readily penetrates body tissues and fluids including CSF and saliva; lipid soluble; interferes with P450 system; enters well into leukocytes, macrophages and peripheral nerves; crosses placenta in pregnancy and enters fetus; **enterohepatic circulation** t ½ = 3 hours	**Pregnancy category C**; asymptomatic liver enzyme elevations may occur, overt hepatitis in < 1%; rarely see: thrombocytopenia, leukopenia, hemolytic anemia, acute renal failure, and purpura; **Red-orange discoloration of urine and secretions;** may interfere with oral contraceptive efficacy (barrier method recommended during Rifampin therapy)	1st Line Agent Part of Anti-Leprosy Regimen Chemoprophylaxis for meningitis caused by *N. gonorrhea* and *H. Influenzae*
STREPTOMYCIN	First effective antituberculous agent available; an aminoglycoside antibiotic active against *M. Tuberculosis* and *M. Kansasii*; does not enter macrophages; use of Streptomycin alone causes secondary resistance	Daily single IM dose t ½ = 5-6 hours	Ototoxicity, usually seen as vertigo and ataxia, but hearing loss may occur; nephrotoxicity; **Pregnancy category D**	1st Line Agent

URINARY ANALGESICS:

AGENT	ORGAN SYSTEM EFFECTS	PHARMACOKINETICS	ADVERSE REACTIONS	THERAPEUTIC USE
PHENAZOPYRIDINE (Pyridium)	Phenazopyridine is urine excreted and has topical analgesic effect on urinary tract mucosa; relieves pain, burning, urgency and frequency; mechanism of action is not known	Urine excretion; 65% excreted unmetabolized	**Orange/red urine discolorization** that may stain fabric; headache, rash, pruritus, occasional GI upset; **Pregnancy category B**	Urinary tract pain, burning, frequency, and discomfort caused by infection, trauma, surgery, or catheter passage

URINARY ANTI-INFECTIVES:

AGENT	ORGAN SYSTEM EFFECTS	PHARMACOKINETICS	ADVERSE REACTIONS	THERAPEUTIC USE
CINOXACIN (Cinobac)	Synthetic antibacterial; activity against many gram negative aerobic bacteria especially *Enterobacter* species, *Escherichia coli, Klebsiella* species, *Proteus mirabilis, Proteus vulgaris;* inhibits bacterial DNA sythesis	Rapidly absorbed po; 97% urine excretion; peak absorption not affected by food	Nausea, anorexia, vomiting, headache, dizziness, rash, urticaria, pruritus; **Pregnancy category C**	Urinary Tract Infection in adults
CIPROFLOXACIN (Cipro)	Synthetic broad spectrum antibacterial agent; has activity against a wide range of gram negative and gram positive organisms; interferes with bacterial DNA gyrase	Well absorbed from GI tract; peak plasma levels 1-2 hours after po dose; 50% excreted unchanged in urine $t \frac{1}{2}$ = 5-6 hours	Nausea, diarrhea, vomiting, abdominal pain/discomfort, headache, restlessness, and rash, CNS disturbances, abnormal liver enzymes; safety in pediatric, pregnant and lactating patients not established; **Pregnancy category C**	Urinary Tract Infection in adults
METHENAMINE (Hiprex, Urex)	Methenamine is metabolized to formaldehyde which has antiseptic properties in urine	Prodrug; rapid absorption from GI tract; rapid excretion in urine	Skin rash, dry mouth, flushing, difficulty initiating urination, rapid pulse, dizziness, and blurred vision; **Pregnancy category C**	Lower urinary tract infection caused by organisms which produce an acid urine and are susceptible to formaldehyde
NALIDIXIC ACID (Neg-Gram)	Oral antibacterial with activity against gram negative bacteria including *Proteus miribilis, P. Morganii, P. Vulgaris, and P. Rettgeri; Escherichia coli;* Enterobacter and Klebsiella	Rapid GI absorption, partially metabolized by liver, then rapidly excreted through the kidneys; peak plasma levels 1-2 hours after po dose; peak urine levels 3-4 hours after po dose	Headache, vertigo, photophobia, abdominal pain, rash; safety in 1st trimester of pregnancy not established	Urinary Tract Infections

269

URINARY ANTI-INFECTIVES:

AGENT	ORGAN SYSTEM EFFECTS	PHARMACOKINETICS	ADVERSE REACTIONS	THERAPEUTIC USE
NITROFURANTOIN (Macrobid, Macrodantin)	Bactericidal in urine at therapeutic dose; Nitrofurantoin is reduced by flavoproteins reactive form which inactivates bacterial ribosomal proteins; resistance has not been a problem since its introduction in 1953	Given with food to improve drug absorption; Macrobid is bid; Macrodantin is qid	Pulmonary hypersensitivity reactions, hepatic reactions including hepatitis, peripheral neuropathy, asthenia, vertigo, nystagmus, dizziness, headache, drowsiness, nausea, vomiting, superinfection by resistant organisms; **Pregnancy category B**	Urinary Tract Infections due to susceptible strains of *Escherichia coli*, enterococci, *Staphylococcus aureus*, some *Klebsiella* and *Enterobacter* species
NORFLOXACIN (Noroxin)	Fluoroquinolone antibacterial with similar activity and side effect profile as Ciprofloxacin	po t ½ = 3-5 hours	Conjunctivitis, photophobia, bitter taste; **Pregnancy category C**	Urinary Tract Infection
OFLOXACIN (Floxin)	Fluoroquinolone antibacterial with similar activity and side effect profile as Ciprofloxacin	po t ½ = 5-7 hours	Nausea, vomiting, diarrhea, rash; **Pregnancy category C**	Urinary Tract Infection

URINARY ANTISPASMODICS:

AGENT	ORGAN SYSTEM EFFECTS	PHARMACOKINETICS	ADVERSE REACTIONS	THERAPEUTIC USE
OXYBUTYNIN (Ditropan)	Direct antispasmodic effect on smooth muscle; antimuscarinic activity on smooth muscle; relaxes bladder smooth muscle; anticholinergic	po	Restlessness, tremor, irritability, convulsions, delirium, hallucination; flushing, fever, nausea, vomiting, tachycardia, hypotension or hypertension, respiratory failure, paralysis and coma; **Pregnancy category B**	Relief of bladder instability associated with voiding in patients with neurogenic bladder

VITAMINS AND VITAMIN SUPPLEMENTS:

AGENT	ORGAN SYSTEM EFFECTS	PHARMACOKINETICS	ADVERSE EFFECTS	THERAPEUTIC USE
CALCIFEDIOL (Calderol)	Synthetic 25-OH-vit D3; increases serum calcium; decreases parathyroid hormone (PTH) levels	Oral	Hypercalcemia; hypercalciuria (possible)	Osteomalacia
CALCITRIOL (Rocaltrol)	Synthetic 1,25-di-OH D3; increases serum calcium; decreases PTH levels; stimulates intestinal absorption of calcium and phosphate	Oral, IV		Hypoparathyroidism
DIHYDROTACHYSTEROL (Hytakerol)	Form of vitamin D	Oral	Weakness, headache, diarrhea, hallucinations	Hypoparathyroidism
FOLIC ACID (Folvite)	Alcoholics, tea-toast widows, leukemia and hemolytic anemia patients commonly have macrocytic anemia; taken in polyglutamate form which is then converted to the monoglutamate form which goes into blood or taken in folic acid form which is converted to tetrahydrofolate which goes into blood	Minimum daily requirement is 50 µg/day; RDA is 400 µg/day; need increased folic acid during pregnancy and lactation	NO toxicity; phenytoin and phenobarbital interfere with folic acid absorption	**Macrocytic anemia** Prophylactic in Prenatal Care (decreases risk of open neural tube defects)
LEUCOVORIN {Folinic Acid} (Wellcovorin)	Chemically reduced derivative of Folic acid; useful as an antidote to drugs which act as folic acid antagonists; Leukovorin is NOT proper therapy for pernicious anemia or other megaloblastic anemias due to lack of vitamin B12	Already active form of folic acid, **tetrahydrofolate**, does NOT need to be converted by dihydrofolate reductase	Allergic sensitization including anaphylactoid reactions and urticaria have been reported; **Pregnancy category C**	Indicated after high dose Methotrexate therapy for osteosarcoma, and to decrease toxicity and counteract the effects of impaired methotrexate elimination and of inadvertent overdose of folic acid antagonists
PHYTONADIONE (Mephyton)	Also known as Phylloquinone and Vitamin K1	GI absorption via intestinal lymphatics only in the presence of bile salts; rapidly metabolized; given IM or subQ when possible	Flushing sensation, peculiar taste sensation; **Pregnancy category C**	Coagulation Disorders Secondary Hypoprothrombinemia Prophylaxis for Hemorrhagic Disease of the Newborn
VITAMIN B12 INJECTION (Redisol)	Vitamin B12 is common name for cobalamins; MUST be bound to **intrinsic factor** for absorption	Typical diet will supply 5-30 µg/day; B12 needed for myelin sheath synthesis → deficiency leads to neurological deficits	NO toxicity	Pernicious Anemia Vitamin B12 Ddeficiency

272

Notes

INDEX

A

A/T/S: see Erythromycin
A-200: Pyrethrins, Piperonyl Butoxide Technical, and Related Compounds
ABBOKINASE: see Urokinase
Abuse, Drugs Of: 66
ACCOLATE: see Zafirlukast
ACCUPRIL: see Quinapril
ACCUTANE: see Isotretinoin
ACEBUTOLOL: 74
Acetaminophen: 83, 174
Acetazolamide: 130, 216
Acetohexamide: 232
Acetylcholine: 203
Acetylcysteine: 219
ACHROMYCIN: see Tetracycline
ACHROMYCIN V: see Tetracycline
ACLOVATE: see Alclometasone
ACNOMEL: Sulfur, Resorcinol, and Alcohol
ACTH: 212
ACTIFED PLUS: Pseudoephedrine, Triprolidine, and Acetaminophen
ACTIFED: Triprolidine and Pseudoephedrine
ACTIFED WITH CODEINE: Pseudoephedrine, Triprolidine, Codeine and Alcohol
ACTIVASE: see Alteplase, Recombinant
ACULAR: see Ketorolac
Acyclovir: 184
ADALAT CC: see Nifedipine
ADALAT: see Nifedipine
Adderall: see Amphetamine
ADENOCARD: see Adenosine
Adenosine: 110
ADIPEX-P: see Phentermine
Adrenergic Agonists, Direct Acting: 69-71
Adrenergic Agonists, Mixed Acting: 72
Adrenergic Blockers, Alpha: 73
Adrenergic Blockers, Beta: 74-75
Adrenergic Neuronal Blockers: 76
ADRIAMYCIN: see Doxorubicin
ADVIL: see Ibuprofen
AEROBID: see Flunisolide
AEROLATE: see Theophylline
AEROSPORIN: see Polymyxin B Sulfate
AFRIN SALINE MIST: Sodium Chloride with Sodium Phosphate Buffer
AFRIN: see Oxymetazoline
AFTATE: see Tolnaftate
AGORAL: Mineral Oil and Phenolphthalein
AKINETON: see Biperiden
Albuterol: 69, 195

Alclometasone: 24
Alcohols, The: 77
ALDACTAZIDE: Spironolactone and Hydrochlorothiazide
ALDACTONE: see Spironolactone
Aldesleukin: 24
ALDOCLOR-150: Chlorothiazide and Methyldopa
ALDOCLOR-250: Chlorothiazide and Methyldopa
ALDOMET: see Methyldopa
ALDORIL D30: Hydrochlorothiazide and Methyldopa
ALDORIL D50: Hydrochlorothiazide and Methyldopa
ALDORIL-15: Hydrochlorothiazide and Methyldopa
ALDORIL-25: Hydrochlorothiazide and Methyldopa
Alendronate: 165, 194
ALEVE: see Naproxen Sodium
ALFENTA: see Alfentanil
Alfentanil: 86
ALFERON N: Interferon alfa-n3
ALKERAN: see Melphalan
ALLEGRA: see Fexofenadine
ALLEREST 12 HOUR: Phenylpropanolamine and Chlorpheniramine
ALLEREST HEADACHE STRENGTH: Pseudoephedrine, Chlorpheniramine, and Acetaminophen
ALLEREST MAXIMUM STRENGTH: Pseudoephedrine and Chlorpheniramine
ALLEREST NO DROWSINESS: Pseudoephedrine and Acetaminophen
ALLEREST SINUS PAIN FORMULA: Pseudoephedrine, Chlorpheniramine and Acetaminophen
Allopurinol: 132
ALOMIDE: see Lodoxamide
ALPHAGAN: see Brimonidine
Alprazolam: 105
ALRIMIDEN: see Anastrozole
ALTACE: see Ramipril
Alteplase, Recombinant: 263
ALTERNAGEL: see Aluminum Hydroxide
Altretamine: 155
ALU-CAP: see Aluminum Hydroxide
ALU-TAB: see Aluminum Hydroxide
Aluminum Hydroxide: 98
ALUPENT: see Metaproterenol
Amantadine: 166, 184
AMARYL: see Glimepiride
Ambenonium: 203

D

ERYPED: see Erythromycin
ERYTHROCIN IV: see Erythromycin
Erythromycin: 100, 151
ERYTHROMYCIN BASE FILMTAB: see
        Erythromycin
ESGIC: Acetaminophen, Butalbital, and Caffeine
ESGIC PLUS: Acetaminophen, Butalbital, and
        Caffeine
ESIDRIX: see Hydrochlorothiazide
ESIMIL: Guanethidine and Hydrochlorothiazide
ESKALITH CR: see Lithium Carbonate
ESKALITH: see Lithium Carbonate
Esmolol: 109
Estazolam: 257
ESTINYL: see Ethinyl Estradiol
ESTRACE: see Estradiol
ESTRADERM: see Estradiol
Estradiol: 217
Estramustine: 158
ESTRING: see Estradiol
Estrogen, Conjugated: 217
Estrogens: 217-218
Estrone: 217
Estropipate: 218
ESTROVIS: see Quinestrol
Ethacrynic Acid: 214
Ethambutol: 265
Ethanol: 66, 77
Ethchlorvynol: 257
Ethinyl Estradiol: 210-211, 218
Ethionamide: 265
ETHMOZINE: see Moricizine
Ethosuximide: 124
Ethotoin: 123
Ethylene Glycol: 77
Etidocaine: 96
Etidronate: 165, 194
Etodolac: 83, 144, 243
Etoposide: 158
ETRAFON 2-10: Perphenazine and Amitriptyline
ETRAFON: Perphenazine and Amitriptyline
ETRAFON-FORTE: Perphenazine and
        Amitriptyline
Etretinate: 170
ETS-2%: see Erythromycin
EULEXIN: see Flutamide
EURAX: see Crotamiton
EVAC-U-GEN: see Phenolphthalein
EX-LAX MAXIMUM RELIEF: see Phenolphthalein
EX-LAX: see Phenolphthalein
EXELDERM: see Sulconazole
EXNA: see Benzthiazide

EXPECTORANT WITH CODEINE:
        Phenylpropanolamine, Guaifenesin,
        Codeine, Alcohol
Expectorants: 219
EXSEL: see Selenium Sulfide
EXTENDRYL: Phenylephrine, Chlorpheniramine,
        and Methscopolamine
EXTENDRYL SR: Phenylephrine,
        Chlorpheniramine, and Methscopolamine
EXTRA-STRENGTH TYLENOL: see
        Acetaminophen

F

Famciclovir: 184
Famotidine: 182, 230
FAMVIR: see Famciclovir
FANSIDAR: see Sulfadoxine and Pyrimethamine
FASTIN: see Phentermine
FDA Administration's Pregnancy Categories: 62
FEDAHIST EXPECTORANT: Pseudoephedrine
        and Guaifenesin
FEDAHIST GYROCAPS: Pseudoephedrine and
        Chlorpheniramine
FEDAHIST TIMECAPS: Pseudoephedrine and
        Chlorpheniramine
Felbamate: 124
FELBATROL: see Felbamate
FELDENE: see Piroxicam
Felodipine: 138, 198
FEMARA: see Letrozole
FEMSTAT: see Butoconazole
Fenfluramine: 97
Fenoprofen: 83, 144
Fentanyl: 86, 94
FENTANYL ORALET: see Fentanyl
FEOSOL: see Ferrous Sulfate
FER-IN-SOL: see Ferrous Sulfate
FERANCEE: Ferrous Fumarate and Vitamin C
FERANCEE-HP: Ferrous Fumarate and Vitamin C
FERGON: see Ferrous Gluconate
FERO-FOLIC-500: Ferrous Sulfate, Folic Acid,
        and Sodium Ascorbate
FERO-GRAD-500: Ferrous Sulfate and Sodium
        Ascorbate
FERO-GRADUMET: see Ferrous Sulfate
FERRO-SEQUELS: Ferrous Fumarate and
        Docusate Sodium
Ferrous Sulfate: 227
FEVERALL, JUNIOR STRENGTH: see
        Acetaminophen
Fexofenadine: 134
FIBERALL: see Calcium Polycarbophil

U

ULTIVA: see Remifentanil
ULTRACEF: see Cefadroxil
Ultralente: 237
ULTRALENTE U: Extended Insulin Zinc
      Suspension
ULTRAM: See Tramadol
ULTRAVATE: see Halobetasol
UNASYN: Ampicillin-Sulbactam
UNIPEN: see Nafcillin
UNISOM: see Doxylamine
UNISOM WITH PAIN RELIEF: Acetaminophen
      and Diphenhydramine
UNIVASC: see Moexipril
URECHOLINE: see Bethanechol
UREX: see Methenamine
Urinary Analgesics: 268
Urinary Anti-Infectives: 269-270
Urinary Antispasmodics: 271
URISED: Methenamine, Phenyl Salicylate,
      Methylene Blue, Benzoic Acid, Atropine,
      and Hyoscyamine
UROBIOTIC-250: Oxytetracycline and
      Phenazopyridine
Urokinase: 263
UTICORT: see Betamethasone

V

VAGISTAT-1: see Tioconazole
Valacyclovir: 186
VALISONE REDUCED STRENGTH: see
      Betamethasone
VALISONE: see Betamethasone
VALIUM: see Diazepam
Valproic acid: 126, 149, 154
VALRELEASE: see Diazepam
Valsartan: 142
VALTREX: see Valacyclovir
VANCENASE AQ: see Beclomethasone
VANCENASE: see Beclomethasone
VANCERIL: see Beclomethasone
VANCOCIN HCL: see Vancomycin
Vancomycin: 56
VANOXIDE-HC: Benzoyl Peroxide and
      Hydrocortisone
VANSIL: see Oxamniquine
VANTIN: see Cefpodoxime
VASCOR: see Bepridil
VASERETIC 10-25: Enalapril and
      Hydrochlorothiazide

VASOCIDIN: Sulfacetamide and Prednisolone
VASODILAN: see Isoxsuprine
Vasopressin: 253
VASOTEC I.V.: see Enalapril
VASOTEC: see Enalapril
Vecuronium: 241, 261
VEETIDS: see Penicillin V
VELBAN: see Vinblastine
VELOSEF: see Cephradine
VELOSULIN HUMAN: see Insulin Injection
      (Regular)
Venlafaxine: 117
VENTOLIN NEBULES: see Albuterol
VENTOLIN ROTACAPS: see Albuterol
VELSAR: see Vinblastine
VENTOLIN: see Albuterol
VEPESID: see Etoposide
Verapamil: 104, 110, 142, 199
VERELAN: see Verapamil
VERMOX: see Mebendazole
VERSED: see Midazolam
VIBRA-TAB: see Doxycycline
VIBRAMYCIN INTRAVENOUS: see Doxycycline
VIBRAMYCIN: see Doxycycline
VICKS FORMULA 44 COUGH MEDICINE: see
      Dextromethorphan
VICKS PEDIATRIC FORMULA 44 COUCH
      MEDICINE: see Dextromethorphan
VICKS SINEX LONG-ACTING: see
      Oxymetazoline
VICODIN ES: Hydrocodone and Acetaminophen
VICODIN: Hydrocodone and Acetaminophen
Vidarabine: 186
VIDEX: see Didanosine
Vinblastine: 163
VINCASAR: see Vincristine
Vincristine: 164
Vinorelbine: 164
VIOFORM: see Clioquinol
VIOFORM-HYDROCORTISONE: Clioquinol and
      Hydrocortisone
VIOFORM-HYDROCORTISONE MILD: Clioquinol
      and Hydrocortisone
VIRA-A: see Vidarabine
VIRAMUNE: see Nevirapine
VIROPTIC: see Trifluridine
VISINE L.R.: see Oxymetazoline
VISINE: see Tetrahydrozoline
VISKEN: see Pindolol
VISTARIL: see Hydroxyzine
VISTIDE: see Cidofovir
Vitamin B12 Injection: 272
Vitamins: 272

ORDER FORM FOR HANDBOOKS

TITLE	PRICE x QUANTITY
Drug Charts in Basic Pharmacology, Second Edition (1998), 304 pages ISBN 0-942447-26-3	$ 18.00 x _____ = $ _____.____
Handbook of Commonly Prescribed Drugs, Thirteenth Edition (1998), 294 pages ISBN 0-942447-25-5	$ 18.00 x _____ = $ _____.____
Antimicrobial Therapy in Primary Care Medicine (1997), 382 pages ISBN 0-942447-22-0	$ 16.50 x _____ = $ _____.____
Handbook of Common Orthopaedic Fractures, Third Edition (1997), 270 pages ISBN 0-942447-24-7	$ 17.00 x _____ = $ _____.____
Handbook of Commonly Prescribed Pediatric Drugs, Fifth Edition (1995), 238 pages ISBN 0-942447-17-4	$ 15.50 x _____ = $ _____.____
Warning: Drugs in Sports (1995), 278 pages ISBN 0-942447-16-6	$ 14.50 x _____ = $ _____.____
Handbook of Commonly Prescribed Geriatric Drugs, First Edition (1993), 334 pages ISBN 0-942447-01-8	$ 15.00 x _____ = $ _____.____
	SUB-TOTAL = $ _____.____
Shipping and Handling	= $ 5.50
PA Residents: Add 6% Sales Tax	= $ _____.____
	TOTAL = $ _____.____

For mail orders for Handbooks, please complete the reverse side of this form.

ORDER FORM FOR TEXTBOOK IN PHARMACOLOGY

TITLE	PRICE x QUANTITY
Basic Pharmacology in Medicine, Fourth Edition (1995), 880 pages ISBN 0-942447-04-2	$ 49.95 x _____ = $ _____._____
Shipping and Handling PA Residents: Add 6% Sales Tax	SUB-TOTAL = $ _____._____
	= $ __5.50
	= $ _____._____
	TOTAL = $ _____._____

Send mail orders for Handbooks or Textbook to:

MEDICAL SURVEILLANCE INC.
P.O. Box 1629   West Chester, PA 19380

(PLEASE PRINT)

Name_____Degree_____

Organization_____

Street Address_____

City_____State_____Zip_____

Telephone Number_____

Payment: Check____ VISA_____ MC_____ Discov____ Am. Express_____

Credit Card No._____ Exp. Date_____

Signature_____

FOR FURTHER INFORMATION CALL: 800 - 417-3189 or 610 - 436-8881
FAX: 610 - 436-1803

REQUEST FOR INFORMATION

If you wish to be placed on a mailing list for information concerning new publications and updates, please fill out the form below and mail to:

MEDICAL SURVEILLANCE INC.
P.O. Box 1629   West Chester, PA 19380

(PLEASE PRINT)

Name_____

Organization_____

Street Address_____

City_____State_____

Zip Code_____

Telephone Number (Optional)_____

FOR FURTHER INFORMATION CALL:
800 - 417-3189 or 610 - 436-8881

E-Mail us at **msi@juno.com**

Visit Us on the **World Wide Web** at
hhtp://www.medicalsurveillance.com

Notes

Notes

Notes

Notes